FOOD YOU WANT

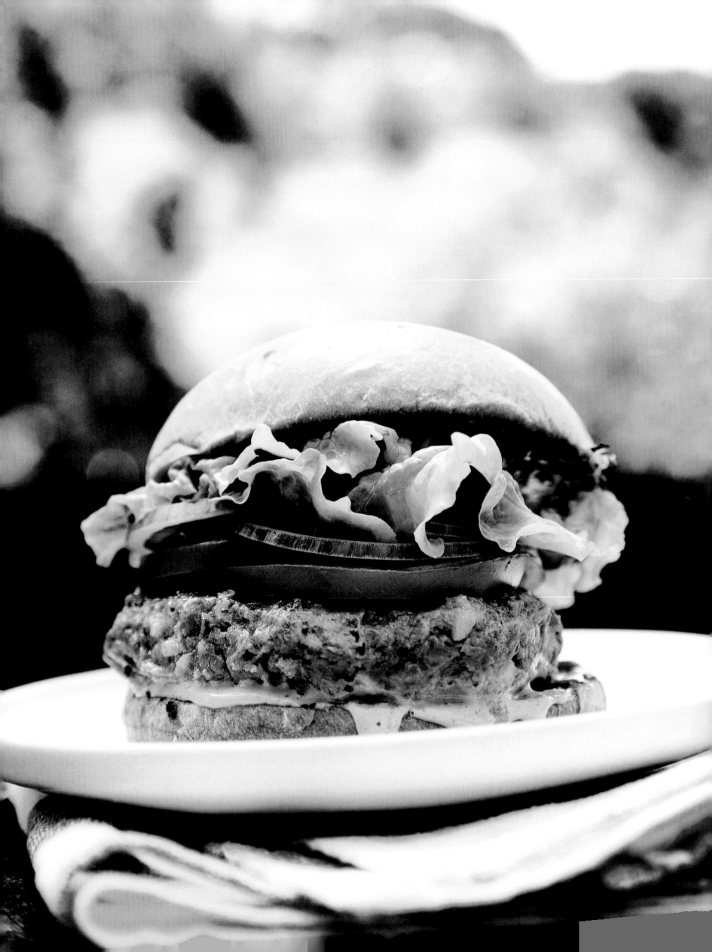

FOOD YOU WANT

FOR THE LIFE YOU CRAVE

100+ HEALTHY, INDULGENT, AND FLEXIBLE RECIPES

BY NEALY FISCHER

THE FLEXIBLE CHEF

PHOTOGRAPHY BY AUBRIE PICK

Da Capo

LIFE
LONG

Da Capo Press
Hachette Book Group
1290 Avenue of the Americas, New York, NY 10104
www.dacapopress.com
@DaCapoPress

Printed in the United States of America

First Edition: April 2019

Published by Da Capo Press, an imprint of Perseus Books, LLC, a subsidiary of Hachette Book Group, Inc.

The Hachette Speakers Bureau provides a wide range of authors for speaking events. To find out more, go to www.hachettespeakersbureau.com or call (866) 376-6591.

The publisher is not responsible for websites (or their content) that are not owned by the publisher.

Writing and recipe development with Ann Volkwein.

Photography by Aubrie Pick.

Print book interior design by Ashley Lima.

Library of Congress Cataloging-in-Publication Data has been applied for.

ISBNs: 978-0-7382-8484-2 (hardcover); 978-0-7382-8485-9 (ebook)

LSC-W

10 9 8 7 6 5 4 3 2 1

FOR BEN, EITAN, AYLA, AND LIAM

You are the best things we've cooked up.

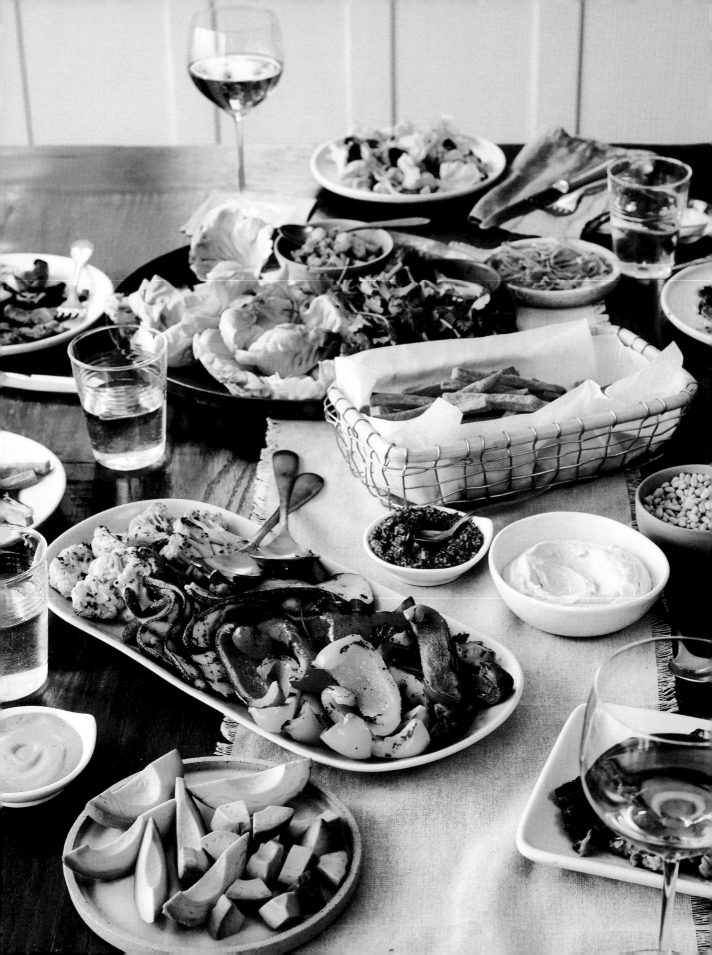

CONTENTS

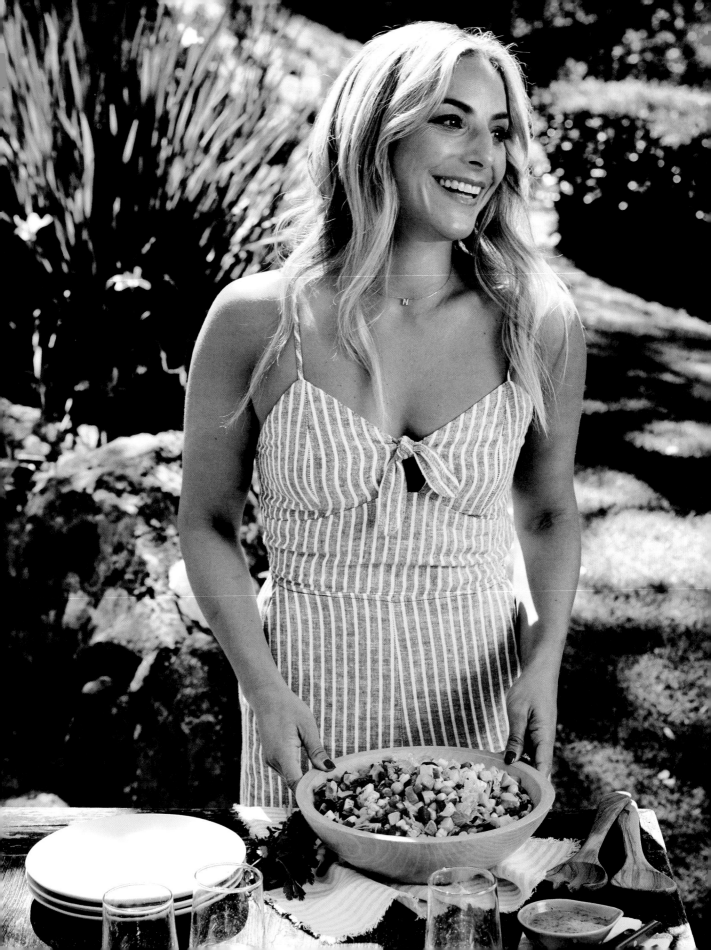

THE FOOD YOU WANT TO EAT

WHAT DO YOU CRAVE?

One day, after leafing through my 300th cookbook, I realized I was hungry for more than just another recipe for chicken or chocolate cake, or another collection of 110 dishes and someone else's formula for success. I wanted more out of those pages—I was hungry for flexible food that satisfied the robust lifestyle I craved.

I wished a recipe would tell me what is most essential, what is absolutely necessary to create the best dish, upfront, to set me up for success. I also yearned for options. What do I do if I don't have an ingredient or the right equipment that a recipe calls for? How do I put gorgeous food on the table without slaving all day in the kitchen? I longed for a cookbook that would help feed me and my family achievable meals, our way.

So I set out to write that book. I'm not interested in just teaching you how to be a cook who can follow my recipes. These pages are designed to help you obtain a simpler recipe for success, both in and out of the kitchen. You'll emerge skilled, confident, and armed with newfound creativity that honors your tastes, your dietary needs, and the preferences of those you're looking to nurture and feed.

Many of us feel bound by the standards we impose on ourselves. The unrelenting pressures of today's world can leave us desperate for a secret ingredient to change all of that. My hope is for this book to serve as a blueprint if you're tired of needing to have it all—but still desire a taste of it. After years of trial and error, I've honed a system (and a way of cooking) that helps make each day less harried and more enjoyable. The key? Flexibility.

BECOMING A FLEXIBLE CHEF: MY STORY

Flexibility is about compromise—how to give yourself a break and still come out on top—in the kitchen and beyond. There's a path available to each of us where excellence (not perfection!) is more readily achieved.

But it's all easier said than done. I know. I've been overweight, overworked, and overwhelmed by the intensity of my own life. Starving for perfection and the notion that I needed to fix myself, I went on my first diet when I was just eleven years old. I spent subsequent years following rules: adhering to strict diets and crazy workout regimens to carve a body and lifestyle that were as close to flawless as possible. If I wasn't sipping my way through the Lemonade Diet then I was crunching my way to perfection on the Carrot Diet (yes, all I ate were carrots until my palms turned orange). I've been macrobiotic, pescatarian, vegetarian, vegan, and iterations in between. And if I fell off a diet, it was into a vat of cookie dough. Sound familiar? After years of bouncing between extremes, I had finally had enough.

My turning point toward a gentler, more constructive path came during my years of practicing and teaching yoga. (Where else do you think the term *flexible* came from?) The practice taught me to slow down, worry less, and appreciate more. While teaching my students how to bend, I came to understand that *strength is the foundation of flexibility.* We first have to be skilled in the rules, and become strong in them, in order to bend. The same principles apply to cooking.

When you think about it, the deep fulfillment we get from our day-to-day routine is intensified in those moments when we're confident enough in our course to veer from it. That's the essence of flexibility, and that's when we are truly free.

THE FOOD IN THIS BOOK

If your family is anything like mine, understanding how to swap key ingredients and throw meals together with limited time and resources is a lifesaver. I'm a kale-eating woman married to a burger-loving man. I cook for four kids whose tastes range from white food only, with nothing touching anything else on the plate, to daily doses of cereals and sweets,

and their preferences change as often as they change their muddy soccer shoes. Their dietary needs have been the catalyst for innovative meal planning.

When we entertain, we cater to guests with diverse tastes and dietary restrictions. If I didn't have my organized but flexible road map down pat (more on that in Chapter 1), I would not feel confident enough to customize and improvise as I go. I apply years of trial and error in that realm, and have lived through and triumphed over some pretty crazy food challenges, including ingredient swapping across continents, raising four children in Asia, and keeping myself and my family healthy while juggling business, motherhood, and marriage.

These pages are infused with craveable global recipes inspired by our life in Asia and Israel, summertime on a ranch in Montana, my Jewish heritage, as well as my curiosity and culinary travels. Recipes often include complementary opposites that combine to create something that's uniquely yours (think Thai spring rolls dipped in Mediterranean tahini—why not?). You'll find the food in this book mostly healthy, sometimes indulgent, and always flexibly delicious.

DOES IT HAVE TO BE GLUTEN FREE?

I stopped eating gluten more than ten years ago in response to some personal health complaints. Back then there was no fad or trend attached to giving up gluten, no labels screaming across the grocery aisle or apples with gluten-free stickers. Now you can find gluten-free versions of virtually everything—

from bagels to cookies to pastas—in designated health food sections, but they're often packed with sugar and other additives. In a way, it was easier back then to eat a natural gluten-free diet because fewer options meant we stuck with mostly fresh and "real" unprocessed foods. It meant that I custom-tailored the school menu for my kids to ensure they were getting veggies and clean protein for lunch (not processed gluten-free nuggets). And thanks to their healthy diets, my kids' medical complaints started to clear up—my son's asthma even disappeared. We experienced renewed vitality from this way of eating; we no longer felt lethargic, heavy, and bloated from processed carbohydrates. (But my husband still sneaks gluten into the house!)

Because of the increasing availability of packaged gluten-free foods, adopting a gluten-free diet alone is no longer a ticket to clear skin, weight loss, or improved health. Unless you suffer from celiac disease, it may not even supply you with increased energy. My advice? Use your life as a laboratory. Test out what types of foods make you feel your best. While I don't do so well with grains, maybe your body can handle them just fine. And if you really don't want to make the chocolate chip cookies gluten free, see page 10 for how to substitute whatever flour you prefer. Regardless, it's wise to reserve any type of cereals, cookies, and crackers to once-in-a-whiles and fill your plate with mostly vegetables, an abundance of healthy proteins, healthy fats, gluten-free grains, and a sprinkling of fruits.

LEARN TO *nail this* AND *flip it*

Throughout the book, recipes are peppered with success strategies (*Nail This*) and flexible flips (*Flip It*) that will elevate you from an elementary cook to an unshackled chef. In *Nail This,* I highlight the most essential elements to master for a dish's success. But while some instructions in a recipe should be followed and nailed, others can (and should) be broken. The *Flip It* tips are crafted to get you started down that road—to encourage you to unleash your creativity and adapt each recipe to suit your preferences and limitations. Think of the flips as tools to transform a hundred recipes into a thousand different dishes!

I also share primers, hacks, and functional strategies, providing real-life solutions to your daily challenges. Learn how to create amazing breakfast menus, how to stock a flexible freezer so you always have a healthy meal an arm's length away, and how to deal with the picky eaters in your life. These adaptable methods will help you be more adventurous with food, creative with meals, and comfortable in the kitchen.

Some of my own culinary adventures have resulted in a few flopped cakes and raw loaves of bread. The many lessons I've learned along the way are shared in this book. It is my deepest desire that you find your way to an enriched, satisfying, and above all flexibly fulfilling life—on your own terms. Let's get cooking!

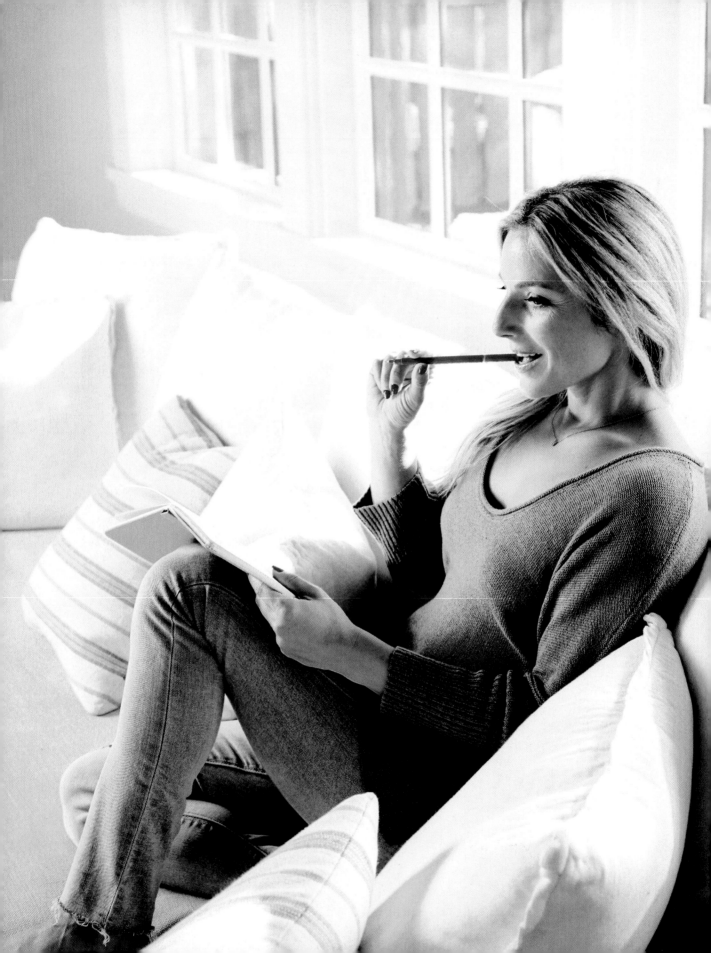

Chapter 1

YOUR FLEXIBLE ROAD MAP

YOUR TEN-STEP GUIDE TO BECOMING A FLEXIBLE CHEF

I'm a rule breaker. A varied, flexible life is so much more rewarding than living solely by rigid dogmas. But to break the rules I first had to master them. Here are my most valuable tips to help empower you on your journey to making your food exquisite, your life efficient, and your healthiest self more attainable.

1 Go deep and find your why

What motivates you to get out of bed in the morning? Most of us deal with a slew of challenges each day. Without clarity about our beliefs and values, managing these demands becomes a chore. But if we identify our deepest inspiration, we can begin to live with purpose. Your "why" will give you answers and act as a pillar when the road gets bumpy. Plus, *knowing what you want makes getting what you want possible.*

2 Make your kitchen and your diet fit your life—not the reverse

Blast away all the noise about "eating and living right," and shape your food choices around your unique needs. After years of extreme dieting, what I really craved was to sit around the dinner table with my kids and be the mom that ate burgers (which I do, bunless). I've since learned how to eat in the middle—that place where food is enjoyable and satisfying without engaging in excess on either end. Also, don't take on more than you can handle. Be realistic when preparing a menu. Ask yourself how much time you really have to marinate, sear, bake, slice, and plate. If you have a full-time job, then undertaking an elaborate dinner-party menu during the week is likely not feasible for you. *Creating strategies that make cooking and eating fit your life, instead of the other way around, will help you avoid exhaustion and frustration and set you up to succeed.*

3 Make a plan to get there

Once you've clearly established your "why," it's time to start thinking about the "how." My secret, and the flexible mind-set that allows me to be spontaneous at times, is *meticulous organization*. I'd be a frazzled mess without my lists, notes, menu plans, and schedules. Organization ensures that you're always prepared for last-minute anythings: surprise dinner guests, forgotten dinner plans, midafternoon snack attacks, picky diners, and rainy Sundays. Here are some ways to consider planning ahead:

- **Stock your pantry:** Think of your pantry as your smart toolbox, containing the ingredients you need to whip up easy sides, mains, snacks, or breakfasts (page 12).
- **Stock your freezer:** That way, you're never without a backup meal (page 12).
- **Plan menus:** Consider how much time you'll have during the week, and shop for your items in advance to avoid a last-minute dinner frenzy.
- **Prep meals in advance:** Stagger your prep so you don't have to cram it in last minute before dinner parties or big meals.
- **Keep a kitchen list:** Note items that need replenishing before you come up empty.
- **Schedule your time:** Slot in your workouts, your "you" time, and your cook time as you would meetings so there's never an urgent excuse to skip what's important.

4 Master the rules

We all have to apprentice as students first. Improving at anything requires perseverance, dedication, and a great deal of hard work, so *get gritty*. When you attempt a recipe for the first time, be sure to first read through the whole recipe and follow the steps meticulously. You might even have to make it numerous times until you get it right. Over time (and perhaps you're already there) the chef in you will be able to apply a critical eye to a recipe and tweak it or choose not to follow it. *You must first master the rules before you can successfully break them.*

5 Forget multitasking—think single-tasking

Can you relate to the idea of trying to do too much, all at once? The myth of multitasking gives us the illusion of productivity, but studies increasingly show that when we multitask, we divide our attention, and the results are poor. When people ask how I am, I've stopped saying, "I'm so busy!" Of course I am, and so are you. Busy does not get us to our destination; it just keeps us buzzed.

Focus is your greatest asset. Eliminate distractions and find ways to prioritize the *important* over the *urgent*. I try not to answer texts, phone calls, or emails when I'm in my zone. I've burnt many cakes because I stepped away from the oven for too long, and I've flopped recipes because I was distracted and forgot a key ingredient. I've even been so preoccupied that in the middle of a conversation with my kids they've asked if I've heard a word they said. Multitasking depletes us in the end because we feel overstretched and compromise the task at hand. *Slow down and focus to become better at everything.*

6 Be prepared for flops

Think about an experience in your life when you didn't quite make it to the finish. Did it lead you somewhere new? Somewhere you couldn't have planned for? In the kitchen, embrace your food flops and turn them into wins. Save the overbaked bread and make garlicky croutons. Or if something absolutely cannot be eaten or recycled, keep trying until you figure out why it failed. And never give up. Some of my best recipes happened by accident as I was trying to salvage a tasteless muffin or transform a botched-up brownie. Real satisfaction lies in turning failure, disappointment, mistakes, and loss into outrageous success. *Sometimes you've got to get it wrong to get it right.*

7 Get creative: Bend the rules

Once you get good, the fun really begins! Graduating from cook to chef gives you freedom and the confidence to use recipes as springboards to create your own unique masterpieces. Spark your creativity here:

- Adapt any recipe to make it your own (page 284).
- Recast your flops into wins (page 207).
- Work with what you have in the fridge (page 12).
- Substitute ingredients (page 10).

Look for ways to work *smarter*, not *harder*. Lemon curd may traditionally need straining, but I skip that process on page 233 because it's unnecessary. Measuring and combining wet and dry ingredients separately might be a cooking rule, but I hate washing an extra bowl, so I whip up one-bowl muffin wonders. One day I even decided to skip the "fry" part of a stir-fry and instead baked the dish in the oven (page 146). Get creative your way, and, hey, you might even write the next best-selling cookbook.

8 Zig and zag: Cheat a little

In order to stay within range of your ideal recipe, diet, and life (and to avoid straying too far from your "why"), be prepared to zig and zag here and there. Veer off course! Cheat a little! I ordered french fries the other night (yes, I really did, my kids were awed). Eating in the middle results in food freedom without deprivation or guilt. It still may mean often saying no. But it also means occasionally saying yes to your favorite splurges. If you've fallen off your ideal way of eating for a week, it's okay. Give yourself a break, and start back on track the next day. I strategically cheat in the kitchen too. In a pinch, I serve store-bought rotisserie chicken next to my freshly roasted veggies, or a store-bought chocolate cake topped with a homemade icing and berries. Guess what? No one knows or cares. Cooking shortcuts preserve your sanity and invite a life beyond slaving all day in the kitchen. And the key to long-term success with any way of eating is moderation, not deprivation. Become a flexible chef by stripping away complexity for the sake of finding a simpler—yet just as craveable—solution. *Flexibility is about learning how to give yourself a break and still come out on top.*

9 Find joy in the process

Cooking was once a chore for me, not the labor of love it is today. Frantically running around to get dinner on the table at six p.m. after a long day of work is almost never enjoyable! These days, however, I've learned to embrace the chaos and to focus on making the cooking process fun—think of it as a form of single-tasking. Yeah, I still sometimes have manic predinner meltdowns, but my kitchen is now a welcoming place to be with my family. Doing chaos with love is better than doing it with resentment. Pour passion into your creations and your diners will be able to taste the difference. Although I often cook with my kids or friends, cooking solo can invoke a spark of creativity and act as a form of inspired meditation. Play your favorite music, pour yourself a glass of wine, and enjoy the art of cooking. *Cooking can be an affair of the heart if you choose to make it so.*

10   Channel your inner chef

You are your own best teacher—nobody knows what is right for you better than you do! What are your unique talents? Challenges? Cravings? I've found it futile to compare my level of success to anyone else's. One-size-fits-all approaches to diets, food, and life, in general, are outdated. Be flexible on your way to the finish line. *You've got this.*

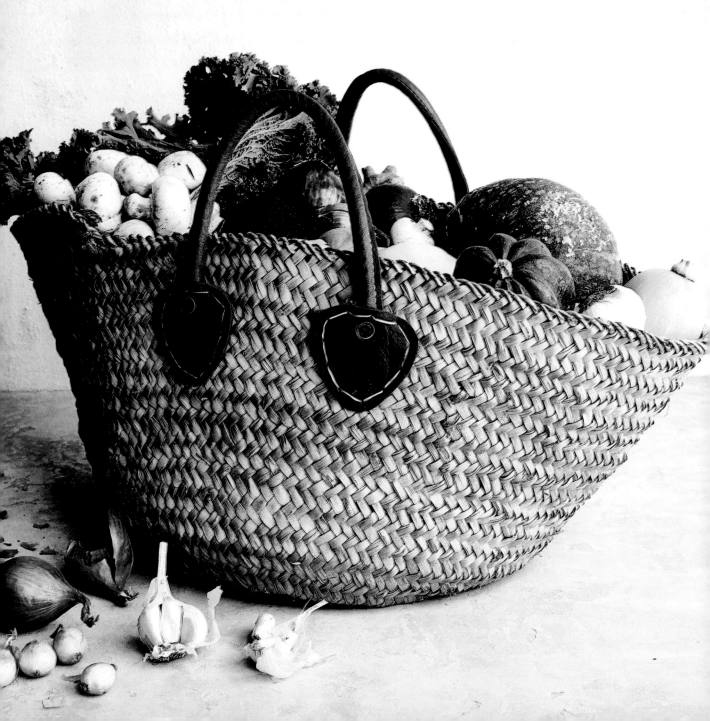

INGREDIENT FLIPS

How often have you gone on a wild-goose chase for an ingredient a recipe calls for, or just skipped over an ingredient entirely, bewildered by where to begin? *Don't flip out. Just flip it!* Many of the ingredient swaps listed below are precise and seamless in effect and flavor, like swapping coconut oil for butter; others are acceptable but produce a different result, like using soy sauce or tamari in place of fish sauce. Soy or tamari will lend a similar saltiness, and they're good swaps for fish sauce if fishiness isn't your thing. Similarly, coconut cream is a wonderful swap for heavy cream; just make sure it is *very* chilled if it must be whipped. The main point here is to stay flexible, adapt, and use what you have!

Baking IN GENERAL, THESE ARE 1:1 SWAPS

- Butter = margarine = coconut oil (Coconut oil can be measured soft or solid.)

- Heavy cream = coconut cream (Make sure it's well chilled if whipping—chill it overnight and use only the solids.)

- Dairy milk = almond milk = any dairy-free milk

- Sugar = brown sugar = date sugar

- 1 cup regular flour = 1 cup gluten-free flour + ½ teaspoon xanthan gum

  (Note: If your gluten-free flour has xanthan added already, omit it in the recipe.)

- 1 12-ounce bag chocolate chips = 2 cups = 1 12-ounce chocolate bar, chopped

- Almond flour = slivered almonds ground into superfine crumbs

- 1 Egg = 3 tablespoons flaxseed meal plus 6 tablespoons water (Mix to make a paste.)

- Arrowroot = cornstarch

- Tapioca starch = potato starch

- Applesauce = mashed banana = cooked pumpkin, sweet potato, or carrot purée

- Grated zucchini = grated carrot

- Spaghetti squash = spiralized raw zucchini noodles = spiralized raw sweet potato noodles

Cooking

- Yellow onions = red onions = pearl onions

- 1 Fresh garlic clove = ½ teaspoon pre-minced bottled garlic

- Olive oil = canola oil = melted coconut oil

- Pine nuts = pili nuts = chopped macadamia nuts = cashews = peanuts

- Almonds = pecans = walnuts

- Soy sauce = tamari

- Hoisin sauce = BBQ sauce

- Fish sauce = soy sauce or tamari (But you will lose the fish's added umami flavor.)

- Minced beef = minced turkey = minced chicken

- Black cod = Chilean sea bass = any fatty fish

- Halibut = flounder = haddock = any flaky white fish

- Chives = green part of scallion

- Basil = cilantro = parsley (For pesto, seasoning eggs, garnishes.)

- Chickpea flour = any rice flour (Works in all the recipes in this book.)

- Capers = chopped pitted green olives

- Sake = mirin

- Kale = romaine lettuce = chicory (Or cabbage or spinach, depending on the recipe.)

- Nutritional yeast = grated Parmesan

- A specific vinegar = any vinegar (Except balsamic, which is unique.)

- Goldenberries = cranberries = raisins = dried cherries

- Pumpkin = acorn squash = butternut squash

- Drizzle of chile oil = pinch of red pepper flakes

- Glass noodles = thin rice noodles

- Mango chutney = apricot or peach jam = citrus marmalade

PANTRY, FRIDGE, AND FREEZER ESSENTIALS

These are the staples to keep on hand. I depend on them for whipping up dinner fast. Make your own personalized lists of staples to cater to your preferences.

In the pantry

- Spices and dried herbs
- Arrowroot or cornstarch
- Chicken broth
- Canned full-fat coconut milk and coconut cream
- Canned tuna in olive oil
- Sardines (I prefer skinless and boneless)
- Canned salmon
- Canned chickpeas
- Canned tomatoes
- Tomato paste
- Bottled marinara sauce
- Roasted red peppers
- Applesauce (single-serving packs)
- Olive oil
- Coconut oil
- Vinegars
- Tamari or soy sauce
- Tahini
- Sriracha
- Dijon mustard, or your favorite
- Salsa
- Honey or maple syrup
- Dried grains, beans, pasta, nuts
- Gluten-free crackers
- Gluten-free pasta
- Brown rice
- Quinoa
- Dried beans or chickpeas
- Assorted nuts
- Onions
- Garlic
- Almond flour, all-purpose gluten-free flour, and assorted gluten-free flours (like oat and sorghum)
- Xanthan gum
- Baking soda and powder
- Good-quality vanilla extract
- Dark chocolate chips
- Natural cocoa powder
- Oats
- Granola
- Boxed mixes (like gluten-free pancakes, brownies, muffins, and cakes)

In the fridge and freezer

- Almond milk
- Eggs
- Fresh, seasonal vegetables
- Fresh, seasonal fruit
- Lemons and limes
- Fresh herbs
- Olives
- Pickles
- Frozen fish, cut into portions to defrost for last-minute dinners
- Raw meat and chicken, cut into portions for last-minute dinners
- Frozen fruit (mango, strawberries, etc.)
- Frozen spinach (for omelets if you run out of fresh vegetables)
- Frozen peas
- Edamame (snacks, protein addition to salads)
- Shredded cheese (lasts a long time)
- Grated Parmesan
- Corn tortillas (to make quesadillas)

COOL GADGETS FOR YOUR WISH LIST

The adventure lies in building your toolbox over time, so don't be in a rush. A purchase should solve a problem for you (when I was tired of hand mixing I invested in a stand-up mixer). Invest in stackables, portables, and multiuse equipment to save on space. I've limited the gadget suggestions below to specialty items or staples beyond the usual frying pan. But remember, even if you have *no* tools you'll still find a way to make your food great.

Bigger

- Immersion or hand blender
- High-speed blender—I prefer the Vitamix
- Food processor
- Dehydrator (for special nuts, raw crackers and cookies, onions, granola, bread crumbs, or crisping stale things)
- Waffle maker with attachments
- Toaster oven
- Whirley Pop Popcorn Popper
- Stand mixer

Smaller

- Small and large wire whisks
- Stainless steel bowls for mixing
- A good set of knives
- Oven donut pan
- Mini and regular muffin pans plus liners
- Mini and regular loaf pans
- 10-inch springform pan
- Glass pie pan
- Large baking sheets and half sheets
- Wire racks for cooling baked goods
- Cutting boards
- Graduated set of round cookie cutters
- Salad spinner
- Garlic press
- A sharp peeler
- Microplane fine zester/ grater
- Instant-read oven thermometer
- Ice-pop tray or molds
- Plastic squeeze bottle
- Silicone baking pans
- Silicone challah bread baking mold

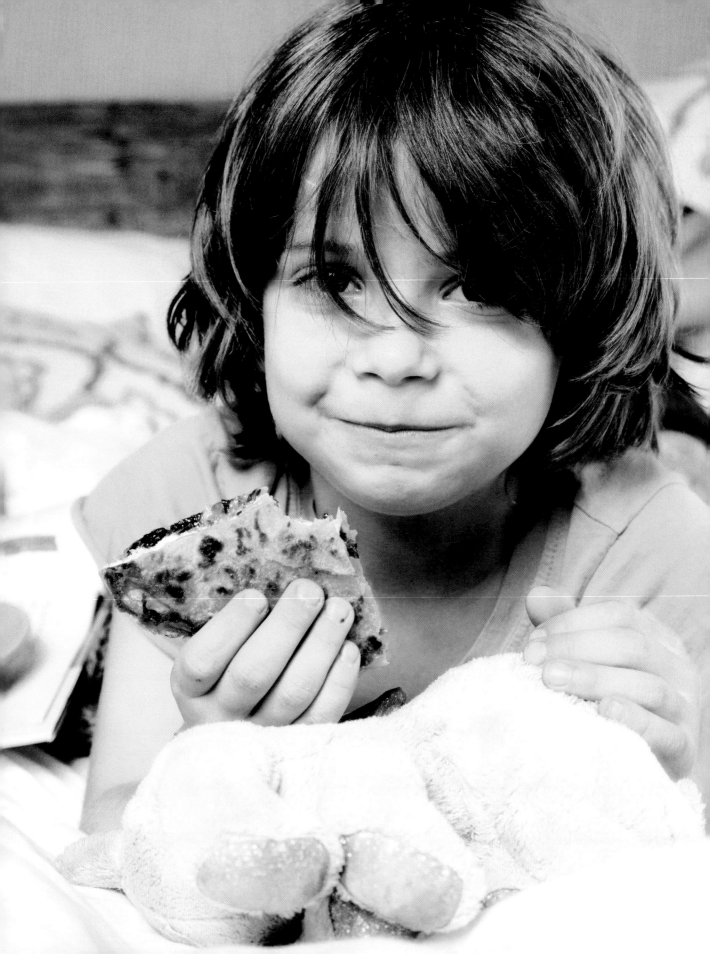

Chapter 2

ALL-DAY BREAKFAST

Breakfast sounds like a great idea until you wake up and actually have to make it. Between getting the kids out the door for school, rushing to work, and maybe squeezing in a workout, preparing a meal on top of it all seems like a chore. But it doesn't have to be. If you plan ahead and apply some time-saving techniques, it may just become your new favorite meal of the day (at any time of the day because why not have eggs for lunch or dinner?).

Take the guesswork out of "What's for breakfast?" during rush hour by posting a weekly breakfast menu in a place everyone can see. It helps combat breakfast fatigue (cereal, again?) and stops picky cereal-only eaters from complaining (sorry, kids, it's eggs today!). Whenever possible, prepare the following day's menu the night before—premeasure dry ingredients for waffles, make the salad dressing, or sauté the veggies for your omelet. You'll find all these morning hacks in the pages ahead.

In my house, we have a few egg days, a pancake day, a muesli or yogurt day, a savory day, and a special breakfast-treat day with muffins and sweet baked goods. Yet, frankly, most days I just crave two eggs and a bowlful of veggies. What do *you* crave that will fuel you for the day ahead? Get creative and adapt these recipes to suit *your* morning routine, taste buds, and lifestyle. Good morning!

GRAINLESS BANANA PANCAKES

STEPS: MASH, BLEND, FLIP, SERVE! / **Makes 18 3-inch pancakes**

Healthy and delicious pancakes, for real? These bad boys have nothing bad about them. They're pretty much like eating bananas and eggs for breakfast, so it's kind of sneaky of me to even sell them as pancakes but, well, they are! So splurge and have a few.

Tools: Nonstick frying pan

2 medium, ripe bananas

3 large eggs

1 cup almond flour

1 tablespoon flaxseeds, ground

2 teaspoons vanilla extract

1 teaspoon raw honey

½ teaspoon ground cinnamon

Pinch of salt

Coconut oil or oil spray, for frying

Maple syrup or butter, for serving (optional)

1 In a medium bowl, mash the bananas with a fork until smooth.

2 Add the eggs, almond flour, flaxseeds, vanilla, honey, cinnamon, and salt, and blend thoroughly. Allow the mixture to sit for 5 minutes to thicken slightly.

3 Heat a griddle or nonstick pan over low heat (to avoid burning) with a touch of coconut oil, or lightly spray the pan.

4 Spoon the desired amount of batter onto the pan. (Because the batter is delicate, smaller pancakes tend to flip more easily without breaking.) Cook until the edges are firm, about 4 to 5 minutes, then flip the pancakes and cook on the other side until cooked through, 2 or 3 more minutes.

5 Serve with maple syrup or butter, if desired.

> *nail this*

The only important measurement is the banana–egg–almond flour ratio. The rest is for added flavoring and sweetness.

» *flip it*

If you prefer a thinner batter, add ¼ cup almond milk.

Pressed for time? Bake them! Spoon the batter into greased mini muffin pans and bake at 350°F for 5 minutes, or until set. Serve with maple syrup.

Stir into the batter: nuts, chocolate chips, blueberries, or extra chunks of banana.

I always peel then freeze extra-ripe bananas—if you have frozen ones, use them.

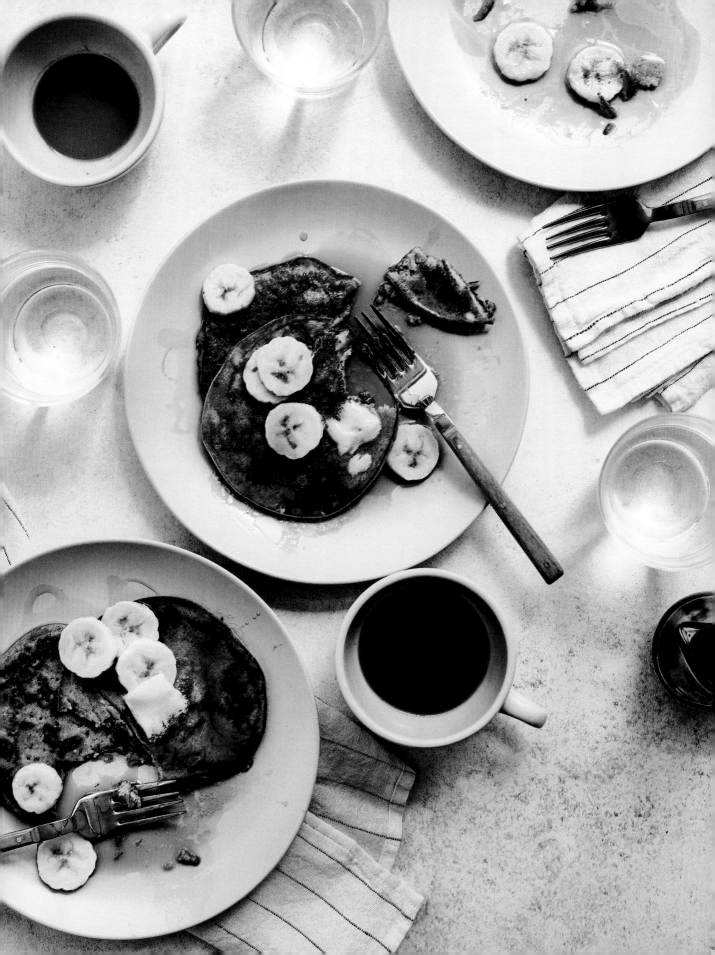

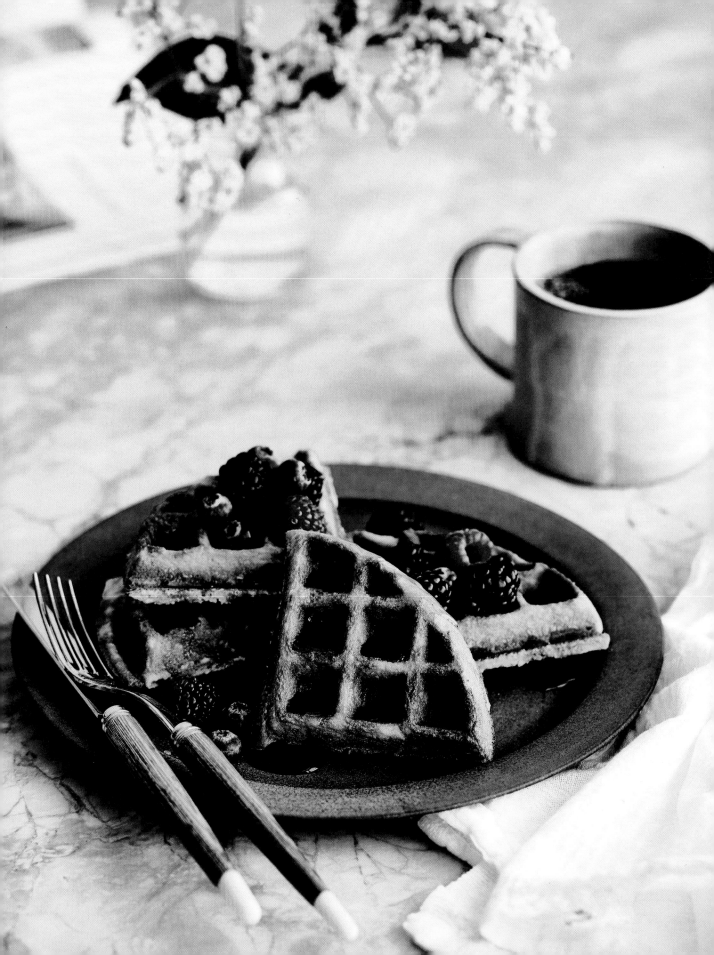

MY FAVORITE HEALTHIFIED WAFFLES

STEPS: WHISK, STIR, COOK! / **Makes 6 large waffles or 22 mini donut waffles (my personal preference)**

It's taken me far too many failed attempts (but that's how we get good!) to create amazing waffles—the batter for which, coincidentally, doubles as the ultimate pancake batter. My healthified twist on a waffle uses a good amount of almond flour and sneaks in some hemp seeds. (Don't worry, the seeds disappear, and even the pickiest eaters won't notice them.) Thanks to the vanilla, cinnamon, and butter, these waffles are flavorful and moist—and may become your favorite way to waffle.

Tools: Waffle maker

DRY INGREDIENTS
1 cup almond flour

½ cup all-purpose gluten-free flour

2 tablespoons granulated sugar

2 tablespoons hemp seeds

1 tablespoon baking powder

½ teaspoon ground cinnamon

¼ teaspoon salt

WET INGREDIENTS
¾ cup almond milk (or a splash more, as needed)

1 large egg

3 tablespoons unsalted butter, melted

1 teaspoon vanilla extract

TO SERVE
Maple syrup

Mixed berries

1 Whisk the dry ingredients together in a large bowl. Set aside.

2 Whisk the wet ingredients together in a small bowl. Stir the wet mix into the dry mix. Consistency should be similar to that of a cake batter. Add more almond milk, if needed, to thin.

3 Preheat and lightly grease the waffle maker. If it has a temperature dial, set it to medium high.

4 Pour the batter into the desired waffle shape (regular or mini donut size). Cook each waffle until it is light golden brown and set; the timing will depend on your machine.

5 Serve the waffles with maple syrup and berries.

> nail this

For a successful stress-free morning, premeasure your dry mix the night before—or even better, double it up and stash half in the freezer for another time.

Some waffle makers turn out waffles that are so massive that after eating one you're stuffed. I prefer a smaller waffle maker that includes a donut attachment, so you can splurge on more than one without feeling overly full.

>> flip it

Eliminate the hemp seeds if you don't have or want them; they just add flavor and nutrition.

Use any milk you prefer.

For a "donut" treat: Top the mini-donut-shaped version with chocolate ganache or a vanilla glaze, decorate with nuts, shredded coconut, or sprinkles, and serve.

Alternatively, make these into pancakes and add any fun ingredients you like; follow the pancake-cooking instructions on page 16.

GREEN SMOOTHIE MILKSHAKE

STEPS: BLEND, SIP!! / **Makes 2 to 4 servings**

I'm not a breakfast-smoothie kind of girl; I prefer my morning nutrients in solid form. But I do have a soft spot for milkshakes. This creamy "smoothie milkshake" tastes so decadent you'd never guess it's actually super good for you...and what mom wouldn't be thrilled when her kids sip away on kale for breakfast? Packed with good fats, protein, and enough sweetness to help the veggies go down unnoticed, it's a no-brainer way to start your day.

Tools: High-speed blender

1 cup chopped raw kale leaves

½ to 1 cup unsweetened almond milk

2 small ripe bananas (I like them frozen), peeled and roughly chopped

2 to 3 heaping tablespoons raw almond butter

1 tablespoon hemp seeds

2 to 3 teaspoons raw honey

1 teaspoon vanilla extract

1 Place the kale, ½ cup almond milk, bananas, almond butter, hemp seeds, 2 teaspoons honey, and vanilla in a blender. You can add more almond milk to achieve your desired consistency and more honey according to your sweet tooth (it will depend on how ripe the bananas are). As for the kale, add more if you can stuff more in!

2 Blend until smooth.

› nail this

If you're making this smoothie for kids, don't you dare let them spot the kale leaves!

Serve cold! Use frozen bananas if you have them, or add ice to final stage of blending.

» flip it

Use any greens you can find: spinach, chard, and bok choy work equally well.

Swap peanut butter or any nut butter for the almond butter. Swap coconut milk or water for the almond milk.

Add a scoop of vanilla protein powder.

Add a spoonful of raw cacao powder, or any cocoa powder, and a bit of extra honey to make this a chocolate-banana-butter milkshake!

Serve this for a party in champagne glasses, topped with shaved chocolate.

Freeze leftovers into popsicles (see page 23 for popsicles—you can freeze any smoothie into a popsicle). They're a great way to stash a fast breakfast or snack in the freezer.

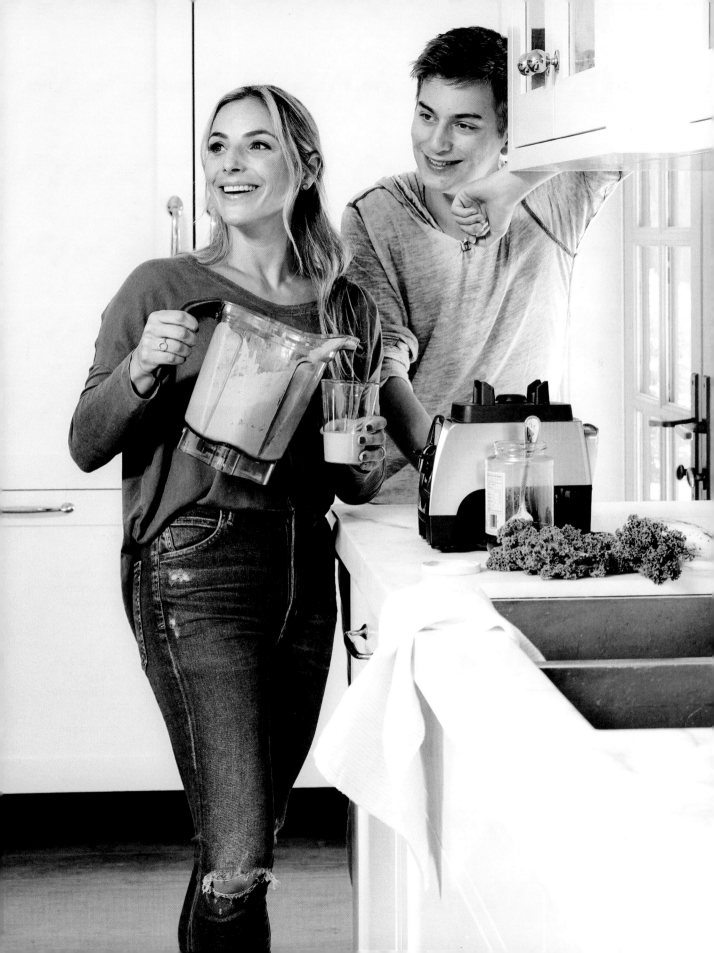

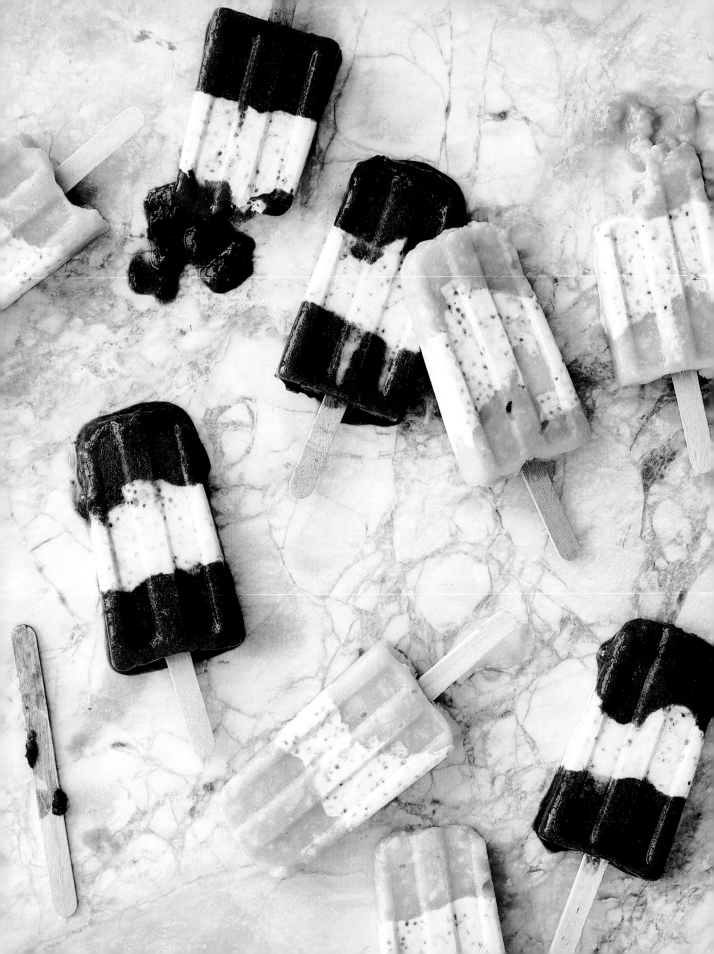

FRUITY COCONUT BREAKFAST POPSICLES

STEPS: BLEND AND FREEZE! / **Makes about 10 small pops**

I usually enjoy making breakfast—except on the days that I don't. That's when the idea of a premade, frozen breakfast is most appealing. These pops, however, have more than convenience going for them. They're massively Instagram-worthy and completely flexible. Keep some in the freezer for an after-school snack or to satisfy a frozen-pop craving.

Tools: Blender, popsicle molds, and sticks

BASE

1 15.5-ounce can full-fat coconut milk

2 tablespoons chia seeds

2 tablespoons maple syrup

2 teaspoons vanilla extract

FRUIT PURÉE

1½ cups diced ripe mango or strawberries, fresh or frozen

1 to 2 tablespoons raw honey (optional, depending on how sweet the fruit is)

1 Make the base: In a medium bowl, stir together the coconut milk, chia seeds, maple syrup, and vanilla. Set aside until the chia seeds expand and the mixture thickens, about 1 hour.

2 Make the fruit purée: In a blender, blend the fruit and the honey, if using, until almost smooth; retain some smaller chunks. Set aside.

3 Assemble the layers: Pour about half of the fruit purée by the spoonful into popsicle molds. Spoon in the coconut mixture. Finish with the remaining purée.

4 Freeze overnight, until the popsicles are firm, then unmold and serve. If you have trouble unmolding, place the molds into a warm glass of water for a few seconds.

» *flip it*

Dairy option: In place of the coconut milk, use 1 cup vanilla yogurt (or use plain yogurt and sweeten it with honey and vanilla).

Fast track: Skip the chia seeds and simply blend together the coconut milk, maple syrup, vanilla, and fruit. You'll lose the beauty and the added nutrition of the chia, but you'll gain a whole hour to work out instead!

Make a decadent smoothie: Pop all the ingredients in a blender. Add protein powder, flax, or hemp to boost nutrition.

Make a few mini pops with the coconut-milk mixture only. Freeze to set, then dip in melted chocolate for a fun treat!

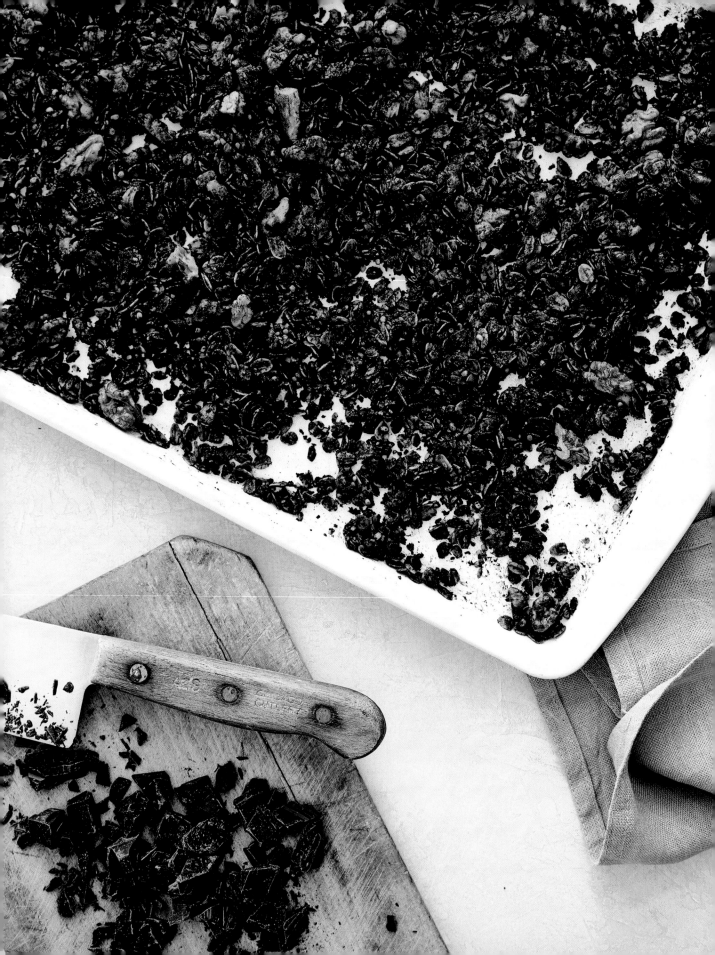

INDULGENT CHOCOLATE GRANOLA

STEPS: STIR, BAKE, CHILL! / **Makes about 4 cups**

Chocolate for breakfast—why not? And don't stop at serving this delectable sweet and salty granola in the morning. Snack on this treat straight from the fridge. (Store it somewhere safe or it's a hazard to your waistline.) Although my secret to making the best granola ever is letting it do its magic in a dehydrator, I created this insanely addicting oven-baked recipe because not everyone owns a dehydrator. After slow-roasting the oat mixture, the magic continues with a final drizzle of dark chocolate at the end of baking. The result is nutty, crunchy, chocolatey heaven.

Tools: Large baking sheet, parchment paper

DRY INGREDIENTS

3 cups old-fashioned rolled oats

1 heaping cup walnuts (or any nuts), chopped

⅓ cup high-quality cocoa powder

¼ cup dark brown sugar

¼ cup flax meal

2 tablespoons hemp seeds

1 teaspoon salt (or use my Rosemary Salt, page 268, for added flavor)

½ teaspoon ground cinnamon

WET INGREDIENTS

¼ cup maple syrup

¼ cup coconut oil, melted

¼ cup (half a stick) unsalted butter, melted

1 tablespoon vanilla extract

1 Preheat the oven to 160°F, or your lowest oven setting. Line a baking sheet with parchment paper.

2 In a large bowl, toss the dry ingredients. Stir in the wet ingredients.

3 Pour the granola onto the prepared baking sheet, and spread it into an even, thick layer. Bake for 2 hours. Check every 20 minutes, and stir to ensure even baking. Baking at a low temperature ensures that it won't burn and the flavors slowly infuse the oats.

4 Remove the granola from the oven, and increase the oven temperature to 350°F.

5 To make the topping: Crumble the chocolate bars into pieces, or coarsely chop them with a large chef's knife. Sprinkle the chocolate over the granola. Return the pan to the oven, and bake until the chocolate is melted, 3 to 5 minutes. Remove the pan from the oven, and stir the melted chocolate into the granola until evenly distributed. Sprinkle with the slightest bit of salt.

6 Transfer the granola to the refrigerator to cool and harden the chocolate, about 30 minutes. Store in an airtight container in the refrigerator for one month (or more, though it probably won't last that long!).

CONTINUED

TOPPING (OPTIONAL)

1½ bars (2 ounces total) of dark chocolate, or ½ cup chocolate chips

pinches of salt

VARIATION: DEHYDRATOR METHOD

1 Spread the tossed granola mixture on a dehydrator sheet in a flat layer. Dehydrate at 120°F for 24 hours.

2 Preheat the oven to 350°F.

3 Continue as above from step 5 to make topping.

> *nail this*

Keep the oven low and watch closely so the granola doesn't burn. Bake the granola in the coolest section of the oven, not next to direct heat.

Pack the granola tightly on the baking sheet so it gets clumpy during baking.

Good cocoa makes all the difference. Hershey's produces a good-enough option, and Valrhona is a splurge. Get the best stuff you can find.

>> *flip it*

The suggested amount of chocolate is my personal preference. If you like things more chocolatey, then add more, and vice versa.

Want to transform this into an even more indulgent snack? Use ½ cup cocoa, and ⅓ cup each maple syrup, coconut oil, and butter.

RAWLICIOUS MUESLI

STEPS: MIX, STIR, SERVE! / **Makes 6 servings**

I make an exception to my usual eggs for breakfast when this scrumptious, no-rules, grain-free muesli is on the menu at home. Crunchy nuts and seeds are complemented by shredded apples infused with citrus and vanilla, then topped with a generous pour of almond milk. Assemble the nuts and spices the night before to make your morning breakfast a delicious breeze.

Tools: Food processor

FOR THE NIGHT BEFORE

½ cup raw almonds

¼ cup pumpkin seeds

¼ cup chopped dried dates

¼ cup chia seeds

2 tablespoons flax meal

2 teaspoons ground cinnamon

¼ teaspoon ground nutmeg

Pinch of salt

IN THE MORNING

2 red apples, grated

1 cup fresh blueberries

1 tablespoon freshly grated orange zest

1 teaspoon vanilla extract

1 cup almond or full-fat coconut milk, or to taste

Drizzle of raw honey, to serve

Fresh mint, to garnish

1 Pulse the almonds, pumpkin seeds, and dates in a food processor. Transfer the mixture to a medium bowl and add the chia, flax, cinnamon, nutmeg, and salt. Store overnight in an airtight container.

2 In the morning, add the apples, blueberries, orange zest, and vanilla to the mixture.

3 Serve the muesli with milk, a drizzle of honey, and fresh mint, if desired.

› *nail this*

If you have a dehydrator, soak then dehydrate your almonds and seeds to make them crunchy. Otherwise, use super-fresh and crispy raw almonds. You can toast them slightly to achieve the desired crispness, if need be.

›› *flip it*

Use any variety of nut and fruits. Great additions include toasted coconut, shredded pears, raspberries, blackberries, cubed mango, or chopped fresh pineapple.

No food processor? Chop the ingredients by hand (but it's more time-consuming, so add a food processor to your holiday-gift wish list).

Turn this into oatmeal by adding 1 cup of old-fashioned oats. Simmer the mixture on the stovetop, and follow the instructions on the package of oats. (I suggest omitting the orange zest for optimal flavor.)

> *nail this*

Don't skip the second layer of cheese to sandwich the vegetables; it will help the quesadilla stick together.

>> *flip it*

Picky eaters? Use finely diced onion and cauliflower or peeled zucchini instead of spinach and mushrooms—those white veggies remain hidden, out of sight between the two layers of cheese!

Are you feeding a non–cheese lover? Mash up the avocado so that it's the "glue," spread it on a warmed tortilla, stuff all the veggies inside, and roll it up as a burrito.

Make cheesy pizza quesadillas: Substitute Veggie-Full Marinara (page 282) or another ready-made marinara sauce for the vegetables. Add a generous amount of sauce so that the cheese and sauce ooze, like the perfect slice of pizza. Why *not* serve healthified "pizza" for breakfast?

Make the veggies ahead of time so that breakfast is a breeze. Or make a few batches of veggies so you have extra for the next day's omelet.

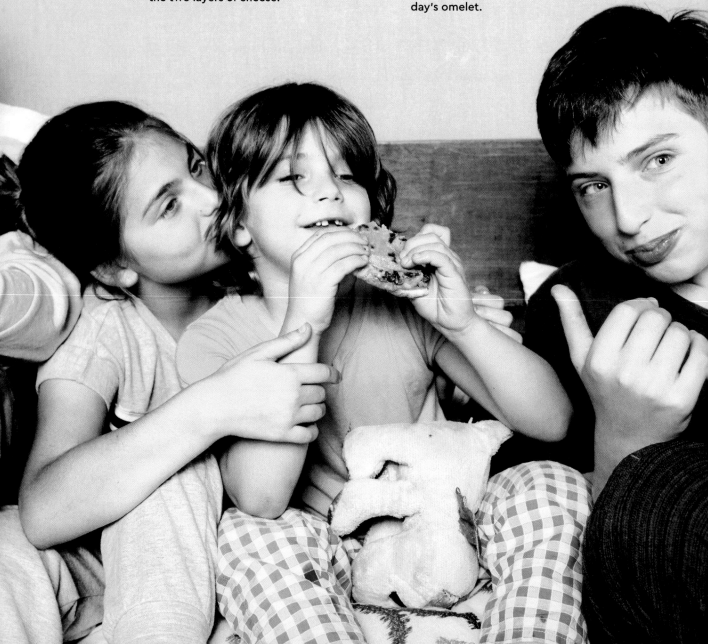

KID-APPROVED BREAKFAST QUESADILLAS

STEPS: SAUTÉ, SCRAMBLE, LAYER, FLIP! / *Makes enough for 3 starving kids or 6 moderately hungry ones*

When my kids were younger (and I was less experienced), I used to worry that they weren't eating enough greens. These quesadillas became my secret way to add vegetables to their meals—sandwiched between layers of cheese and corn tortillas. We still make variations of these for any meal of the day. Sometimes (often) I have no idea what to make for dinner. I literally brain freeze. When I ask my kids what they want to eat, nine times out of ten they ask for these versatile quesadillas. Phew, because nothing could be easier.

2 tablespoons olive oil or unsalted butter

1 small yellow onion, chopped

½ cup diced assorted mushrooms

2 cups fresh spinach, julienned

1 jalapeño pepper, seeded and finely diced (optional)

Salt and freshly ground black pepper, to taste

6 large eggs

1½ cups shredded melting cheese (such as Cheddar, Monterey Jack, or mozzarella)

6 corn tortillas (6 inch)

Oil spray, for pan

Guacamole, for serving (optional)

1 In a large frying pan over medium heat, heat the oil or butter and cook the onion, stirring frequently, until translucent, about 5 minutes.

2 Add the mushrooms and cook over medium-high heat until they are browned and have released their juices, about 8 more minutes. It's essential to sweat them long enough to evaporate the juices so that the quesadilla isn't too wet.

3 Add the spinach and jalapeño, if using, and cook, stirring, until the spinach is wilted, 2 to 3 minutes. Season with salt and pepper.

4 Remove the vegetables from the pan onto a plate, and quickly scramble the eggs in the same pan, over medium heat, or cook them as an omelet.

5 To assemble the quesadillas, layer one tortilla with some cheese, then add some cooked veggies and scrambled eggs, and top with more cheese. Cover with a second tortilla.

6 Wipe out the pan and spray it lightly with oil spray. Heat the pan over medium heat, and cook one of the quesadillas until it is lightly browned and the cheese is melted, about 3 minutes. Carefully flip the quesadilla and finish the other side, cooking until browned, about 2 more minutes. Repeat with the other two quesadillas. Note: You can preheat the oven to 350°F, place all three quesadillas on a baking sheet that has been lightly sprayed with oil, and bake them until the cheese is melted, about 10 minutes.

7 To serve, cut each in half and top with guacamole, if desired.

SMOKED SALMON AND ONION FRITTATA MUFFINS

STEPS: BROWN, STIR, BAKE! / **Makes 8 to 10 servings**

If I have a lot of mouths to feed in the morning, this is a dish I turn to. Instead of standing at my stovetop making ten individual omelets, I just bake these the night before and then reheat before serving. If smoked salmon isn't your thing, don't flip the page just yet—you can totally skip the whole smoky thing and make any vegetable frittata muffin flavor you dream up.

Tools: 12-cup muffin pan

1 tablespoon olive oil, plus more for greasing

2 tablespoons unsalted butter

1 small red onion, finely chopped

3 ounces smoked salmon, lox style or your favorite

8 large eggs, lightly beaten

½ cup chopped chives

¼ teaspoon salt

Freshly ground black pepper, to taste

1 Preheat the oven to 400°F. Grease the muffin cups with olive oil or cooking spray.

2 In a large skillet over medium to medium-high heat, heat 1 tablespoon olive oil with the butter. Add the onion and cook, stirring, until lightly browned, about 8 minutes.

3 Move the onions to one side of the skillet, and fry the smoked salmon, using a spatula to flip, until the edges are crisped, about 1 minute total. Break up the salmon into smaller pieces.

4 Remove the skillet from the heat, transfer the onion and salmon to a bowl, and allow them to cool for a few minutes.

5 Add the eggs, chives, salt, and pepper to the bowl, whisking to combine.

6 Pour the egg mixture into the prepared muffin cups, dividing the mixture evenly and filling each cup almost to the top. Bake for 20 to 25 minutes, or until the eggs are set in the center. Allow to cool for 1 minute before removing the muffins from the pan.

> *nail this*

Crisp up your smoked salmon well; this step makes it extra yummy.

A silicone muffin pan will ensure that these do not stick.

>> *flip it*

If you prefer, make this into a few omelets or a baked frittata.

Skip the smoked salmon and instead sauté some veggies; top with some mozzarella for extra oomph.

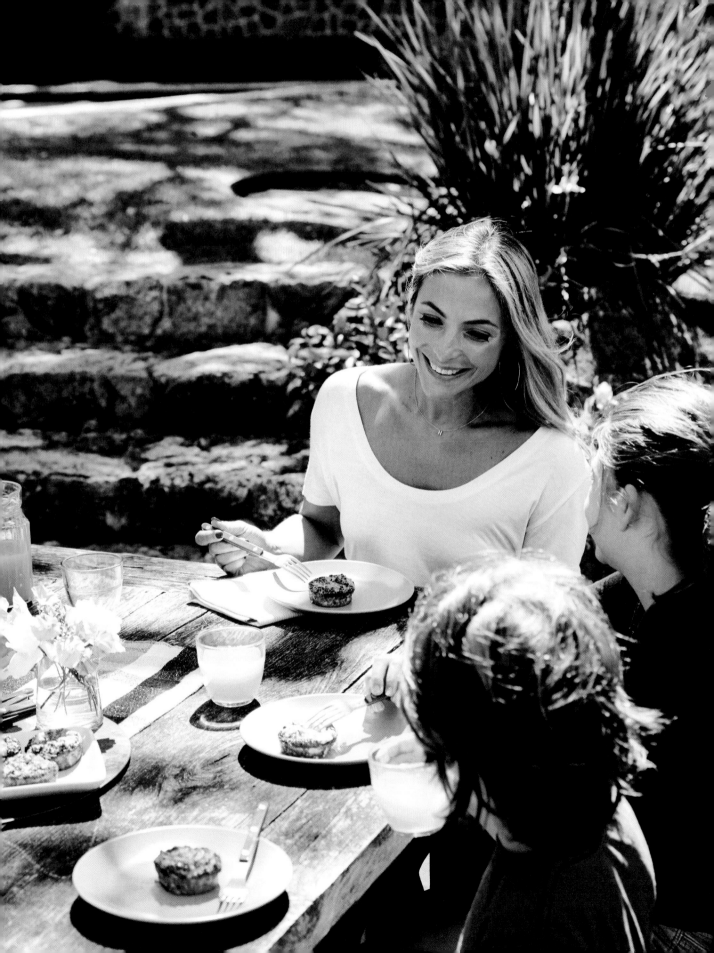

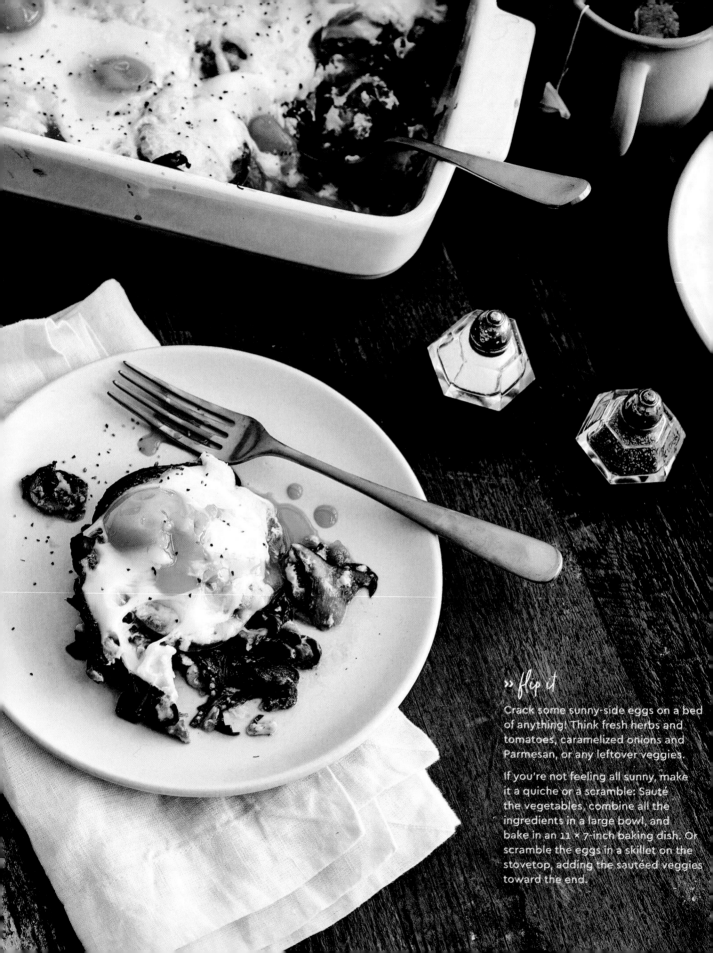

» flip it

Crack some sunny-side eggs on a bed of anything! Think fresh herbs and tomatoes, caramelized onions and Parmesan, or any leftover veggies.

If you're not feeling all sunny, make it a quiche or a scramble: Sauté the vegetables, combine all the ingredients in a large bowl, and bake in an 11 × 7-inch baking dish. Or scramble the eggs in a skillet on the stovetop, adding the sautéed veggies toward the end.

SUNNY-SIDE MUSHROOM BAKE

STEPS: SAUTÉ, COOL, BAKE! / *Makes 4 to 6 servings*

I thought I'd tried making eggs every which way...until this breakfast happened. I had sautéed a batch of veggies the night before for a planned breakfast quiche. Then, a stroke of total genius arrived in the early morning: Cook the quiche ingredients in layers for a fun way to mix things up. Holy yum! The soft veggies are gooey with cheese, and as you dig in, the yolks ooze a bit over the veggies—oh breakfast, I just love you.

Tools: 11 × 7-inch baking dish

2 tablespoons olive oil, plus more if needed

1 tablespoon unsalted butter

1 medium yellow onion, finely chopped

4 cups assorted sliced mushrooms

Salt, to taste

1 cup fresh spinach, chopped

A few basil leaves

2 medium tomatoes, thinly sliced

¾ cup shredded mozzarella cheese

6 large eggs

Freshly ground black pepper, to taste

1 In a large sauté pan over medium heat, heat the olive oil and butter, and cook the onion, stirring frequently, until translucent, about 5 minutes.

2 Add the mushrooms, season them with salt, and cook, stirring frequently, until they've released their juices and browned, about 10 minutes.

3 Add another splash of olive oil, if needed, then stir in the spinach and basil and cook until wilted, about 2 minutes.

4 Remove the vegetables from the heat and spoon them into a baking dish. Cool the mixture for 10 minutes or overnight.

5 When ready to cook, preheat the oven to 350°F.

6 If you've chilled the mushroom mixture overnight, warm it in the oven for 15 minutes before proceeding. Arrange the tomatoes over the mushroom mixture, then sprinkle the cheese over the veggies. Crack the eggs on top of the mixture, keeping the yolks intact. Season with salt and pepper.

7 Bake until the egg whites are set and the yolks are still runny, about 15 to 20 minutes. Note that the eggs will continue cooking a bit more once removed from the oven.

> *nail this*

Watch the eggs in the oven carefully—there's a sweet spot when the whites are set but the yolks remain runny. If you cook a minute too long the yolks will harden, and that's a bummer.

ONE-PAN CARAMELIZED CABBAGE AND EGGS

STEPS: CARAMELIZE, FRY, EAT! / **Makes 2 servings (or 1 if you're me)**

One-pan breakfasts are the wave of the future, and this recipe uses the highly neglected but all-star cabbage. When cabbage and onions cook together for long enough, they turn into a buttery, delicious, and oh-so-light veggie medley. When you serve the cabbage side by side with eggs cooked sunny-side up, the yolks run into the cabbage and bring the dish to life. I eat a version of this efficient breakfast almost every morning, sometimes at the countertop and always straight from the skillet so I don't even dirty a plate.

2 tablespoons plus 1½ teaspoons olive oil

¼ yellow onion, chopped

½ medium head green cabbage, shredded

Salt and freshly ground black pepper, to taste

4 large eggs

Grated Parmesan cheese, to garnish

Fresh parsley leaves, to garnish (optional)

1 Heat the olive oil in a large skillet over low heat. Add the onions and cook until translucent, about 6 minutes.

2 Add the cabbage and cook slowly until the vegetables are caramelized, 15 to 20 minutes. Season with salt and pepper.

3 Move the vegetables to one side of the pan to make room for the eggs. Spray the pan with more oil if it looks dry, so the eggs don't stick. Crack the eggs into the pan and cook them until the whites set, about 3 minutes.

4 Sprinkle the eggs with Parmesan, and season them with additional salt and pepper, if desired. Garnish with parsley, if desired.

> *nail this*

Time is cabbage's best friend. Allow the cabbage and onion to caramelize sufficiently to create the melt-away effect.

» *flip it*

Add greens, for color and nutrition, by tossing in julienned fresh spinach right before you add the eggs.

You can ditch the cabbage if it's not your thing and cook up any veggies as a side to your one-pan hash.

Cook the cabbage as a side dish for dinner. Allow it to caramelize and wilt for the full flavor to emerge, then finish with a splash of lemon juice.

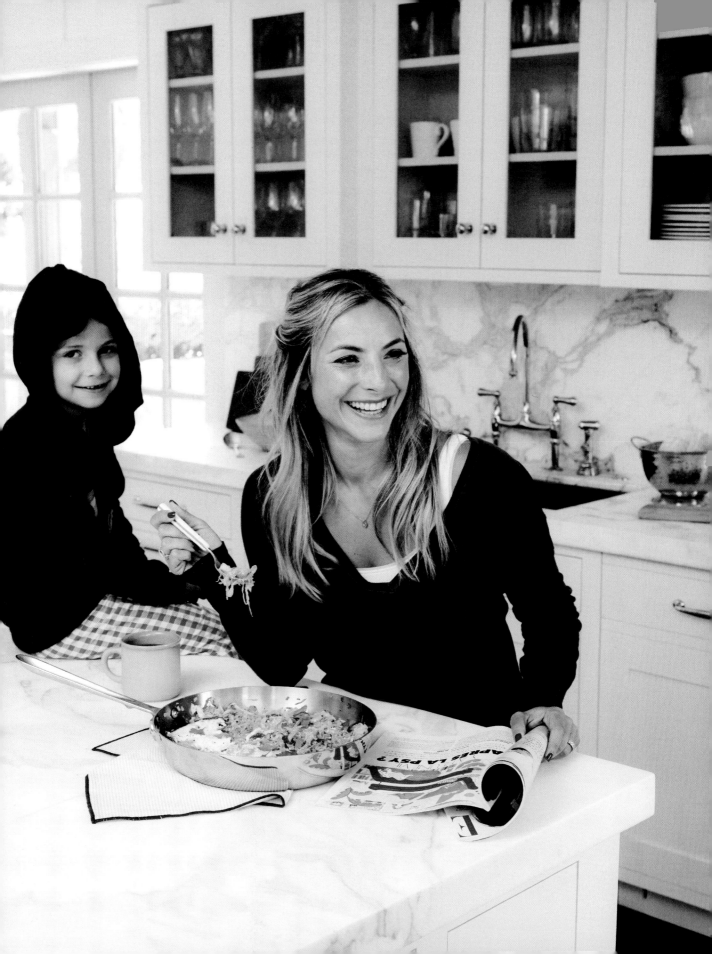

» flip it

Robust-flavored greens like arugula or frisée are terrific in this salad.

Serve with Tangy Mustard Vinaigrette (page 122), Outrageous Lemon Caper Dressing (page 124), or any other dressing from the salad chapter.

Use any veggies or fruits that you like. Consider varieties that will add a pop of color, such as cooked, sliced beetroot, segmented oranges, or pomegranate seeds.

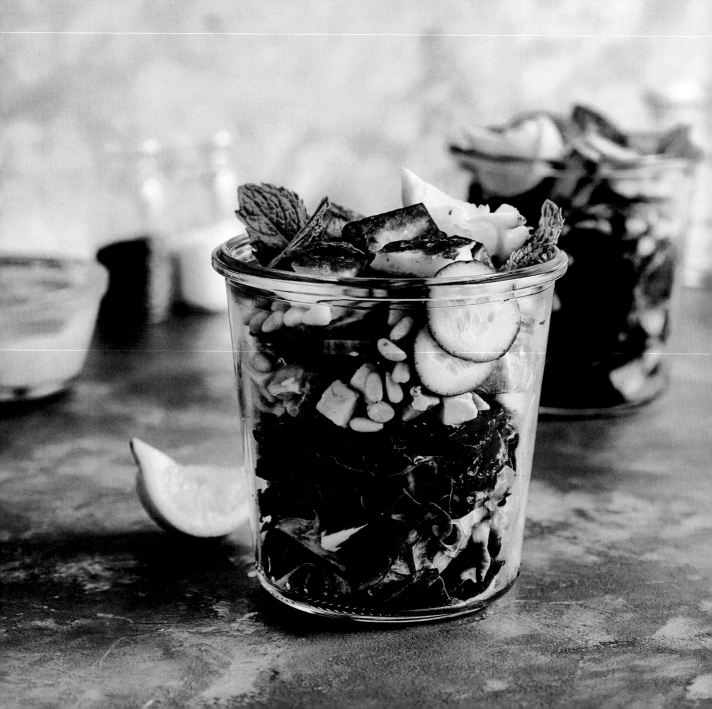

LAYERED HALOUMI BREAKFAST SALAD

STEPS: BROWN, BLEND, LAYER! / **Makes 4 servings**

Dear haloumi, I'm obsessed with you. Good luck having any of this firm and delicious cheese left for your salad after you pan-fry it to a delicious crisp—you may gobble it right out of the pan. After a good morning workout, this satisfying haloumi salad pairs exquisitely with a fresh and lively lemon dressing that really hits the spot. If starting your day with a salad sounds too extreme, ditch the greens and serve pan-fried haloumi with avocado, strawberries, and some sliced gluten-free bread. That's how my daughter Ayla likes it. Keep a batch of the creamy dressing in your fridge (like, all the time, to pour on *anything*).

Tools: Blender, 4 mason jars, small Ziploc bags (I use snack-size bags)

1 8-ounce package of haloumi cheese

Oil, for spraying pan

3 cups packed mixed salad greens, chopped

1 cup strawberries, sliced

2 avocados, peeled and diced

2 small Persian cucumbers, skin on, thinly sliced

⅓ cup pine nuts, lightly toasted

Handful of fresh mint, chopped, to garnish

1 lemon, sliced into 4 wedges

CREAMY LEMON VINAIGRETTE

¾ cup extra-virgin olive oil

½ cup pine nuts

¼ cup lemon juice

1 small shallot, peeled

Grated zest from ½ lemon

1 teaspoon Dijon mustard

1 teaspoon raw honey

Salt and freshly ground black pepper, to taste

1 Cut the haloumi into squares. I like to slice it thinly, to give it more surface area so that it crisps all over.

2 In a lightly oiled frying pan over medium heat, brown each piece of haloumi on both sides, about 6 minutes total. Transfer to a plate. (The cheese can be browned in advance and reheated later.)

3 Make the vinaigrette: In a blender, combine the olive oil, pine nuts, lemon juice, shallot, lemon zest, mustard, and honey. Blend to purée, then season to taste with salt and pepper.

4 In each mason jar, layer some greens, strawberries, avocado, and cucumber. Add the pine nuts and some mint, then the haloumi. Top with a lemon wedge (for color and to squeeze for extra flavor).

5 If you're packing this to go, pour the desired amount of dressing into a small Ziploc bag and place on top of the ingredients in the jar before closing. (If you're serving this salad in a large glass bowl, layer all the ingredients, and then drizzle with the dressing just before serving.)

> *nail this*

If you're packing this for later, let the haloumi cool before you seal the jar or the piping-hot cheese will steam your mixed greens.

SAVORY QUINOA BOWL

STEPS: STEAM, CHOP, FRY, ASSEMBLE! / **Makes 4 to 6 servings**

The combo of quinoa and chopped raw veggies makes for a hearty departure from what you'd expect of the typical breakfast—with a perfectly fried egg on top, naturally. This fun meal-in-a-bowl provides an energy boost that will keep you fueled all morning. Thanks to the abundance of fresh herbs and vegetables, it's surprisingly light, too. Consider making breakfast an all-day affair, and serve this dish for lunch or dinner too!

½ cup red or white quinoa, rinsed (makes 2 heaping cups cooked)

2 small Persian or Kirby cucumbers, skin on, chopped (about 1½ cups)

2 tomatoes, chopped (about 1 cup)

1 avocado, peeled and chopped (about 1 cup)

1 cup arugula

½ cup chopped green onion (about 4)

½ cup chopped fresh mint

¼ cup finely chopped shallots

3 tablespoons lemon juice

4 tablespoons extra-virgin olive oil, plus more for frying

Salt and freshly ground black pepper, to taste

6 large eggs

1 Cook the quinoa: Mix it with 1 cup water in a saucepan over medium-low heat. Bring to a simmer and cook, covered, for 10 minutes. Check to see if it's done or if it needs a tad more liquid. Depending on the level of humidity in the air where you live, quinoa may need a little more or less time and water. Once it's tender but still has some tooth, drain any excess water. Set aside to cool.

2 Toss the cucumber, tomatoes, avocado, arugula, green onion, mint, and shallots in a large bowl.

3 Add the cooled quinoa to the veggie bowl, then season with lemon juice, olive oil, salt, and pepper. Adjust seasoning to taste.

4 Divide the mixture between 6 bowls. If you are serving a hungrier crowd, divide into 4 bowls (you can increase the number of eggs you cook, too).

5 Fry the eggs in a lightly oiled frying pan over medium heat until the whites have set (sunny-side up), or to desired doneness. Season the eggs with salt and pepper to taste, then carefully slide them on top of the quinoa bowls.

> *nail this*

To save time in the morning, cook your quinoa and chop your vegetables (except the avocado) the night before.

If you prefer this dish more veggie heavy, only add as much quinoa as you feel like!

» *flip it*

To serve as a side dish, replace the raw veggies with Any Veggie Sauté (page 281). Just fold the cooked vegetables into the quinoa and season. Stir in a scrambled egg to make the dish even heartier.

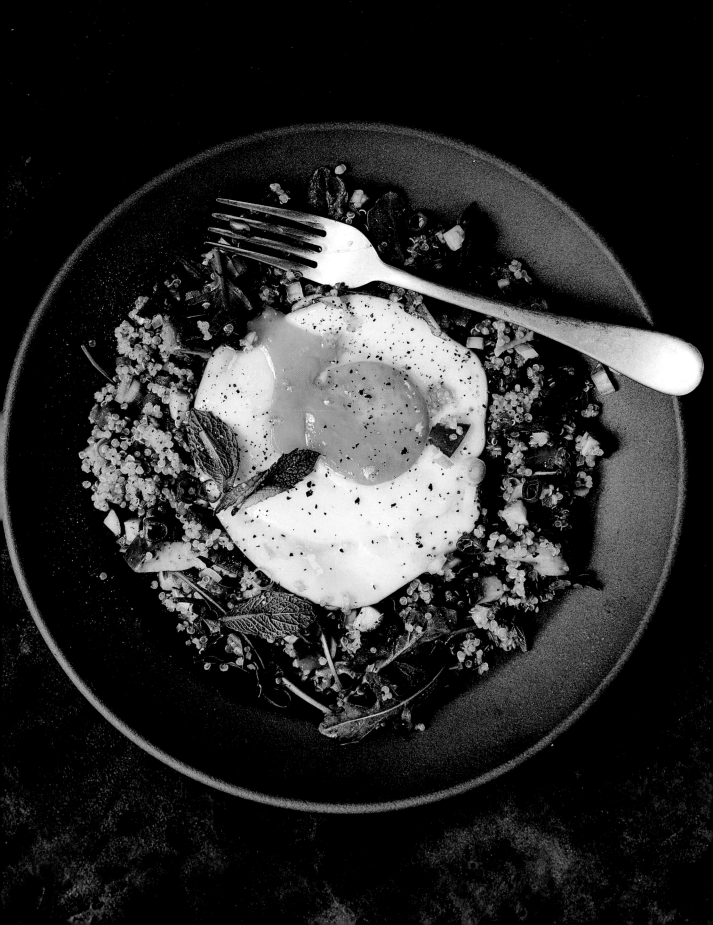

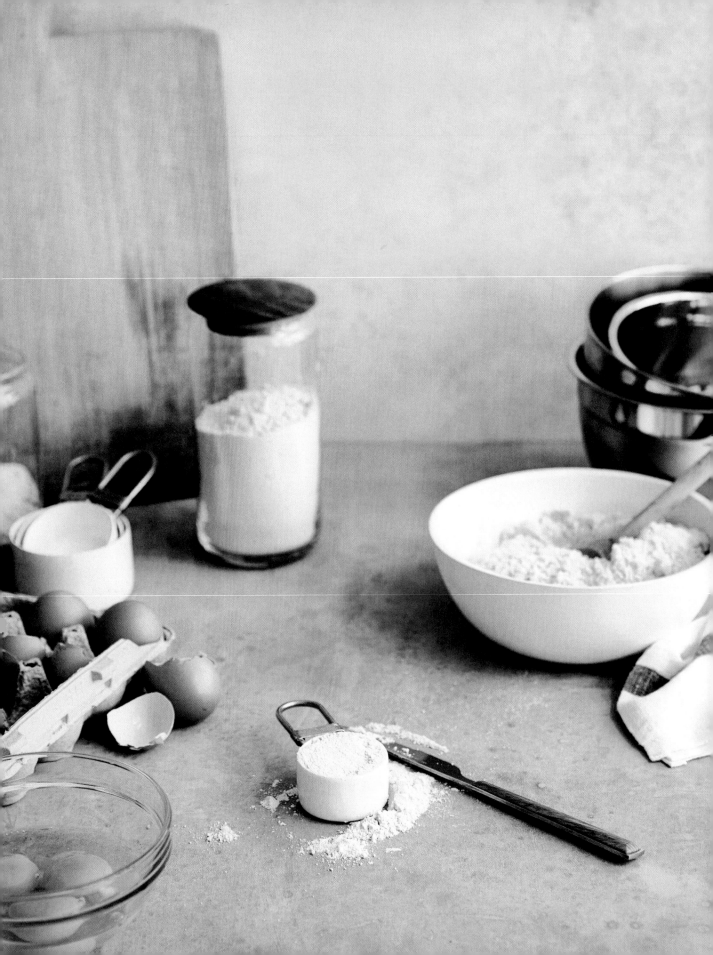

Chapter 3

BREADS AND MUFFINS

You're about to discover that better-for-you, lightened-up breads and muffins can be as delectable and mouthwatering as their gluten- and sugar-filled cousins. When your friends bite into your Best-Ever Gluten-Free Challah (page 47) or soft Craveable Banana Bread (page 55) they'll be shocked to learn that they're gluten free. To me, that's the test of a covetable recipe!

Although it's wise to avoid a muffin a day (to keep your muffin top away), keeping breads and muffins stashed in the freezer can save the day. I serve a quick bread or a muffin once a week as a weekend breakfast treat (alongside eggs and berries). I also always have sliced bread on hand for company, sandwiches, after school, and travel snacks. Since baking often demands attention to detail and requires precision, plan to bake on a day that's stress free (if you have one). Eliminate any distractions and focus on the task at hand. To make it easy, one of my favorite things to do is create homemade muffin and bread mixes. Premeasure and combine the dry ingredients for any recipe, and store the mix in an airtight, labeled container for when the craving hits. This helps make baking a breeze because often the most time-consuming aspects of baking are taking out the ingredients and carefully measuring them.

Baking is a process, and sometimes it's more of a science than the art of cooking can be. Be patient, try and fail, experiment, and learn.

Strategies for Baking Success

The best bread recipes in the world are only as good as the TLC you give them, and mastering some essential baking rules is the key to becoming a baking goddess. I bet you can add a few rules of your own, but here are mine:

Measure precisely! Using a measuring cup with a handle (or a measuring spoon for ingredients used in small quantities, like baking powder), scoop your dry ingredients from the container, and level them off with a knife. Don't pack the flour, oats, etc., into the measuring cup—scoop lightly. Measure wet ingredients in a glass measuring cup—one that looks like a pitcher—and duck your head down to countertop level to check that you've measured correctly (lifting the cup with your hand to eye level can be deceiving as liquid is not level).

Watch your breads and muffins carefully. Stay alert during baking. Don't ever rely on the stated bake time, because no two ovens are the same. If the time says "30 minutes or until lightly browned on the edges," start checking at the 25-minute mark.

Know your oven. Do things burn on the top or bottom? Where's your heat source? Put your bread on the middle rack to avoid top or bottom burn. If you want to go even further, invest in an oven thermometer that will measure your oven's real temperature, as the dial is often inaccurate. But don't freak out—just watch carefully.

Err on the side of underbaking. Particularly for soft breads and muffins, never overbake (unless you like your baked goods drier and crunchier). A banana bread recipe is only as good as how well you bake it, and any banana bread will be blah if it's burnt and dry! Remember, you can always remove your bread too soon, realize it needs another few minutes, and pop it back in the oven.

Troubleshoot your sweet-bread flops. If you do overbake something, transform it! Cut it into cubes, layer the cubes with yogurt or coconut cream and fruit, and turn it into a trifle. Or make cake pops! I once mistakenly undersweetened a batch of muffins, and they tasted really bland. So I sliced the muffins in half, warmed them up in a frying pan coated with a little coconut oil, then drizzled maple syrup on top to make crispy muffin pancakes. (For more flop fixes see page 207.)

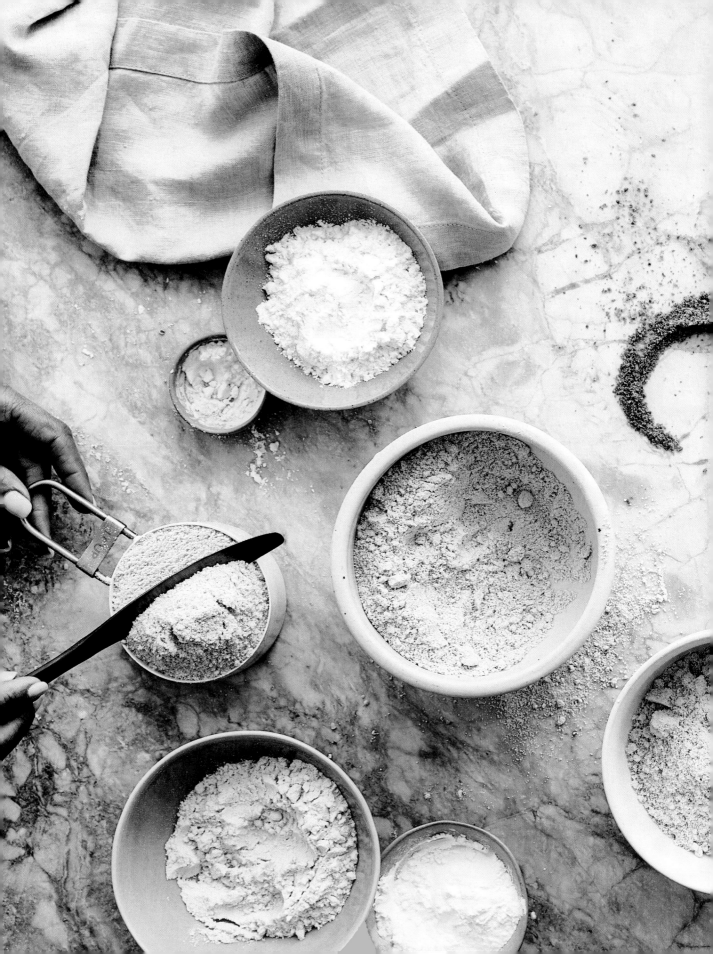

Cool it down. Allow breads and muffins to cool slightly in their baking pans before removing them, so that the shape stays intact. If you remove them too soon, when they are soft, they may drop in the center or stick to the pan. And always cool completely before freezing anything; otherwise the slight heat given off from the bread will form condensation and turn into ice crystals (tastes like freezer burn).

If you plan to stock your freezer with baked goods, always underbake them. That way, when you're ready to serve, you just pop them back in the oven to finish cooking, and they taste freshly baked. I do this with all my breads and loaves that are destined for the freezer. Underbake by about 5 minutes, cool completely, wrap, and slide them into the freezer!

Keep a good supply of essential baking ingredients on hand. You can find most items in the natural or gluten-free aisle of your local supermarket. For more specialty items, like certain flours or hemp seeds, you may need to make a trip to your health food store, or buy them online and have them delivered straight to your door. I don't use anything too weird or complicated, but you will have to stock your pantry. It's worth it, I promise.

To add or not to add xanthan gum? Xanthan gum is an ingredient that's often used in gluten-free baked goods to mimic the elasticity of gluten. I've included it in some recipes when I've found it's necessary (including some in the dessert chapter). However, many all-purpose gluten-free flours, like my favorite, Cup4Cup, already have xanthan gum added. Check the label of the flour you're using, and omit xanthan from a recipe if it's included in your flour.

A note on salt. Salt is salt, right? Actually, no. It turns out that some salts are more or less "salty" than others. (I'm looking at you, iodized table salt!) Bummer, because wouldn't it be nice if some things in life were predictable? These recipes have been tested using fine sea salt, but if they—or any other items you bake—need more salt, then add an extra pinch next time you make it. Remember: salt enhances the flavor of all foods; that's why it's an essential ingredient in baked goods.

Lining with parchment paper. Most recipes in this chapter call for lining the baking pan with parchment paper. While this isn't necessarily a rule, it does make releasing loaves and breads a breeze. For round pans: Trace the bottom of the pan onto the parchment, and cut the paper to a perfect fit. For springform pans: Use a sheet that is larger than the pan, wrap the round base with parchment, put it inside the contraption, seal the sides closed, and cut away the excess—it will fit like a glove. For loaf pans: Cut a piece of parchment that extends the length of the pan and up each end, so that about an inch or so of paper peeks above the top rim on the ends. Then, after baking, you simply grasp the parchment to pull (or lever) the loaf up and out.

Pick a pan, any pan. So, you're about to bake a cake or a loaf, and you discover that you don't have the exact pan size called for in the recipe. Don't panic. The last thing I want you to do is spend your day chasing after a mini loaf pan that is exactly like mine (6.5 × 3 × 2.5-inch). Sizes for those can vary. All you need to do is change the timing of the recipe and divide the batter between pans if you're going from larger to smaller. Whether you're using mini muffin pans instead of full size, or a 9-inch cake pan instead of an 8-inch, just be careful not to overfill. Do some cowboy math on the time estimate, adding more time if you're using a single bigger pan, subtracting time if you're using multiple smaller pans. Then, once it's in the oven, watch it like a hawk, checking well before the time you estimated, and follow my visual direction in the recipe as to when it will be done (and see "Err on the side of underbaking," above). Experiment and adapt.

Rising with yeast. When you're activating yeast, the temperature of the water must be between 110 and 115°F. Any lower and the yeast won't bubble; any higher and you may just kill it off! I always use a finger to test—it should feel like the temperature of a baby's bath, not too hot but warm enough to be comfortable. How long it takes for a yeasted bread to rise can vary quite a bit. If your kitchen is on the cool side, it might take longer than the recipe indicates. Always follow the visual cue, and wait for it to rise to the right level before baking.

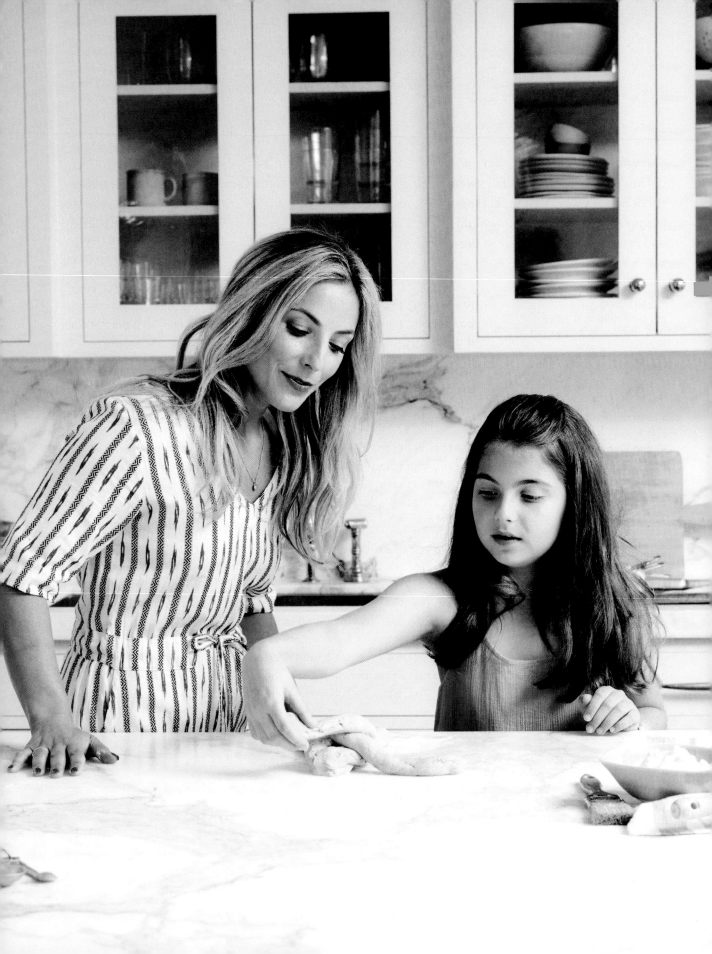

BEST-EVER GLUTEN-FREE CHALLAH

STEPS: WHISK, STIR, BAKE! / **Makes 2 mini loaves or braided loaves**

I grew up baking challah with my mom every week, and my most delicious memories involve baking (and then eating!) her sweetly vanilla-infused loaf. I've been testing my own lightened-up version for over a decade, and now my kids and I create similar memories each week—and we no longer miss gluten on Friday nights. Don't wait for a Jewish occasion to bake this dense, sweet, and insanely delicious challah bread.

Tools: Two 6.5 × 3 x 2.5-inch mini loaf pans or a sheet pan if braiding, parchment paper

YEAST

1 packet (¼ ounce) active dry yeast (2¼ teaspoons)

1 teaspoon granulated sugar

⅓ cup warm water (110 to 115°F)

DRY INGREDIENTS

2 cups all-purpose gluten-free flour

1 cup potato starch

2 teaspoons xanthan gum (omit if contained in flour)

¾ teaspoon salt

WET INGREDIENTS

½ cup almond milk

¼ cup granulated sugar

2 large eggs (plus 1 more, beaten, for brushing)

3 tablespoons extra-virgin olive oil

2 tablespoons coconut oil, melted

2 teaspoons vanilla extract

½ teaspoon rice vinegar

If braiding: 1 tablespoon flour and 1 tablespoon sugar, or more if needed, for rolling

1 Prepare the loaf pans by greasing them and lining them with parchment. If braiding, grease the sheet pan and line with parchment, if desired.

2 In a large bowl, mix the yeast and sugar with the warm water; let it stand for 8 minutes or until the yeast bubbles.

3 In a separate medium bowl, whisk together the dry ingredients.

4 Stir the wet ingredients into the bowl with the yeast mixture. Add the dry ingredient mixture and mix well. The dough will be wet. Allow it to rise in the bowl, covered and in a warm place, until it approximately doubles in height, about 70 to 90 minutes, depending on the humidity where you live (drier conditions take longer).

5 If using loaf pans: Divide the dough in half, and transfer each half to a pan. Brush the tops of the loaves with the beaten egg.

If braiding: Divide the dough in half, then divide each half into three pieces. The dough will be very soft; you'll want to barely touch it as you roll. Gently roll each piece on a floured and sugared surface until they're each about 8 inches by 1 inch. Pinch the ends of three of the strands together, then braid them. Repeat, then transfer the two braided loaves to the greased sheet pan. Brush them each with the beaten egg.

CONTINUED

6 Let the loaves stand, covered and in a warm place, for an additional 30 minutes or until slightly puffy and bulkier in size (longer if your kitchen is cool).

7 Preheat the oven to 350°F.

8 Bake the bread for 20 to 25 minutes or until each loaf is lightly golden and set in the center. Cool the bread completely before removing from the pan (if using) and slicing. Reheat before serving. The loaves may be double wrapped and frozen once cool.

› nail this

This challah tends to be more successful when made in small loaves, to ensure even baking. Do not overbake or the bread will dry out.

If braiding, work with a light touch as dough is soft. Practice makes perfect.

» flip it

Make variations: Add chocolate chips for fun; top with one of the crumbles on page 61, 65, or 205; make into rolls; or use a challah mold (see page 51 for tools).

Top with cinnamon sugar, sesame seeds, or poppy seeds.

Fake It Till You Bake It

Lifesaver: Fake your way to great baked goods by jazzing up cake, muffin, and pancake mixes. Read labels carefully, and choose mixes with less junk when possible. Use the directions on the box for measurement guidelines, but spice up the mix to make it taste homemade. Nobody will be able to tell that you've cheated.

Add nuts. Chopped and toasted walnuts, pecans, and almonds are fun additions that give your baked goods more taste, texture, and good-for-you fats.

Add nutrition. Sneak in some hemp seeds, flax meal (ground flaxseeds), or chia seeds. Hemp seeds and flax meal will impart a slightly nutty flavor, while chia seeds are flavorless. A quick note: Chia seeds absorb a lot of liquid, so if you add them to a boxed mix, then you may need a splash more liquid.

Add extra chocolate to brownies. Chips or chopped chocolate goes a long way.

Add fruit and vegetables. Add berries or chopped stone fruits, shredded apples, carrots, or zucchini to boost flavor and moisture.

Spice it up. Add cinnamon or vanilla extract to spice up almost any mix.

Don't use water. Instead, swap out the recommended amount of water with coconut, almond, or soy milk. This will give your cake a much richer taste and texture.

Add moisture. Create a denser baked good (versus a light and fluffy treat) by adding mashed banana, pumpkin purée, applesauce, or cooked carrot purée.

Swap out the oil. A lot of times boxed mixes will call for vegetable or corn oil. Replace these less healthy fats with something like coconut or olive oil. If you need the oil to be liquid, just melt the coconut oil gently on the stovetop.

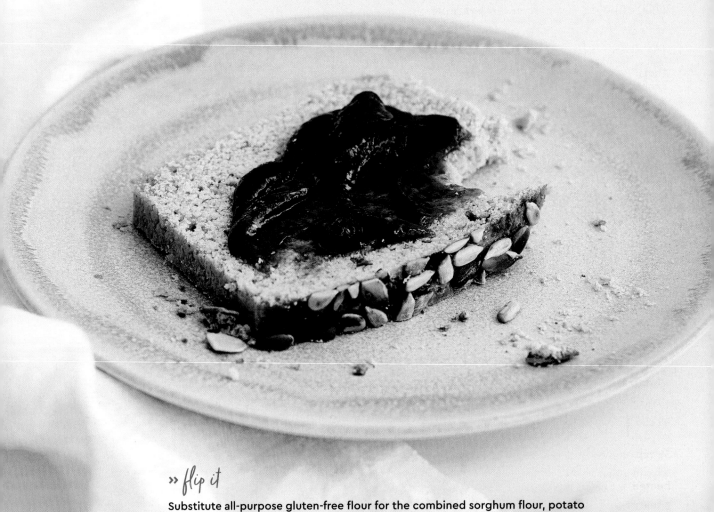

» flip it

Substitute all-purpose gluten-free flour for the combined sorghum flour, potato starch, and millet flour. But not all gluten-free flours are the same. The popular Bob's Red Mill brand, for example, is too heavy for this recipe. Cup4Cup or Manhattan Blends by Orly works very well.

If you prefer a savory cornbread, use water instead of almond milk, reduce the sugar a tad, and omit the vanilla.

Slice before freezing if you want to use the bread for morning toast (divine).

VANILLA-INFUSED CORNBREAD CHALLAH

STEPS: BUBBLE, WHISK, STIR, RISE, BAKE! / **Makes 2 challahs or 2 mini loaves or 1 large loaf**

My friend Paula Shoyer, aka the Kosher Baker, shared this recipe with me one Thanksgiving. The bread was such a hit that it's no longer reserved for holidays. My gluten-free adaptation has added vanilla and almond milk to kick this yeasted cornbread up an extra notch. Lightly rather than overly sweet, it's great as an accompaniment to a breakfast salad or omelet, as a side with chili, or however you'd serve a regular challah.

Tools: Two silicone challah molds or two 6.5 x 3 × 2.5-inch mini loaf pans or one 8.5 × 4.5-inch loaf pan, parchment paper

YEAST

2 packets (½ ounce) active dry yeast

1 teaspoon sugar

⅓ cup warm water (110 to 115°F)

DRY INGREDIENTS

1½ cups cornmeal

1 cup sorghum flour

1 cup potato starch

¾ cup millet flour

⅔ cup sugar

2 teaspoons salt

1 teaspoon xanthan gum

WET INGREDIENTS

½ cup extra-virgin olive oil

½ cup almond milk

2 large eggs (plus 1 more, beaten, for brushing)

3 teaspoons vanilla extract

TOPPING

Pumpkin or sunflower seeds (optional)

1 In a large bowl, mix the yeast and sugar with the warm water; let it stand until the yeast bubbles, about 8 minutes.

2 In a separate medium bowl, whisk together all the dry ingredients.

3 Stir the wet ingredients into the bowl with the yeast mixture. Add the dry ingredient mixture and mix well.

4 Roll the dough into a ball and cover it with a cloth. Allow it to rise in a warm place for 1½ hours.

5 Meanwhile, line the loaf pans, if using, with parchment paper.

6 If using two pans, divide the dough in half. Place the dough in the pans and let them rise in a warm place, covered, for 1 more hour. Dough will puff and increase in size.

7 Preheat the oven to 350°F.

8 Brush the tops of the loaves with the remaining beaten egg, and sprinkle with pumpkin or sunflower seeds, if desired.

9 Bake the bread for 25 minutes for smaller loaves, 35 to 40 minutes for a larger loaf, or until lightly golden and set in the center. Check often to avoid overbaking. Cool the bread completely before removing from the pan and slicing. Reheat before serving. Or, make these ahead of time, as they may be double wrapped and frozen once cool.

> nail this

This bread is denser than a traditional challah (thanks, cornmeal), so don't skimp on letting both the dough and the loaf rise sufficiently.

Err on the side of slightly underbaking for best results.

BULGE-FREE BLUEBERRY MUFFINS

STEPS: WHISK, MIX, TOP, BAKE! / **Makes 12 muffins**

These grain-free muffins don't bear any resemblance to the sugar- and gluten-filled monster-sized versions of my youth. They are light, fluffy, and massively flavorful, with a heavenly cinnamon topping. Even my husband, Seth (who wishes we had gluten at home), devours them! Keep a batch in the freezer—lifesaver.

Tools: 12-cup muffin pan, paper liners (if using)

DRY INGREDIENTS

2 cups almond flour

2 tablespoons hemp seeds

1 teaspoon baking soda

½ teaspoon ground cinnamon

¼ teaspoon salt

WET INGREDIENTS

¼ cup olive oil

¼ cup maple syrup

¼ cup dark brown sugar

3 large eggs

2 teaspoons vanilla extract

1½ cups fresh blueberries

CINNAMON TOPPING

⅓ cup almond flour

¼ cup dark brown sugar

1 teaspoon ground cinnamon

2 tablespoons coconut oil

1 Preheat the oven to 350°F. Lightly grease the muffin cups with coconut oil. Or use paper liners if possible.

2 In a large mixing bowl, whisk together the dry ingredients.

3 Add the oil, syrup, brown sugar, eggs, and vanilla to the dry ingredients, and mix well. Fold in the blueberries.

4 Make the cinnamon topping: Mix the almond flour, brown sugar, cinnamon, and oil in a small bowl.

5 Pour the batter into the prepared muffin cups, dividing evenly and filling each about ¾ full. The muffins will rise, so it's important to leave room at the top or they love to overflow! Sprinkle the muffins with the topping.

6 Bake for 18 to 20 minutes, or until they're set and lightly golden. Check them every 5 minutes toward the end (through the oven window) to ensure that they don't burn.

7 Remove the muffins from the oven and allow them to cool for about 10 minutes, or until they are ready to handle and serve. Or cool completely and freeze them in airtight containers or Ziploc freezer bags; they will keep for a few months.

> *nail this*

Do not open the oven while these are baking or they may flop!

These muffins are very soft; it's best to use paper liners so they release cleanly from the pan.

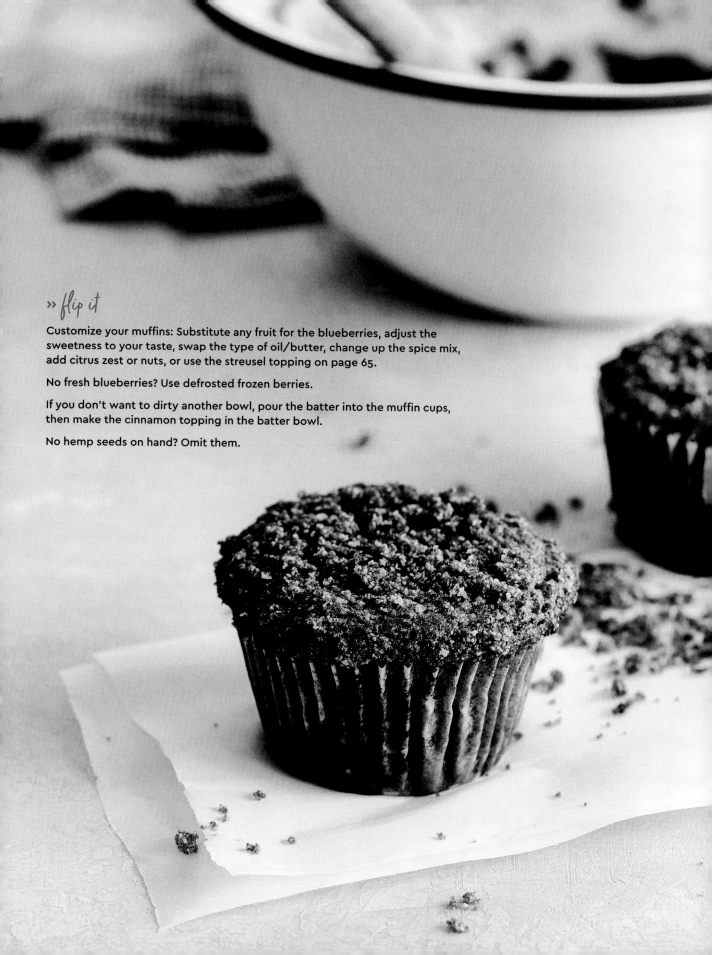

›› flip it

Customize your muffins: Substitute any fruit for the blueberries, adjust the sweetness to your taste, swap the type of oil/butter, change up the spice mix, add citrus zest or nuts, or use the streusel topping on page 65.

No fresh blueberries? Use defrosted frozen berries.

If you don't want to dirty another bowl, pour the batter into the muffin cups, then make the cinnamon topping in the batter bowl.

No hemp seeds on hand? Omit them.

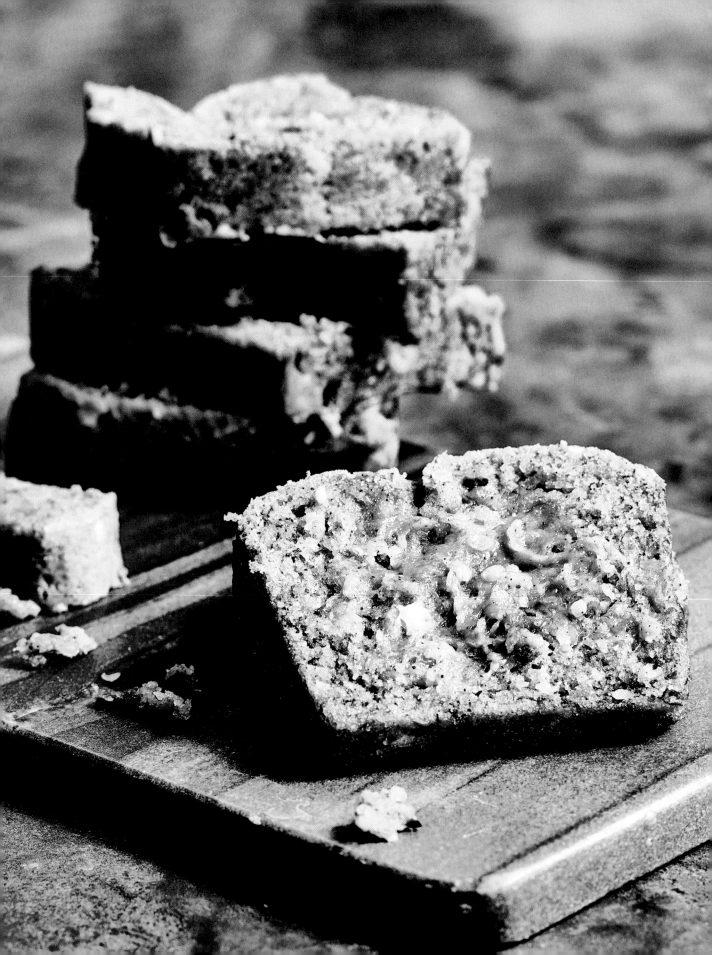

CRAVEABLE BANANA BREAD

STEPS: STIR, MIX, BAKE! / **Makes 1 loaf or 2 mini loaves**

Gooey, flavorful, light, and delish—need I say more? The original inspiration for this recipe came from one of my visits to Canyon Ranch Spa. They serve their version of this bread every morning at their breakfast buffet (if it's healthy enough for a spa...). Here is my spiced-up and flexible version that's been a staple on our table for years. It is addictingly irresistible.

Tools: One 8.5 × 4.5-inch loaf pan or two 6.5 × 3 x 2.5-inch mini loaf pans, parchment paper

DRY INGREDIENTS
1¼ cups all-purpose gluten-free flour

2 tablespoons hemp seeds

1 teaspoon baking powder

½ teaspoon baking soda

½ teaspoon xanthan gum (omit if already in flour)

½ teaspoon ground cinnamon

Pinch of salt

⅓ cup chopped walnuts or pecans, toasted (optional)

WET INGREDIENTS
1 cup mashed ripe banana (about 2 medium bananas)

⅓ cup coconut oil, melted, plus more for greasing the pan(s)

½ cup maple syrup

1 large egg

2 teaspoons vanilla extract

1 Preheat the oven to 350°F. Grease or lightly spray the pan(s) with oil. Line the pan(s) with parchment paper for easy release.

2 Whisk the dry ingredients together in a large bowl.

3 Add the wet ingredients directly into the same bowl. Mix well to incorporate. Pour the batter into the prepared pan(s).

4 Bake the larger loaf for 35 to 45 minutes or the smaller loaves for about 25 minutes. Whichever size you're making, check regularly and remove when the center is set and the loaf is very slightly brown on the edges. Do *not* overbake. These freeze very well: Double wrap them, and keep them in the freezer for up to 5 months.

› nail this

This bread is best when the center is a tad mushy. Don't leave the kitchen during the second half of the baking time so that you can remove it from the oven promptly when needed.

Measure well. Even a tablespoon of extra flour will create a different result (see page 42 for more on successful measuring).

You can totally nail this without hemp.

›› flip it

Fold in chocolate chips, extra banana chunks, or your favorite add-ins. Sprinkle with nuts or a crumble topping of your choice (pages 61, 65, and 205).

Serve as a banana parfait for breakfast (this is especially good if you've either underbaked or overbaked your loaf). Just arrange cubed pieces of the bread in pretty bowls, and top with vanilla yogurt, sliced bananas, and berries.

Make muffins: Use a 12-cup pan with liners, and bake for 15 to 20 minutes.

This batter is so versatile. Add one more egg, and make decadent pancakes or banana-bread waffles.

CHUNKY APPLE CINNAMON LOAF

STEPS: ROAST, WHISK, STIR, BAKE! / **Makes 1 loaf or 2 mini loaves**

This moist, sweet loaf is actually a gluten-free apple cake in disguise—*shhh!* Cut it into thin slices so everyone at the table has an excuse to enjoy a second helping. My inspiration was Erin McKenna's Vegan Apple Cinnamon Toasty, which I've revised over the years. The result may become your favorite sweet bread ever. Plan this recipe ahead of time, because you'll need to roast the apples before you're ready to mix and bake.

Tools: One 8.5 × 4.5-inch loaf pan or two 6.5 × 3 x 2.5-inch mini loaf pans

DRY INGREDIENTS

1 cup all-purpose gluten-free flour

½ cup potato starch

¼ cup arrowroot

1 tablespoon ground cinnamon

2 teaspoons baking powder

½ teaspoon xanthan gum (omit if already in flour)

½ teaspoon salt

¼ teaspoon baking soda

WET INGREDIENTS

⅔ cup maple syrup

½ cup applesauce (4-ounce tub)

½ cup coconut oil, melted

1 large egg

1 tablespoon vanilla extract

2 cups roasted apples (see recipe below)

TOPPING

1 tablespoon dark brown sugar

1 teaspoon ground cinnamon

1 Prepare the roasted apples (recipe follows). Set aside to cool.

2 Preheat the oven to 350°F and grease the loaf pan(s).

3 In a large bowl, whisk all of the dry ingredients together.

4 Stir in the maple syrup, applesauce, oil, egg, and vanilla.

5 In a separate bowl, mix half of the batter with all of the roasted apples. Pour the batter with the apples into greased loaf pan(s), and top with the remaining apple-less batter, dividing evenly if using two pans. Sprinkle the sugar and cinnamon on top.

6 Bake until set, about 45 minutes for the large loaf or 25 to 30 minutes for the small loaves. Keep an eye on them, and do not overbake. Cool completely before slicing, or cool and freeze in an airtight container or Ziploc freezer bags.

CONTINUED

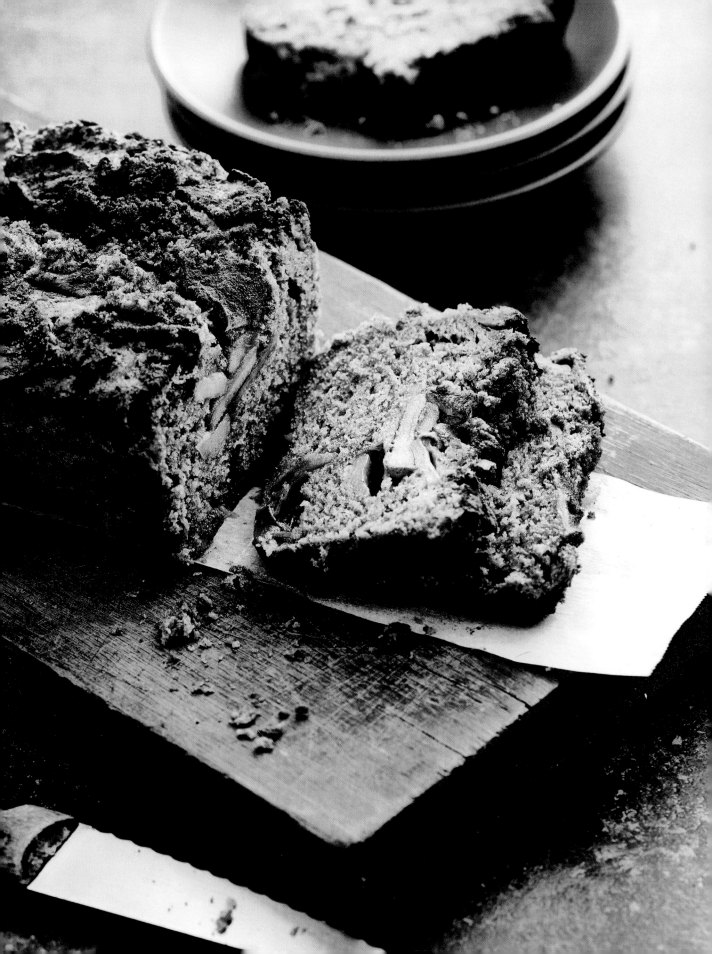

ROASTED APPLES

Makes about 2 cups

2 large apples (your choice; I like Granny Smith), peeled, cored, thinly sliced, then slices cut in half

3 tablespoons maple syrup

2 teaspoons ground cinnamon

1 teaspoon lemon juice

½ teaspoon vanilla extract

1 Preheat the oven to 375°F.

2 In a small baking dish, toss the apples with the maple syrup, cinnamon, lemon juice, and vanilla.

3 Spread the apples on a parchment-lined baking sheet, and roast them in the oven for 20 minutes, or until the apples are soft. Alternatively, you can cook the apples on the stovetop in a sauté pan over medium heat, until soft. But the oven method (favorable here) brings out the cinnamon flavor and caramelizes the apples slightly.

> *nail this*

It's essential to mix half the batter with the apples and spread it into the loaf pan(s) *first* to achieve a bottom that's creamy and apple-y—so don't skip this step.

This recipe bakes better in two mini loaf pans than in one large one. But, as always, use the pan you've got, and adjust the bake time accordingly.

>> *flip it*

Try it with roasted pears or peaches.

Top it with a cinnamon topping (page 52).

Double batch the roasted apples (they will keep in the refrigerator for up to a week), and fold the extras into muffins, pancakes, or waffles. Serve them on their own with a scoop of vanilla ice cream, or purée them into applesauce for another use.

HEALTHY-ISH ZUCCHINI MUFFINS

STEPS: MIX, WHISK, BAKE! / **Makes 12 muffins**

It's amazing how a vegetable can just melt into baked batter, leaving behind no veggie flavor, just an incredibly moist muffin. Serve these sneakily healthy, not-too-sweet goodies as a sidekick to a sunny-side-up egg breakfast or as a snack on the go. Add a few chocolate chips, top with any streusel topping, or swap veggies to make carrot or sweet potato variations. Whatever you do, keep this recipe in your back pocket for that end-of-summer zucchini harvest.

Tools: 12-cup muffin pan, liners (if using)

DRY INGREDIENTS

1½ cups all-purpose gluten-free flour

½ cup almond flour

¼ cup flax meal

1 teaspoon xanthan gum (omit if already in flour)

1 teaspoon baking powder

1 teaspoon baking soda

½ teaspoon salt

2 teaspoons ground cinnamon

½ teaspoon ground ginger

WET INGREDIENTS

¾ cup maple syrup

½ cup coconut oil, melted

2 large eggs

1 tablespoon vanilla extract

2 cups shredded zucchini (about 2 small to medium zucchini)

½ cup raisins (optional)

⅓ cup finely chopped walnuts (optional)

1 Preheat the oven to 350°F. Grease the muffin cups with a little bit of coconut oil, or line with the liners, if using.

2 In a large bowl, whisk together all the dry ingredients.

3 Stir the syrup, oil, eggs, and vanilla into the dry ingredients.

4 Fold in the zucchini, raisins, and walnuts, if using.

5 Fill the prepared muffin cups with the batter, each about ¾ full.

6 Bake for approximately 20 minutes, or until set. Do not overbake. Allow the muffins to cool for 10 minutes, then remove them from the pan and serve. These freeze very well, for up to 5 months.

> *nail this*

During baking, check the muffins regularly, and remove them when the centers are set and they are very slightly brown on the edges.

Make a double batch, double Ziploc them, freeze, and label the bag with the name and date.

» *flip it*

Make loaves instead of muffins: Line the pan(s) with parchment paper for easy removal; bake a larger loaf for 35 to 45 minutes, and mini loaves for about 20 minutes.

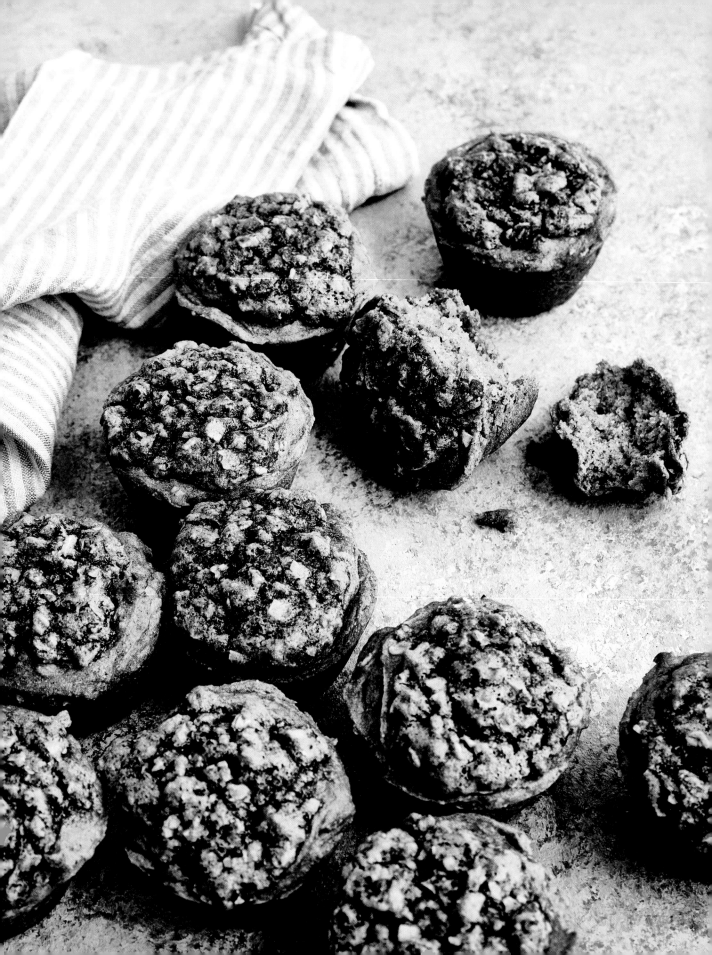

PUMPKIN CRUNCH MUFFINS

STEPS: WHISK, TOP, BAKE! / **Makes about 12 muffins**

There's nothing ordinary about these jazzed, spiced, and crumble-topped gluten-free pumpkin muffins. Don't skimp on the topping...it's the kicker. Brown sugar and pecans are mixed with the batter to form yummy crumbles that bake into an irresistible crisp.

Tools: 12-cup muffin pan, liners (if using)

DRY INGREDIENTS

1 cup all-purpose gluten-free flour

1 cup granulated sugar

¾ cup almond flour

½ cup old-fashioned rolled oats

1 teaspoon baking soda

1 teaspoon xanthan gum (omit if already in flour)

1 teaspoon ground cinnamon

¾ teaspoon salt

½ teaspoon ground nutmeg

¼ teaspoon ground ginger

WET INGREDIENTS

1¾ cups (15-ounce can) pumpkin purée

½ cup olive oil or melted coconut oil

2 large eggs

2 teaspoons vanilla extract

½ teaspoon apple cider vinegar

CRUNCH TOPPING

¾ cup pecans, finely chopped

⅓ cup muffin batter, reserved from above

¼ cup dark brown sugar

1 Preheat the oven to 350°F. Grease or lightly spray the muffin cups with oil. Or line them with liners, if using.

2 In a large bowl, combine all of the dry ingredients. Whisk well to combine.

3 Stir in the wet ingredients. Mix to combine well. (Don't bother measuring the wet ingredients in a separate bowl as is traditionally done. This works equally well in one bowl!)

4 Reserve ⅓ cup of the batter for the topping. (Or you can eyeball ⅓ cup and leave this amount in the bowl to avoid dirtying a measuring cup.) Pour the remaining batter into the prepared muffin cups, dividing evenly and filling each about ¾ full.

5 Make the topping: To the reserved batter add the chopped pecans and brown sugar. Spread the topping over the batter in each muffin cup, dividing evenly.

6 Bake for 25 minutes or until golden on top but still soft inside. Do not overbake. Allow the muffins to cool for 10 minutes, then remove them from the pan and serve. These freeze very well: Double seal, and keep them in the freezer for up to 5 months.

» *flip it*

Serve these for dessert: Frost them with the Marshmallowy Frosting on page 211, or whip up a cream cheese frosting.

Make pumpkin bread. Use a long (12 × 4-inch) lined loaf pan (bake for 50 minutes) or two 6.5 × 3 × 2.5-inch mini loaf pans (bake for 40 minutes).

Use fresh pumpkin purée, or substitute butternut squash, sweet potato, or carrot purée.

Use this topping method (mixing chopped nuts and brown sugar with a bit of batter) for any quick bread; it's the quickest way to add crunch.

HERBED EVERYDAY BREAD

STEPS: BUBBLE, WHISK, STIR, BAKE! / **Makes 2 mini loaves or 1 large loaf**

I used to eat bread and bagels every day, and I had a belly to prove it. But this light, flavorful bread hits the spot when you're craving a slice of toast in the morning minus the after-bloat. I'm partial to baking mini loaves, so the slices are petite—just the size you need to satisfy your hunger for carbs. Bake a few loaves in advance, then cut, wrap, and freeze for a slice of bread in a pinch.

Tools: Two 6.5 × 3 × 2.5-inch mini loaf pans or one 8.5 × 4.5-inch loaf pan, parchment paper

YEAST
1 packet active dry yeast (2¼ teaspoons)

1¼ cups warm water (110 to 115°F)

DRY INGREDIENTS
1 cup all-purpose gluten-free flour

1 cup oat flour

¼ cup almond flour

¼ cup flax meal

2 teaspoons xanthan gum (omit if already in flour)

1½ teaspoons dried rosemary

1 teaspoon salt

WET INGREDIENTS
¼ cup extra-virgin olive oil

2 large eggs (plus 1 more, beaten, for brushing)

2 tablespoons raw honey

½ teaspoon rice vinegar

1. In a large bowl, mix the yeast with the warm water; let stand until the yeast bubbles, about 8 minutes.

2. In a separate medium bowl, whisk together the dry ingredients.

3. Stir the wet ingredients into the yeast mixture. Stir the dry ingredient mixture into the wet. Mix well; the dough will be wet.

4. Transfer the dough to the parchment-lined loaf pan(s) and let stand, covered in a warm place, until the bread rises to double its height, about 45 minutes.

5. Preheat the oven to 350°F.

6. Brush the top with the remaining beaten egg.

7. Bake the bread until it is golden and set in the center, 30 to 35 minutes for mini loaves, or about 45 minutes for a larger loaf. Cool the bread completely before removing from the pan(s) and slicing. The loaves may be double wrapped and frozen once cool.

> *nail this*

For total precision, use a thermometer for any bread you bake: The bread is done when the center temperature reaches 200°F.

If you choose to use smaller pans than the ones suggested, be sure not to fill them more than ⅔ full or they will overflow!

 flip it

Not a fan of rosemary? Swap it out for dried thyme or tarragon, or even mix in a small handful of chopped black olives or sunflower seeds.

These make great rolls to accompany soup or a hearty main dish. Divide the dough into 6 pieces and shape into rolls. Bake on a parchment-lined baking sheet for about 20 minutes or until golden and set in the center.

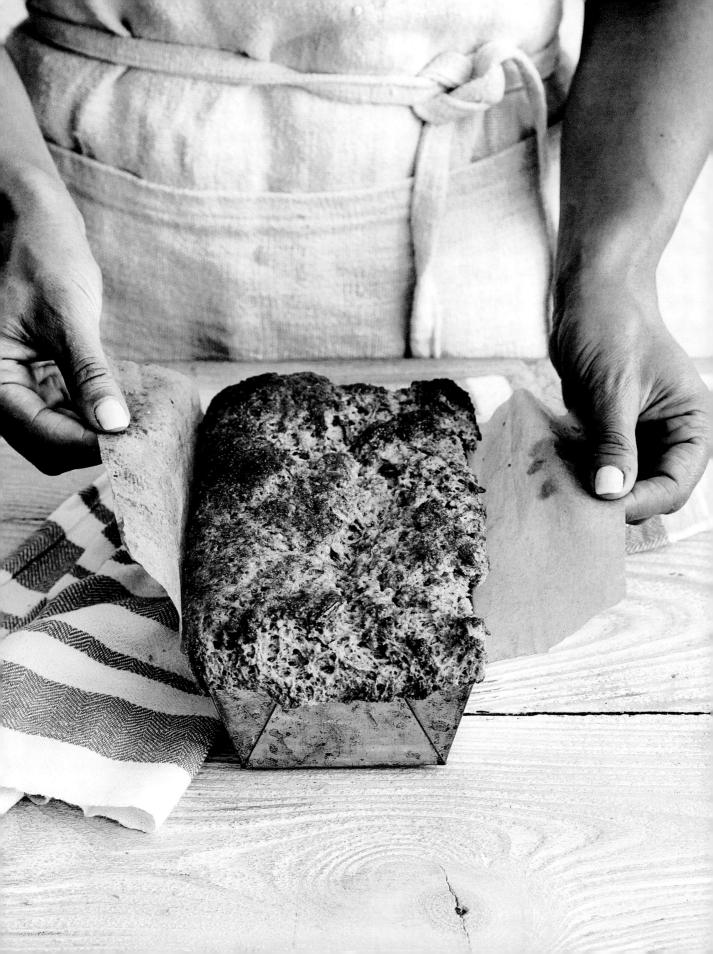

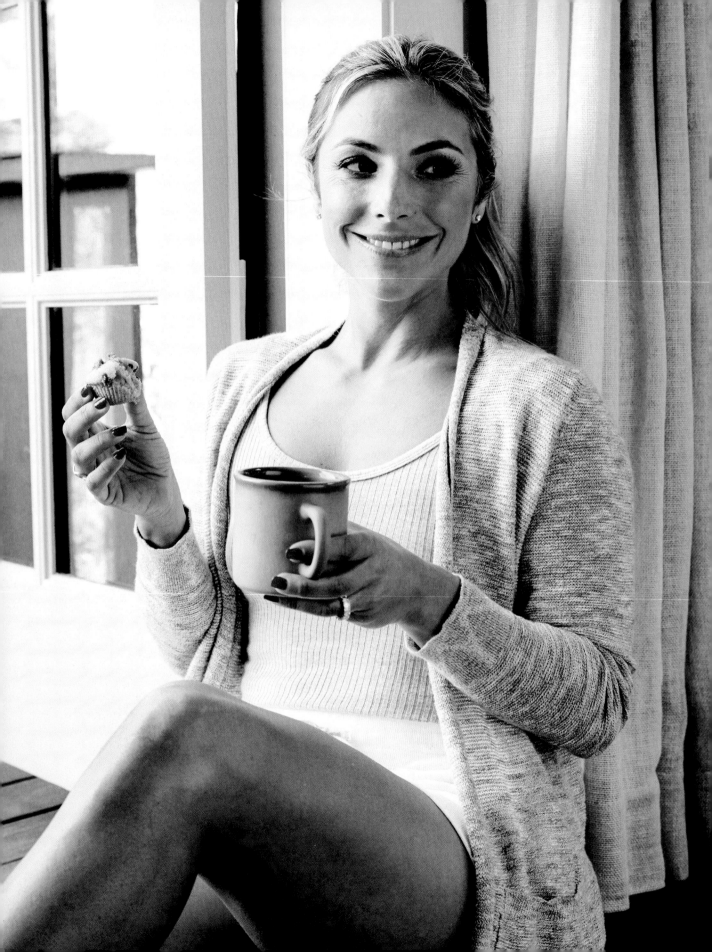

MINI COFFEE CAKE MUFFINS

STEPS: WHISK, MIX, TOP, BAKE! / **Makes about 30 mini muffins**

While dreaming up this recipe I was craving a streusel coffee cake. I created this lightened-up version with a base that doubles as a basic vanilla cupcake. Oh boy, are you in for a versatile and yummy treat! I make these in mini size, so they are the perfect coffee cake bite, but you could make regular-sized muffins too. Plus, you know all the batter left in your bowl that you need a spatula to get out? Leave it in, and add the topping ingredients straight into the bowl to incorporate that little bit of batter into the cinnamon crumble. Saves on dirtying a dish, and tastes delish!

Tools: Mini muffin pans, liners (if using)

DRY INGREDIENTS

1 cup all-purpose gluten-free flour

¼ cup almond flour

½ teaspoon baking powder

½ teaspoon baking soda

½ teaspoon xanthan gum (omit if already in flour)

Pinch of salt

WET INGREDIENTS

⅓ cup coconut oil, melted

¼ cup maple syrup

¼ cup granulated sugar

2 large eggs

2 teaspoons vanilla extract

STREUSEL TOPPING

¼ cup granulated sugar

¼ cup all-purpose gluten-free flour

2 tablespoons unsalted butter or coconut oil, at room temperature

2 teaspoons ground cinnamon

Pinch of salt

1 Preheat the oven to 350°F. Grease the muffin cups with a little bit of coconut oil, if using. I prefer to use paper liners as these grain-free muffins are very soft.

2 Whisk the dry ingredients together in a large bowl.

3 Add the wet ingredients directly into the same bowl. Mix well to incorporate. Spoon the batter into the prepared muffin cups, dividing it evenly and filling each cup to about ¾ full.

4 In the batter bowl (which should still have some batter stuck to the sides), stir together the topping ingredients, incorporating any remnants of batter. Sprinkle the topping over the batter, dividing evenly among the muffin cups.

5 Bake the muffins for 12 minutes, or until set. Do not overbake. Remove the muffins from the oven, and allow them to cool for 10 minutes, or until cool enough to handle.

> *nail this*

Do not fill the muffin cups or they will flop in the center and overflow while baking.

The muffins will be dry if you overbake them. Remove them from the oven when the centers are set, but *before* the edges fully brown.

>> *flip it*

Baked without the streusel, these make great vanilla cupcakes! Ice with Marshmallowy Frosting (page 211).

Make larger muffins: Use a 12-cup muffin pan, double the topping, fill the cups halfway, spoon some topping in, top with more batter, then finish with more topping. Double crumble goodness.

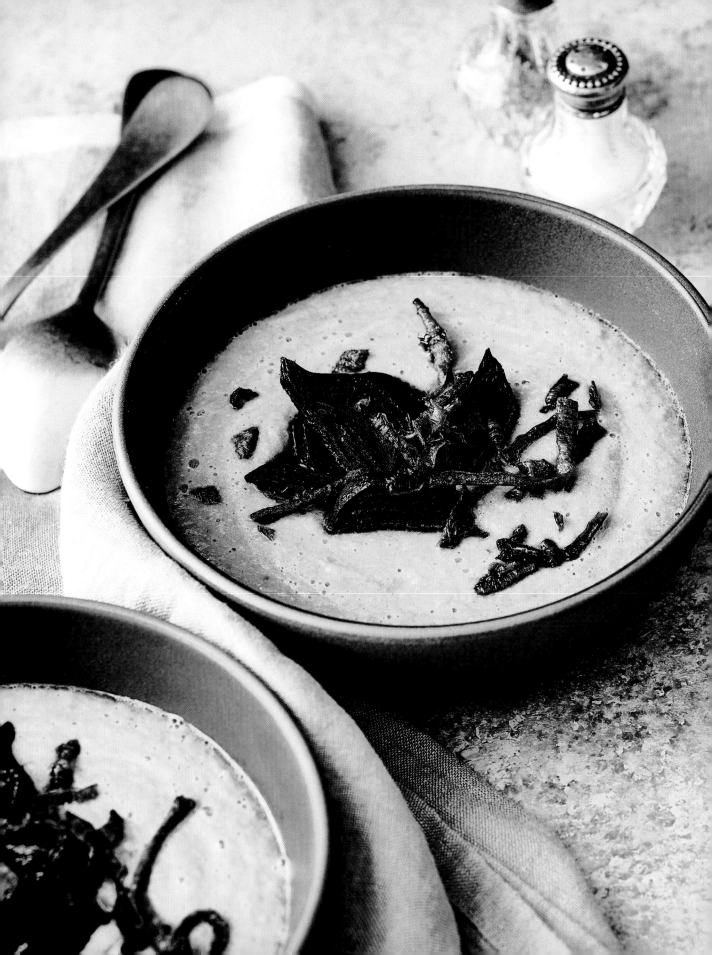

Chapter 4

SOUPS AND SMALL PLATES

Some occasions call for smaller portions and prettier bites. Here's my arsenal of uncomplicated soups and jaw-dropping appetizers (that can double as party bites or finger foods). It's possible to wow your diners without having to slave away in the kitchen all day. Read on to make your soups and small plates look great and taste amazing, plated just the right size so they won't fill you up and spoil the main dish. Need to serve more than just a tasty tease? Go ahead and transform soups and small plates into complete, flexible meals. Soups fill you up with loads of nutrition without making you feel heavy—and I've even been known to serve my main dishes on smaller plates to ensure that I don't eat too much, yet they still look and feel abundant!

TOMATO PIZZA SOUP

STEPS: SAUTÉ, SIMMER, BLEND! / **Makes 10 servings**

This soup tastes like pizza. For real. The key is to start by cooking your onions in butter—oh yeah, I said butter. The recipe calls for only a little bit, and it makes all the difference. After puréeing the soup and topping it off with grated Parmesan cheese, you'll be in liquid pizza heaven. If you're serving this to picky eaters, don't call it tomato soup—tell them it's pizza soup. (That's how I first got my kids to try it.)

Tools: Hand blender

4 tablespoons unsalted butter

1 tablespoon olive oil

1 medium yellow onion, chopped

2 to 3 medium carrots, chopped

2 celery stalks, chopped

4 garlic cloves, pressed or minced

2 28-ounce cans whole tomatoes with juice

2 6-ounce cans tomato paste

3 cups vegetable broth or water

1½ teaspoons salt

12 fresh basil leaves (a small handful), plus more to garnish

Freshly ground black pepper, to taste

Shredded Parmesan, to garnish

1 In a large soup pot over medium heat, melt the butter together with the oil. Add the onions, and cook, stirring frequently, until browned, about 7 minutes.

2 Add the carrots, celery, and garlic, and cook, stirring, until the vegetables are softened and the flavors have melded, 8 to 10 minutes.

3 Add the canned tomatoes, tomato paste, broth, and salt. Bring to a boil, then reduce the heat and simmer for about 40 minutes.

4 Dilute the soup with a touch more liquid, if needed. I like to wait to do so until after simmering because as the soup cooks, the tomatoes release their own juices—and you definitely don't want the soup to be too watery. Add the basil leaves.

5 Using a hand blender, blend the soup until smooth. Season to taste with salt and pepper.

6 To serve, ladle into warmed soup bowls or mugs, and top with a touch of shredded Parmesan cheese and a fresh basil leaf or two.

> nail this

The best parts of this soup are the butter and the Parmesan. Something magical happens when butter meets tomatoes and when the Parmesan melts into the soup.

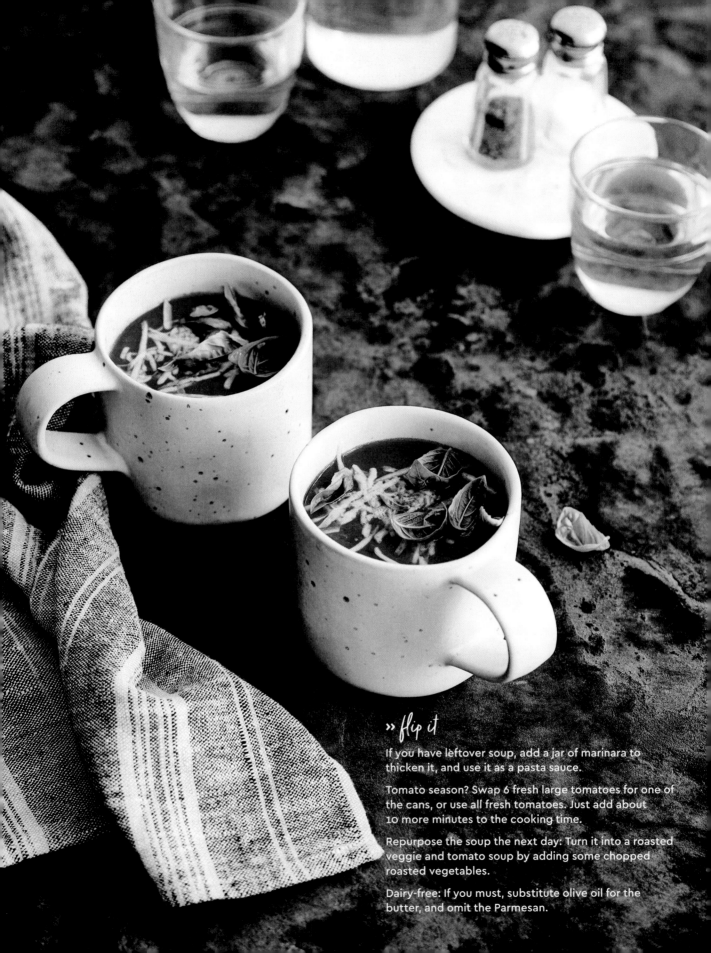

» flip it

If you have leftover soup, add a jar of marinara to thicken it, and use it as a pasta sauce.

Tomato season? Swap 6 fresh large tomatoes for one of the cans, or use all fresh tomatoes. Just add about 10 more minutes to the cooking time.

Repurpose the soup the next day: Turn it into a roasted veggie and tomato soup by adding some chopped roasted vegetables.

Dairy-free: If you must, substitute olive oil for the butter, and omit the Parmesan.

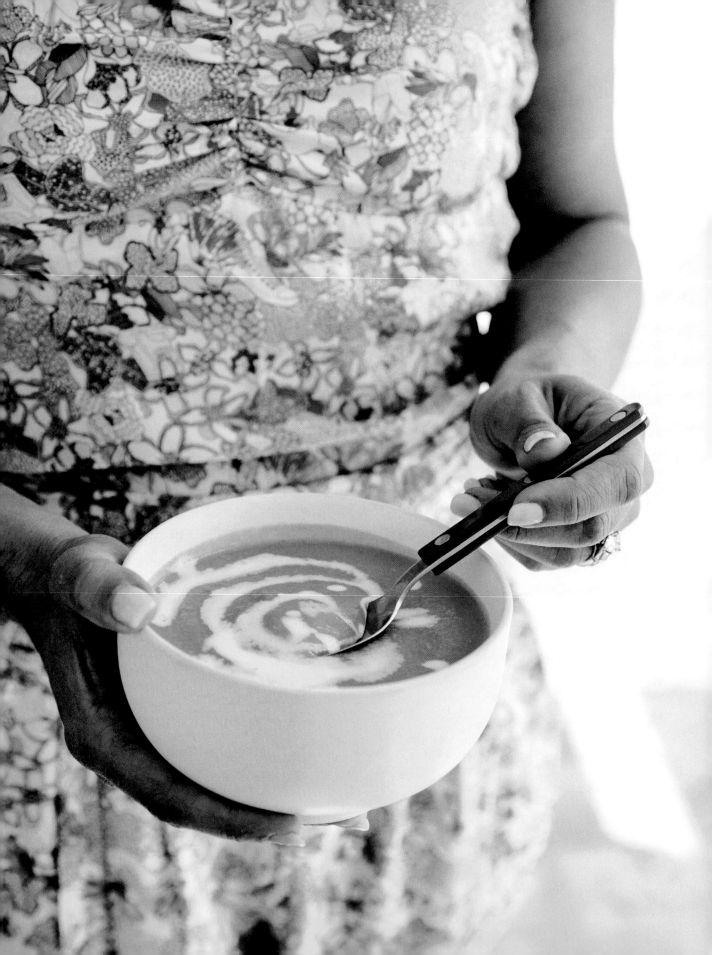

VELVETY CARROT SOUP

When I was a teenager I went completely bonkers for carrots—so much so that in my attempt to lose a few pounds all I ate for a few weeks were carrots, until my hands and feet turned bright orange. How crazy! I look back now with the perspective that there's a gentler, more constructive way to find your ideal weight (and your ideal life) that doesn't require extremes. Meanwhile, to this day carrots remain my best friend, and I'm completely obsessed (in a healthy way, I promise) with this nutrient-dense, delicious, creamy carrot soup. Thanks to coconut milk, cashews, and a whole lot of TLC to caramelize the vegetables, this soup may well become your new fave.

Tools: Hand blender

¼ cup olive oil

1 large yellow onion, chopped

2 stalks celery, chopped

4 garlic cloves, minced

2-inch piece fresh ginger, peeled and minced

1 teaspoon cumin

1 teaspoon curry powder

10 medium carrots, chopped (about 8 cups)

8 cups chicken or vegetable broth, or water

¼ teaspoon salt, plus more to taste

¼ teaspoon freshly ground black pepper, plus more to taste

½ cup raw, unsalted cashews, chopped

1 cup full-fat coconut milk, for garnish

1 In a large soup pot over medium heat, heat the olive oil and cook the onion, stirring, until translucent, about 5 minutes.

2 Add the celery, garlic, ginger, cumin, and curry, and cook, stirring, until fragrant, roughly 1 minute.

3 Add the carrots, and toss to coat. Add the broth, salt, and pepper. Bring the mixture to a boil. Reduce the heat and simmer the soup until the carrots soften, about 30 minutes.

4 Add the cashews and cook an additional 10 minutes.

5 Using a hand blender, purée the soup until it's combined but still chunky. Taste and reseason, if needed.

6 To serve, ladle into warmed soup bowls, and drizzle coconut milk on top. This soup freezes perfectly! Make ahead, and reheat to serve.

> *nail this*

For a dinner party, nail a killer presentation by serving the soup in espresso cups. For a cocktail party, serve it in shot glasses arranged on a tray.

>> *flip it*

If you aren't a coconut fan, stir in a bit of butter and milk instead, or ditch the added creaminess altogether.

For a lighter (or nut-free) variation, skip the cashews completely.

Get creative with garnishes: Top each bowl with roasted cauliflower, fresh herbs, fried onions, or assorted nuts and seeds for crunch.

MINTED PEA SOUP WITH ROASTED BEETROOT

STEPS: BROWN, SIMMER, ROAST, PURÉE! / **Makes 8 to 10 servings**

Tasty food is great, but tasty *and* pretty-looking food is extraordinary! This soup evolved from being a dull-looking bowl of green to a dish that's bursting with color and texture. The sweet, purple beets are stunning on top of the creamy green-pea purée, and the savory shallots balance out the naturally sweet soup. All in all, it's a pretty and memorable way to begin a meal.

Tools: Hand blender

2 tablespoons olive oil

2 medium yellow onions, chopped

½ cup diced celery

1 medium carrot, diced

2 garlic cloves, minced

3 16-ounce bags frozen green peas

6 cups chicken or vegetable broth, or water (enough to cover)

⅓ cup fresh mint leaves, plus more for garnish

Salt and freshly ground black pepper, to taste

Roasted beet cubes, to garnish (see sidebar)

Crispy Onions or shallots, to garnish (page 269; optional)

1 In a large soup pot over medium heat, heat the olive oil. Add the onions and cook, stirring frequently, until they're golden brown and caramelized, about 10 minutes.

2 Add the celery, carrot, and garlic, and cook until the vegetables have softened and the flavors have melded, roughly 10 minutes.

3 Stir in the frozen peas. Add just enough broth to cover the veggies. If you add too much, the soup will be too watery. Cover the pot and simmer on low heat for 30 minutes. Add the mint leaves toward the end of cooking, just to heat through.

4 Remove the soup from the heat. Using a hand blender, purée the soup until it's smooth. Add salt and pepper and more fresh mint, if needed, to taste.

5 To serve: Ladle the soup into bowls, and garnish with mint, beets, and onions, if desired. Can be made a day ahead and reheated before serving.

» *flip it*

When making soup, practice eyeballing the veggie quantities so that eventually you don't have to measure exactly ½ cup of celery. Soups are less a science and more an art.

Replace the peas with corn to make a corn soup—omitting the mint—and use butter instead of oil for an indulgent complement to the sweet corn.

This is delicious garnished with Flexible Green Pesto (page 272).

How to Roast Beets

2 medium beets, peeled and cut into ½-inch cubes
1 tablespoon olive oil
Salt and freshly ground black pepper, to taste

1 Preheat the oven to 350°F.

2 In a small roasting pan, drizzle the beets with the oil and bake, tossing occasionally, for 30 minutes, or until tender. Season with salt and pepper. Set aside.

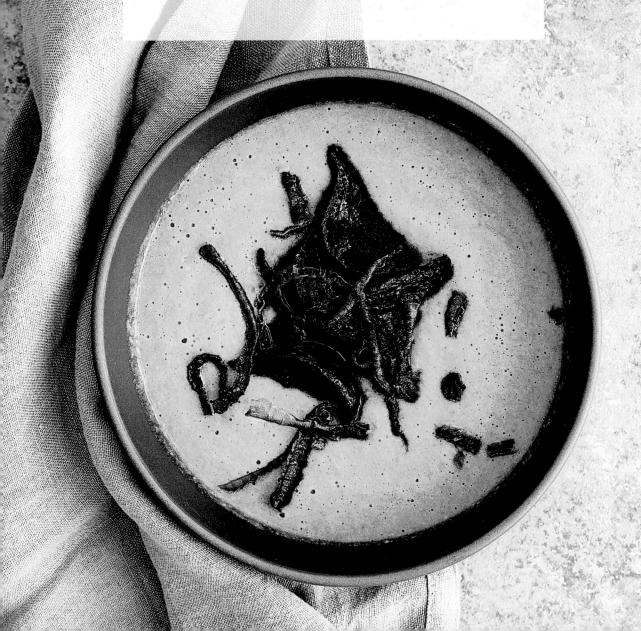

MY MOM'S COMFORTING CHICKEN SOUP

There's nothing quite like my mom's chicken soup. She has a few secrets that elevate it to extraordinary. First, she simmers her vegetable peels in water, so she starts with a flavorful foundation. Later, she adds the chicken alone, and simmers it long enough for the fatty bits to float to the surface for easy removal. Then the veggies go in for an hour-plus simmer to transform the mixture into the most flavorful soup you've ever tried. Throwing in a few turkey necks adds even more depth of flavor—and simmering it with love doesn't hurt either.

Tools: Very large pot, serrated grater or mandolin (optional)

4 medium carrots

4 small or 2 large zucchini (about 11 ounces)

1 medium parsnip

5 teaspoons salt

1 teaspoon ground white pepper

3 medium celery stalks with lots of leaves

½ butternut squash (about 1 pound), peeled, seeds removed

1 or 2 medium turnips

1 large (4½-pound) chicken, cut into eighths

3 or 4 turkey necks (optional)

1 whole medium yellow onion, peeled

1 head of garlic, rinsed and outer layers peeled

1 bunch fresh dill

1 In a large stockpot over high heat, bring 1¼ gallons (20 cups) filtered water to a boil.

2 While the water is reaching temperature, wash and peel the carrots, zucchini, and parsnip, reserving the peels.

3 Add the vegetable peels, salt, and white pepper to the pot. Reduce the heat to a simmer. Simmer the vegetable peels at least 10 to 15 minutes, then scoop them out with a fine-mesh strainer and discard.

4 Meanwhile, continue to prep the veggies: Cut the carrots, zucchini, parsnip, and celery (reserve the leaves) into thick slices—using a serrated grater or mandolin to create a wave pattern, if desired. Cut the butternut squash and the turnip(s) into 1-inch cubes.

5 Add the chicken pieces and turkey necks, if using, to the pot, and simmer another 10 to 15 minutes or until you can start skimming the scum that rises to the top.

6 Add all the sliced and cubed vegetables (including the celery leaves), the whole onion, and the whole garlic head to the pot, and simmer for 90 minutes, occasionally skimming any scum off the top.

7 Stir in the dill, and remove the pot from the heat.

8 Optional: Allow the soup to cool to room temperature, then refrigerate it, covered, for 24 to 48 hours. Remove the pot from the refrigerator, and skim off and discard any congealed fat from the top.

Quick Broth or Stock

For a quick veggie broth, throw whatever chopped veggies (and their peels) you have from the recipe above—carrots, zucchini, parsnips, celery, onion, and garlic ideally—into a large soup pot, and add filtered water, salt, pepper, and dill (optional). To make it a chicken stock, add 4 to 5 pounds chicken necks, backs, wings, and/or legs to the mix. For an extra-rich stock, throw in a few beef bones, too. Simmer on low for 2 hours, strain, and use right away, or let it cool completely and freeze.

9 Discard the celery leaves, onion, garlic, and dill before serving, if desired. You can either serve the chicken pieces on the bone or remove the chicken skin and bones and add the chicken meat back to the pot. Leave the turkey necks in—someone inevitably devours them. If freezing, remove the herbs and bones first. When defrosting, skim off the fat layer that has risen to the top.

> ## nail this

Mom's rule of thumb for making any soup is 1 teaspoon salt for every 4 cups water.

Simmering the peels adds a distinct level of flavor to this soup. You can certainly omit this step if needed, but if you have the time it's worth the effort.

>> ## flip it

Use Quick Broth or Stock (see sidebar) to make Asian Hot and Sour Soup (page 78).

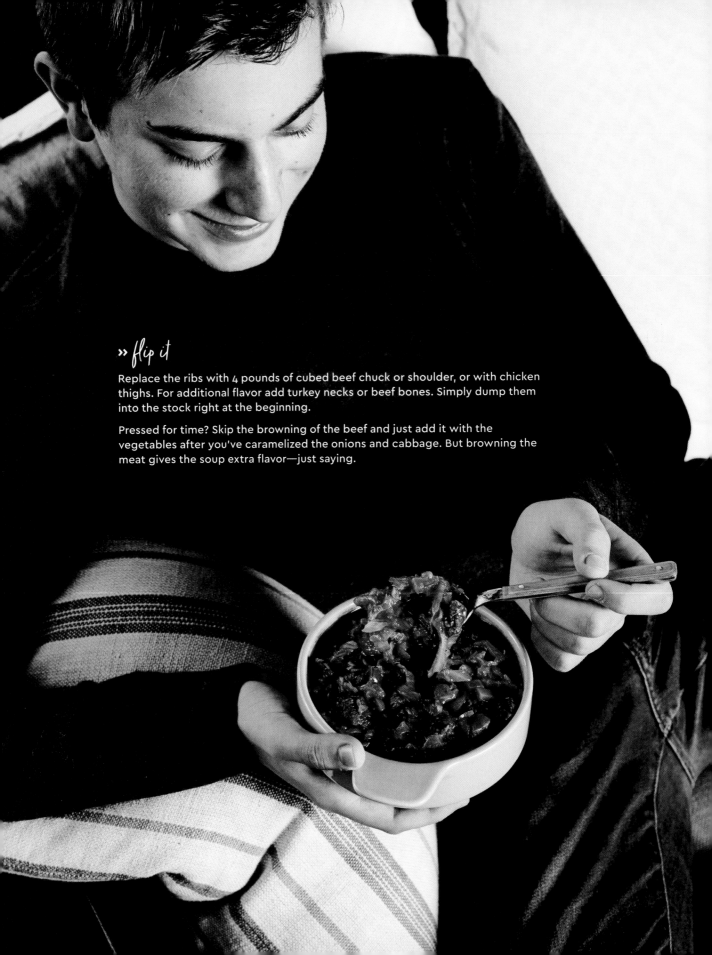

» flip it

Replace the ribs with 4 pounds of cubed beef chuck or shoulder, or with chicken thighs. For additional flavor add turkey necks or beef bones. Simply dump them into the stock right at the beginning.

Pressed for time? Skip the browning of the beef and just add it with the vegetables after you've caramelized the onions and cabbage. But browning the meat gives the soup extra flavor—just saying.

HUG-IN-A-BOWL CABBAGE SOUP

STEPS: SEAR, SAUTÉ, SIMMER!! / **Makes 12 servings**

I kid you not, on a cold day (or in summertime, in an overly air-conditioned dining room) this soup is like a warm hug in a bowl. Soft and succulent cabbage is paired with meltingly tender beef, which may make you want to sink even deeper into your cozy sweats and help yourself to another bowl. At home my kids devour this alone for dinner because it serves as a full meal in a bowl. For guests, serve this filling soup as part of a menu that's on the lighter side.

6 tablespoons olive oil, divided

12 beef spare ribs or short ribs

2 medium yellow onions, thinly sliced

1½ heads green cabbage, shredded

3 carrots, diced

3 stalks celery, diced

5 garlic cloves, crushed

1 14.5-ounce can diced tomatoes with juice

2 6-ounce cans tomato paste

3 cubes Family Secret Red Spread (Salat Adom) (page 271; optional)

8 to 10 cups chicken or beef broth

3 teaspoons salt

Freshly ground black pepper, to taste

1 Sear the ribs: In a soup pot, heat 1 tablespoon oil over medium heat, and brown the ribs on all sides, for about 5 minutes. Remove the ribs and set aside, reserving the beef drippings.

2 In the same pot, heat the remaining 5 tablespoons oil over medium heat. Add the onions and cabbage, and cook, stirring, until the onions are translucent and the cabbage has begun to caramelize, about 10 to 15 minutes. Stir in the carrots, celery, and garlic, and cook until the flavors have melded, another 8 to 10 minutes.

3 Add the canned tomatoes, tomato paste, and red spread, if desired. Stir the mixture to coat the cabbage with the tomatoes and veggies.

4 Return the beef ribs to the pot, and add just enough broth to cover the meat and veggies. (You can always add more broth later; if the cabbage heads are small, the soup requires less liquid.) Add the salt and pepper, and bring to a boil.

5 Lower the heat to a simmer, and cook for 2 to 2½ hours. The meat should fall off the bone. Taste and reseason, or add more stock if needed. You may wish to cook the soup for a tad longer to intensify the flavors. Remove the bones before serving—or leave them in, that's how my boys like it.

> nail this

The soup is better when you properly sweat and caramelize the cabbage.

Sometimes midway into simmering I'll add another small can of tomato paste to make the soup richer and more tomatoey.

Red Spread isn't necessary and you can completely omit it, but if you happen to have some in your freezer it gives the soup a real kick.

ASIAN HOT AND SOUR SOUP

STEPS: SOAK, BOIL, SWIRL, SERVE! / **Makes 12 servings**

We've lived in Asia for so many years that this recipe has become a familiar and crowd-pleasing treasure to share with you. Bursting with veggies and oomph, it's devoured by all at dinnertime. You'll need to start with a homemade chicken stock, so check out My Mom's Comforting Chicken Soup (page 74) or Quick Broth or Stock (page 75), and get that stock nailed. Serve this in the winter as a starter for a hearty meal with friends or on a weeknight as a one-pot dinner.

5 medium dried shiitake mushrooms, rinsed well

8 cups chicken stock (recipe page 75)

½ cup rice vinegar

⅓ cup soy sauce

3 chicken breast cutlets (about ½ pound), cut into thin strips

½ cup cornstarch, divided

1 small carrot, peeled and finely julienned

½ cup sliced baby corn (about 5 from a can)

4 garlic cloves, minced

1 tablespoon peeled and minced fresh ginger

¼ cup finely julienned snow peas

¼ cup enoki mushrooms (about ¾ ounce)

8 ounces firm tofu, cut into ¼-inch cubes

1 large egg, beaten

½ cup bean sprouts

3 green onions, thinly sliced

½ teaspoon hot chile oil, or to taste

Salt and freshly ground black pepper, to taste

1 In a small bowl, soak the shiitake mushrooms in about 1 cup of warm water for 1 hour, to soften.

2 Drain the mushrooms, reserving the liquid for later use. Discard the tough stems, and thinly slice the caps. Set aside.

3 In a large pot over medium-high heat, combine the chicken stock, vinegar, and soy sauce, and bring to a boil.

4 Dredge the chicken strips in ¼ cup of the cornstarch, and drop into the boiling soup.

5 Stir in the shiitake mushrooms, carrots, baby corn, garlic, ginger, snow peas, and enoki mushrooms. Return the soup to a boil. Reduce the heat, and simmer gently for 8 minutes.

6 In a small bowl, combine the remaining ¼ cup cornstarch with the reserved mushroom-soaking water, and stir to dissolve the cornstarch. Stir the slurry into the soup slowly and gently, to thicken the broth. Stir in the tofu. Bring the mixture briefly to a boil to ensure that the cornstarch is cooked.

7 Just before serving, add the egg, gently swirling it into the soup. Add the bean sprouts, green onions, chile oil, and salt and pepper to taste.

▸ nail this

This is best freshly made, just before serving. If it is made in advance, the veggies wilt.

Use any chicken stock recipe you have; just avoid using canned broth, as the homemade stock is an essential part of the dish's flavor.

Warning: Never add dry cornstarch to hot liquid or it'll clump and make a mess! Make sure it's mixed into a cold liquid before stirring it into the hot soup.

▸▸ flip it

Use leftover cooked chicken, dropping it directly into the soup broth, or substitute beef strips for the chicken.

All of the veggies can be played around with or removed entirely. If you don't have enoki mushrooms, any mushroom will do.

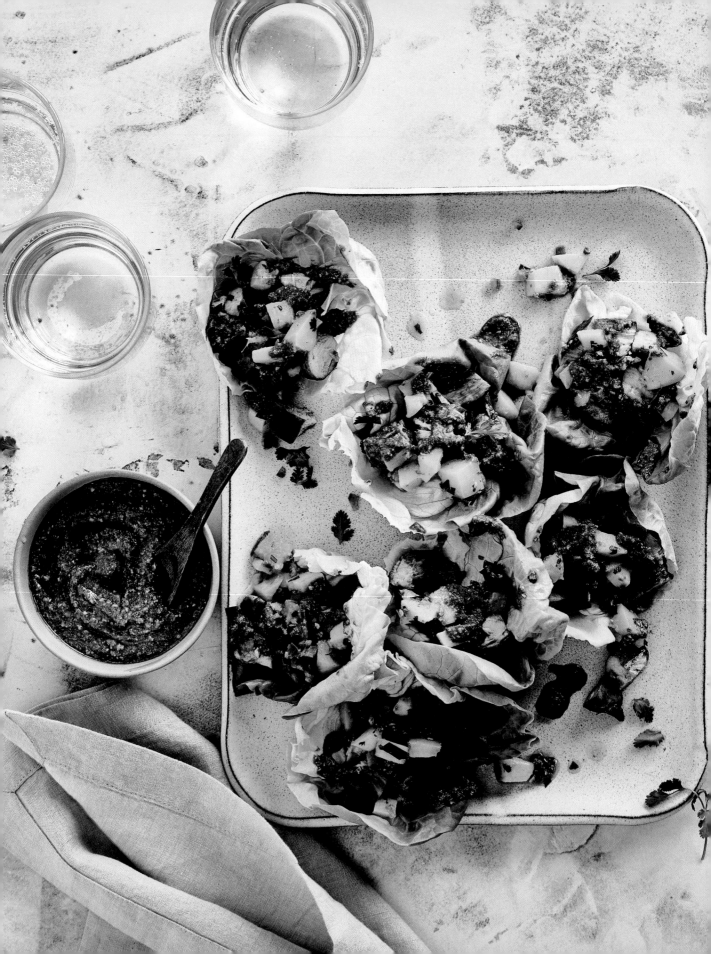

CHICKEN LETTUCE CUPS WITH GREEN PESTO AND MANGO SALSA

STEPS: MARINATE, GRILL, ASSEMBLE! / **Makes 4 to 6 servings**

I have a slight obsession with loaded butter-lettuce cups. I stuff them with a bite of just about anything, but I'm especially addicted to this combo of chicken, pesto, and mango salsa. The succulent chicken thighs marry sweetly with spiced mango, and the salty and fragrant pesto adds a final kick—to create a one-bite party in your mouth! Whip these up as a healthy appetizer for your next gathering, or serve them as finger-food party bites.

MARINADE

⅓ cup extra-virgin olive oil

¼ cup freshly squeezed lemon juice

¼ cup orange juice

3 tablespoons maple syrup

2 tablespoons balsamic vinegar

2 teaspoons Dijon mustard

2 garlic cloves, minced

Grated zest from 2 limes

¼ teaspoon salt

¼ teaspoon freshly ground black pepper

1 pound boneless, skinless chicken thighs

TO ASSEMBLE

1 head butter lettuce, cleaned, leaves separated

1 cup Mango Salsa (recipe follows)

½ cup Flexible Green Pesto (page 272)

1 In a medium bowl, mix together all the marinade ingredients. Pour the mixture over the chicken and allow it to marinate for one hour, or overnight if desired, covered, in the refrigerator.

2 Preheat a grill or broiler to high.

3 Remove the chicken thighs from the marinade. Grill or broil the thighs about 12 minutes total, turning once, until they are cooked through and the centers are no longer pink. Set the thighs aside for a couple of minutes, until they are cool enough to handle.

4 Slice the chicken into bite-sized pieces.

5 To assemble, arrange the individual butter-lettuce leaves side by side on a large platter. If serving as an appetizer, divide the leaves among small plates.

6 Put a few slices of chicken on each lettuce leaf. Top with a spoonful of salsa and a drizzle of pesto. Eat immediately to avoid soggy lettuce.

CONTINUED

MANGO SALSA

Makes about 2 cups

3 fresh, ripe mangoes
or 1 10-ounce bag frozen
mangoes

1 small jalapeño

¼ cup chopped fresh
cilantro leaves, packed

Juice and grated zest
of 1 lime

1-inch piece fresh ginger,
peeled and finely grated

1 tablespoon extra-virgin
olive oil

½ teaspoon cumin

Pinch of salt

Once, while I was in the supermarket shopping for ingredients for this mango salsa, I confess I panicked for a moment. Lo and behold, some supermarkets don't always stock fresh mangoes. Determined to pair chicken and mango, I picked up a bag of frozen organic mangoes and...OMG. Frozen mangoes are AH-mazing. They are perfectly cubed and ready to use, they hold their shape well, and they are reliable and consistent in ripeness and flavor.

1 Peel, seed, and chop the mango into your desired cube size, such as ¼- to ½-inch square. If using frozen mangoes, chop them while frozen (it's easier; when they defrost they are a bit slimy), then set aside to defrost.

2 Remove the seeds and ribs from the jalapeño (or keep them if you like the heat), and mince.

3 In a medium bowl, mix the jalapeño, cilantro, lime juice, lime zest, ginger, olive oil, cumin, and salt. Stir in the mango, and mix to combine. The salsa is best served chilled.

› *nail this*

Choose butter-lettuce leaves that are big enough to hold a few bites and deep enough that your filling will stay inside (see photo).

Taste your salsa and pesto before serving to make sure the flavors are just right.

» *flip it*

Swap the chicken with any meat or grilled fish. I make this dish if we have leftover steak from a BBQ or grilled salmon from the night before.

Lettuce cups too messy for you? Place the chicken, mango salsa, and pesto in the center of a rice-paper wrapper to create a tidier chicken spring roll! (See page 88 for spring roll assembly.)

Make this recipe even easier by doubling the pesto recipe and ditching the other marinade. Use half the pesto to marinate the chicken and the other half for serving.

MAKE-YOUR-OWN BEEF WRAPS

STEPS: BROWN, LAYER! / **Makes 12 appetizer-sized servings**

Mediterranean spiced beef, meet Lao-style beef wraps. The method is simple: Sauté beef with spices, then serve alongside herbs, butter lettuce, and a selection of crunchy garnishes. Diners get to assemble their own beef "wraps" with a drizzle of tahini to finish. The prep is a breeze, and the wraps deliver the ultimate fusion of deliciousness and fun. If you like, serve with sticky rice or steamed short-grain rice for an additional filling.

BEEF

3 tablespoons olive oil

1 large yellow onion, chopped

3 garlic cloves, minced

1 teaspoon cumin

1 teaspoon sweet paprika

1 teaspoon ground coriander

¼ teaspoon cayenne pepper

2 pounds lean or grass-fed ground beef

¾ teaspoon salt, or to taste

Freshly ground black pepper, to taste

TO ASSEMBLE

2 heads butter lettuce, cleaned, leaves separated

2 cups chopped fresh herbs (such as mint, parsley, cilantro, green onion)

½ cup pine nuts, toasted

Pickled Red Onions (recipe follows)

The Ultimate Flexible Tahini (page 273)

1 In a large skillet over medium heat, heat the oil and cook the onions, stirring, until they're soft and lightly browned, about 7 minutes.

2 Add the garlic, cumin, paprika, coriander, and cayenne, and cook, tossing, until the spices are fragrant, about 1 minute.

3 Add the beef and salt and cook, stirring, until cooked through, 6 to 8 minutes. Set the pan aside to cool slightly, reseason if needed with salt and pepper, then spoon the meat into a serving bowl.

4 On a large platter, arrange the butter-lettuce leaves, a bowl each of fresh herbs, pine nuts, pickled red onions, and tahini.

5 Set the platter next to the beef. To serve, scoop some beef into a lettuce cup, top with herbs, pine nuts, onions, and a drizzle of tahini. Repeat.

› nail this

Make sure you use high-quality and well-sourced grass-fed beef to reap the health benefits!

›› flip it

For an Asian twist, replace the cumin, paprika, and coriander with lemongrass, lime leaves, and ginger.

Substitute lean ground turkey. For a veggie option, use tofu in the same method, or swap in my Sheet-Pan Tofu Medley (page 183).

Make a beef salad: Toss all herbs and veggies with torn lettuce, top with beef, and drizzle tahini on top!

To make a quick meat sauce, add a jar of marinara to the seasoned, cooked beef, and simmer for 30 minutes.

PICKLED RED ONIONS

Makes about 2 cups

¾ cup apple cider vinegar

¾ cup red wine vinegar

1 teaspoon sugar

1 teaspoon salt

1 large red onion,
thinly sliced

Pinch of red pepper flakes

1 Combine the vinegars, sugar, and salt in a saucepan over medium-high heat. Bring to a boil, and stir until the sugar is dissolved. Remove from the heat.

2 Stir in the onions and pepper and allow the mixture to steep until cool. Store in an airtight container in the refrigerator for up to 1 month. They're ready for use after 24 hours.

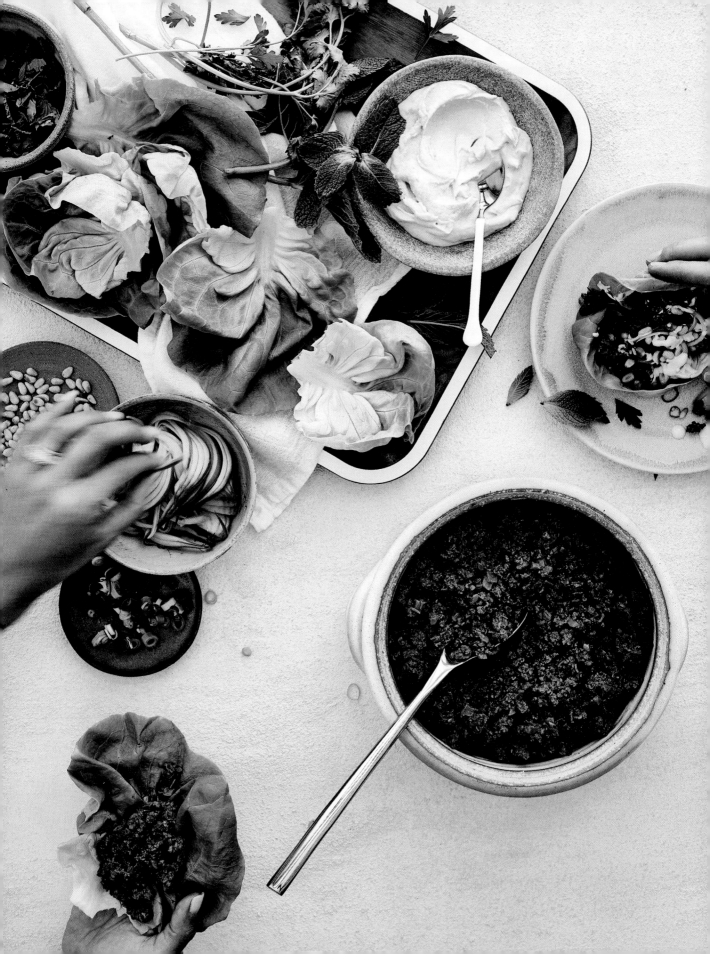

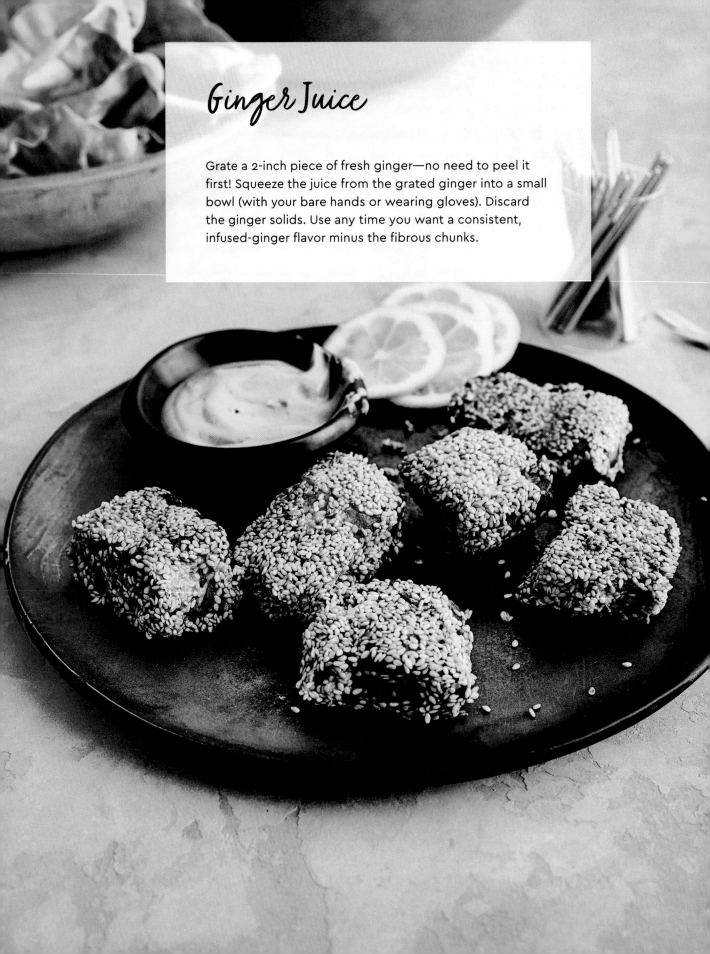

Ginger Juice

Grate a 2-inch piece of fresh ginger—no need to peel it first! Squeeze the juice from the grated ginger into a small bowl (with your bare hands or wearing gloves). Discard the ginger solids. Use any time you want a consistent, infused-ginger flavor minus the fibrous chunks.

SESAME SALMON BITES

STEPS: MARINATE, COAT, SEAR! / **Makes 6 appetizer-sized servings**

I'm hungry just writing about my favorite way to bite into salmon. The ingredient list below is deceptively simple, but the flavor is robust and totally crave-worthy. Sesame pairs exquisitely with salmon, and I serve this with Spicy Sriracha Mayo (page 277) and some fresh greens to complete the dish. Don't just make these as a plated appetizer; serve them as finger food for a dinner party, or add a few to a green salad for lunch.

Tools: Toothpicks, for serving

½ cup tamari

2 tablespoons toasted sesame oil

1 tablespoon Ginger Juice (see sidebar)

1 tablespoon maple syrup

1 pound salmon, skin removed, cut into bite-size (1½-inch) chunks

2 large egg whites

½ cup sesame seeds

3 tablespoons olive oil

TO SERVE

2 lemons, cut into wedges

Mixed green lettuce leaves

Spicy Sriracha Mayo (page 277)

1 In a small bowl, whisk together the tamari, sesame oil, ginger juice, and maple syrup. Pour the marinade over the salmon. Marinate for 4 hours, covered, in the refrigerator. In a pinch, reduce the marinating time to 30 minutes, or omit the marinating entirely. The flavor will be less robust but still delicious.

2 Remove the salmon from the marinade. Dip each piece in egg white, then coat it with sesame seeds. The salmon has been marinating in salty liquid, so it shouldn't need more salt.

3 Heat the olive oil in a large frying pan over medium-high heat. Pan-fry the salmon chunks on all six sides until they are golden and cooked through, about 4 minutes total (depending on the size of your pieces).

4 Serve with lemon wedges, drizzled with Spicy Sriracha Mayo, or serve as party bites on a platter with toothpicks and lemon wedges, using the mayo as a dip.

› nail this

Time-saving tip: Make the salmon in advance and undercook it slightly. Finish it in the oven before serving.

›› flip it

Serve the salmon chunks in a butter-lettuce cup to create a healthy salmon wrap.

Make a salmon hand roll with a nori sheet, cucumber sticks, and avocado. Drizzle with sriracha.

VIETNAMESE VEGGIE SPRING ROLLS

STEPS: SAUTÉ, FILL, ROLL, DIP! / **Makes 20 rolls**

The cities and villages of Vietnam are full of exotic street-food inspiration, and on one of my most recent trips to the region I became utterly obsessed with upgrading fresh spring rolls. Variations on spring rolls abound, with fillings ranging from raw veggies only to cooked meat and seafood. Here I bypass the usual bland vermicelli noodles and replace them with zesty herbs, crispy tofu, and wok-fried julienned veggies that add sweetness to the mix, offsetting the mild bitterness of the raw salad greens for a balanced, robust bite.

Tools: Wok or large frying pan, baking sheet, small fine-mesh strainer

COOKED VEGGIES

2 tablespoons olive oil

8 green onions, white part only, chopped (green part reserved)

2 shallots, thinly sliced

2 cups shredded green cabbage

3-inch piece fresh ginger, peeled and julienned

1 large carrot, julienned

1 jicama, sliced in 3 x ¼-inch sticks

1 cup sliced wood ear mushrooms (or any mushroom you prefer)

Salt and freshly ground black pepper, to taste

CRISPY BAKED TOFU

1 8-ounce block firm tofu, cut into long, thin strips

1 tablespoon tamari or soy sauce

1 tablespoon olive oil

1 tablespoon cornstarch

Salt and freshly ground black pepper, to taste

1 Preheat the oven to 400°F.

2 While the oven is preheating, cook the veggies: In a wok or large frying pan over medium-high heat, heat the oil. Sauté the green onion (white parts) and shallots until fragrant, about 3 minutes. Stir in the cabbage and ginger, and cook until the cabbage is slightly wilted, about 10 minutes.

3 Add the carrot and jicama and cook until softened, about 3 more minutes. Stir in the mushrooms. Season the mixture with salt and pepper and set aside.

4 Bake the tofu: Arrange the tofu strips on a baking sheet, and drizzle all sides of the tofu with the tamari and oil. Using a fine-mesh strainer, sprinkle the cornstarch over the tofu, turning the tofu halfway through to cover all sides. Season with salt and pepper. Bake in the oven, without flipping, for 20 minutes or until crispy.

5 Prepare the wrappers: Wet a small, clean kitchen towel, and squeeze out the extra water. Lay the rice-paper wrappers, a few at a time, on a cutting board, and wipe each wrapper with the dampened towel on both sides to soften it.

6 Fill the rolls: On the bottom third of the wrapper, layer a few tablespoons of the cooked veggies with some of the lettuce, tofu, greens, basil, mint, peanuts, and green onion. Roll from the bottom, tucking the wrapper around the filling. Halfway up, fold the sides of the wrapper into the center, much like you would for a burrito. Continue rolling until closed. Repeat.

TO ASSEMBLE

20 round rice-paper wrappers

2 cups torn butter-lettuce leaves

1 cup chopped mustard greens or arugula

1 cup fresh Thai basil, chopped

1 cup fresh mint, chopped

½ cup roasted and salted peanuts

Reserved green parts from 8 green onions, chopped (see above)

Traditional Fish Dipping Sauce and/or Tangy Peanut Sauce (recipes follow)

7 These may be made up to an hour in advance. Keep them at room temperature. (But they're best eaten immediately.) Serve the rolls with dipping sauce(s).

› nail this

Many methods soften rice-paper wrappers by dipping them in hot water. This makes them overly soggy. The wet-towel method, which is faster and easier to manage, will transform your spring-roll making. Wipe enough water onto the wrapper to make it soft enough to roll.

Be patient and cook your cabbage over low heat to allow it to soften and caramelize—this brings out the best flavor.

›› flip it

If you prefer uncooked rolls, julienne your favorite fresh ingredients—try fresh mint and cilantro, cucumbers and carrots, avocado and mango. Roll using the same method, and serve with one of the dipping sauces or with my Green Tahini (page 273).

I've been lazy and have made this recipe without the rolling! Assemble the filling ingredients on a plate, and top them with sauce for a yummy salad. You could do this with leftover filling, too.

Can't find Thai basil? Substitute any of your favorite green herbs such as cilantro, mint, or regular basil, or just omit it.

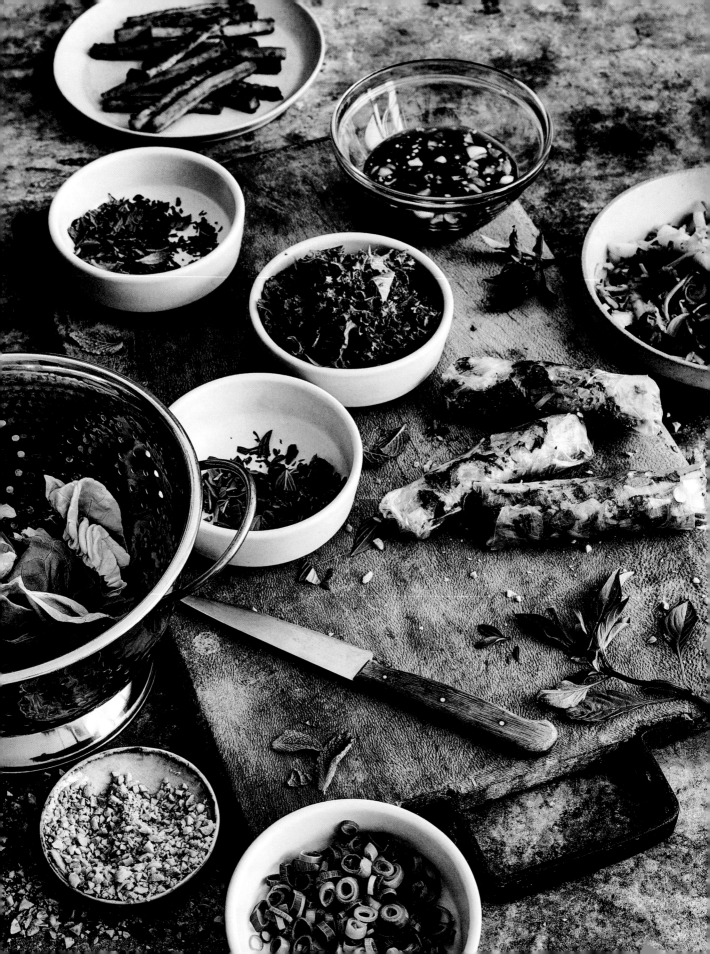

TRADITIONAL FISH DIPPING SAUCE

3 garlic cloves, peeled

1 to 2 fresh red chiles, or to taste

4 tablespoons lime juice

3 tablespoons raw honey

4 teaspoons tamari or soy sauce

4 teaspoons fish sauce

1 Smash the garlic with the back of a large chef's knife.

2 Chop the chiles into small chunks, then smash them using the same method as you did for the garlic.

3 In a bowl, stir the garlic and chiles with the lime juice, honey, tamari, and fish sauce. Keeps in the fridge for a few days.

4 Makes enough for 8 spring-roll servings. Double the recipe if you're serving more. If you don't like fish sauce, you can use more tamari instead, for a different but still good flavor.

TANGY PEANUT SAUCE

½ cup crunchy natural peanut butter

⅓ cup water

1 tablespoon plus 1½ teaspoons maple syrup

1 tablespoon lime juice

1 tablespoon tamari

1 garlic clove, crushed

1 teaspoon red pepper flakes, or more, to taste

1-inch piece lemongrass, if available (tough outer leaves removed)

1 Add all of the ingredients to a food processor and pulse to combine. Alternatively, whisk vigorously by hand, achieving a smooth texture (except for the crunchy peanuts). Keeps in the fridge for a few days.

2 Makes enough sauce for 8 spring-roll servings. Double the recipe if you're serving more.

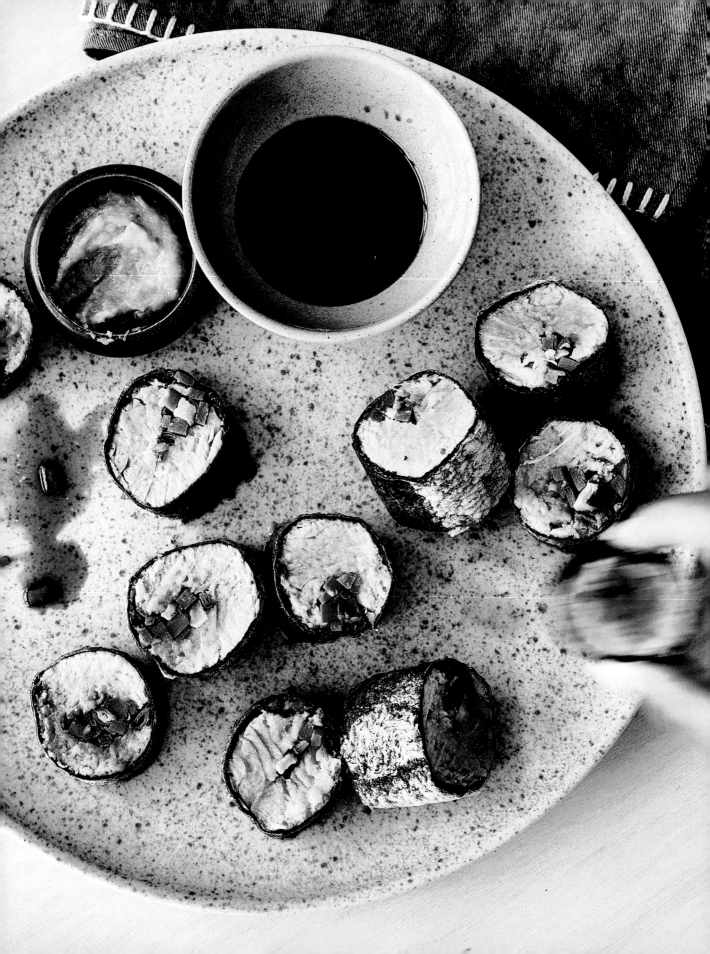

HOT AND CRISPY SUSHI ROLLS

STEPS: SAUTÉ, STUFF, ROLL, CRISP! / **Makes 6 servings**

This is a more time-consuming recipe, but it is so irresistible (and once you master it, very achievable) that I promise it will be worth your while. Raw salmon and cooked veggies are rolled in a combo of rice-paper wrappers and nori sheets, then seared and sliced to serve like sushi, in attractive, bite-size pieces. No rice cooking involved! Every bite is a masterpiece.

Tools: Chopsticks, for serving (optional)

1 pound skinless salmon fillet

Salt and freshly ground black pepper, to taste

2 tablespoons olive oil, for frying

1 tablespoon minced, peeled fresh ginger

½ cup julienned shiitake mushrooms

½ cup julienned carrots

½ cup julienned snow peas

1 teaspoon toasted sesame oil

6 nori sheets

6 rice-paper wrappers

1 large egg white

Micro greens or mixed salad greens drizzled with lemon juice, oil, and salt, for serving

Tamari, for dipping

Wasabi, for serving

1 Cut the salmon into six fillets, each slightly larger than 1 inch thick, trimming the length to the width of a rice-paper wrapper, if needed. Using a paring knife, make a slit down the length of the middle of the top of each piece of salmon, to create a pocket. Do not cut all the way through the fillet on the bottom or sides. Season with salt and pepper; set aside.

2 In a frying pan over medium-high heat, heat the olive oil, and cook the ginger, mushrooms, carrots, and snow peas, stirring, until they begin to soften, 3 or 4 minutes. Toss the vegetables with the sesame oil, and season them with salt and pepper. Set aside to cool.

3 Prep your wraps: Stack the nori sheets, then position a rice-paper round on top, and cut around the nori with kitchen scissors so that the nori sheets are the same size as the rice-paper round.

4 Wet a small, clean kitchen towel, and squeeze out the water. Lay your rice-paper wrappers (two at a time) on a cutting board, and wipe each wrapper on both sides with the damp towel, until they are softened enough to roll.

5 Brush the edges of each nori sheet and rice-paper wrapper with a touch of egg white to cause them to stick together. Layer each nori sheet with a rice-paper wrapper. Place each rice-paper/nori round on a cutting board with the nori side up.

6 Fill each salmon pocket with a small amount of the cooked vegetables. Position the stuffed salmon pocket on the bottom third of a nori/rice paper round. Roll, tucking the wrapper around the salmon, and secure the seam closed with a touch of egg white.

CONTINUED

7 In a large frying pan over medium heat, heat just enough oil to lightly coat the pan. Cook the salmon rolls on all sides (starting with the seam side down) until the salmon is cooked through but still a little pink, about 8 minutes total.

8 When done, cut the rolls into sushi-sized pieces. (If making these ahead, reheat and crisp the pieces in a 400°F oven for 5 minutes before serving.)

9 To serve: Mound some lightly dressed salad greens in the center of a plate. Arrange the sushi alongside, and serve with tamari and wasabi in small dipping-sauce dishes.

› nail this

So that these will remain crispy, they are best consumed immediately. If you do make them in advance, watch them closely while reheating them in the oven, and don't overcook the salmon.

Don't attempt this recipe if you're busy and stressed—plan it as a starter with a menu that's on the simpler side.

Rice paper is not pliable until it is moistened with water. Don't freak out about working with this versatile ingredient; just wet it with a damp kitchen towel until it's flexible.

» flip it

Use cod or sea bass.

Serve with Spicy Sriracha Mayo (page 277), as a party finger food.

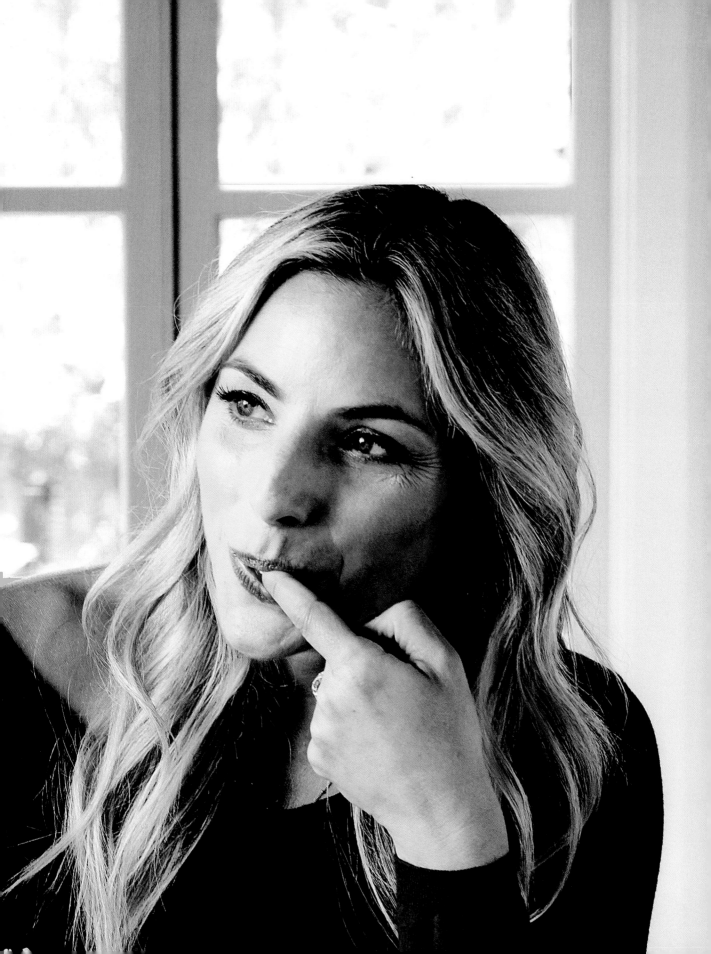

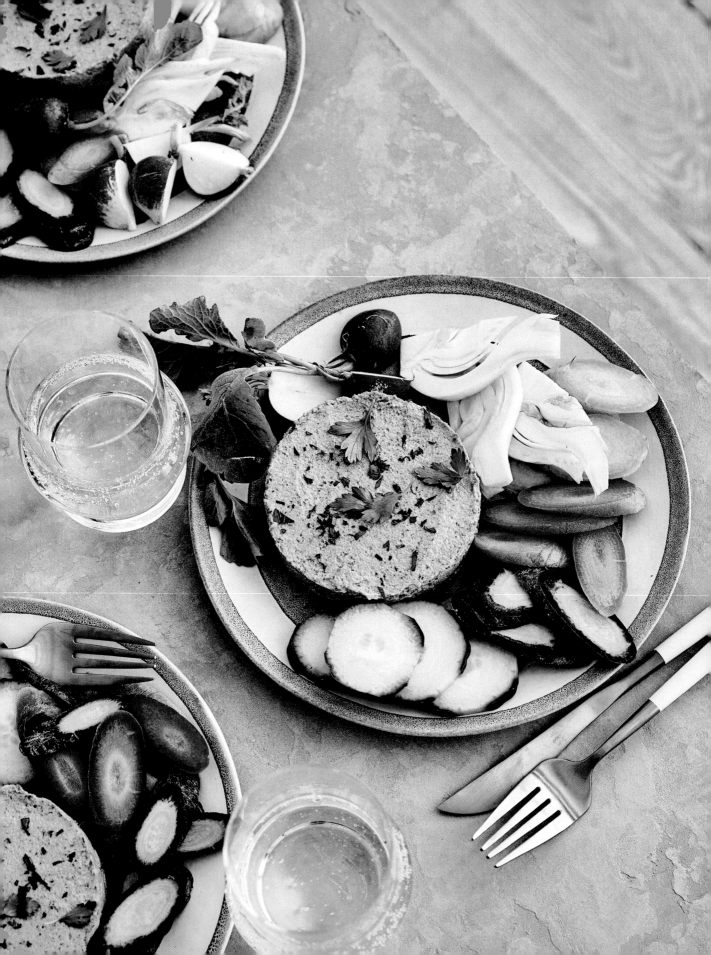

VEGGIE PECAN PATE

STEPS: CARAMELIZE, PULSE! / **Makes 12 appetizer-sized servings**

This veggie version of the classic chopped-liver spread gets equally happy *oohs* and *aahs* from carnivores and vegetarians alike because it is just so darn good. Onions are caramelized forever to produce the deepest golden color, and then they are pulsed with sweet pecans, hard-boiled eggs, and verdant peas. The result? The most delicious and versatile appetizer, which can be plated and molded as shown, used as a sandwich spread, or served as part of a mezze assortment of dips and crackers.

Tools: Food processor, 3-inch round cookie cutter or ring mold

¼ cup olive oil

3 large yellow onions, diced or thinly sliced

1 10-ounce bag frozen peas

1 heaping cup pecan halves, toasted

3 large eggs, hard boiled and peeled

2 tablespoons chopped fresh basil

1 garlic clove, crushed

1 teaspoon salt

1 teaspoon cumin

½ teaspoon freshly ground black pepper

TO SERVE
Basil leaves, to garnish

Raw crackers or tortilla chips and/or a selection of fresh vegetables

1 In a large skillet over low heat, heat the oil and cook the onions, stirring frequently, until deeply browned, about 15 to 20 minutes.

2 Defrost the peas in a bowl of hot water for 5 minutes. Drain well.

3 Grind the pecans to a course meal in a food processor.

4 Add the caramelized onions to the food processor, and mix for another 30 seconds. Add the peas, eggs, basil, garlic, salt, cumin, and pepper. Pulse until combined and smooth, pausing often to check for consistency. Taste for seasoning, and adjust as needed.

5 To serve as a plated appetizer, set the cookie cutter or ring mold on an appetizer plate, and mound a few tablespoons of pate into the mold. Press the pate into the mold firmly with the back of a spoon to eliminate gaps or air pockets. Remove the mold, and top with basil leaves, if desired. Arrange crackers or tortilla chips or vegetables on the plate alongside the pate. To serve a crowd, scoop the pate into a pretty bowl, and serve it with crackers and other dips alongside. The pate keeps in the refrigerator for 3 days.

> *nail this*

The flavor improves with time, so prepare this dip the day before serving.

It's important to cook the onions slowly, for a long time on low heat, to impart the caramelized sweetness. It's the most important flavor of the pate.

>> *flip it*

Use this molded presentation for other dishes—for party dips like guacamole, chunky salsa, or bean dip, or to plate rice, quinoa, or smashed sweet potato as a side or base for a plated main dish.

Substitute toasted walnuts or almonds for the pecans.

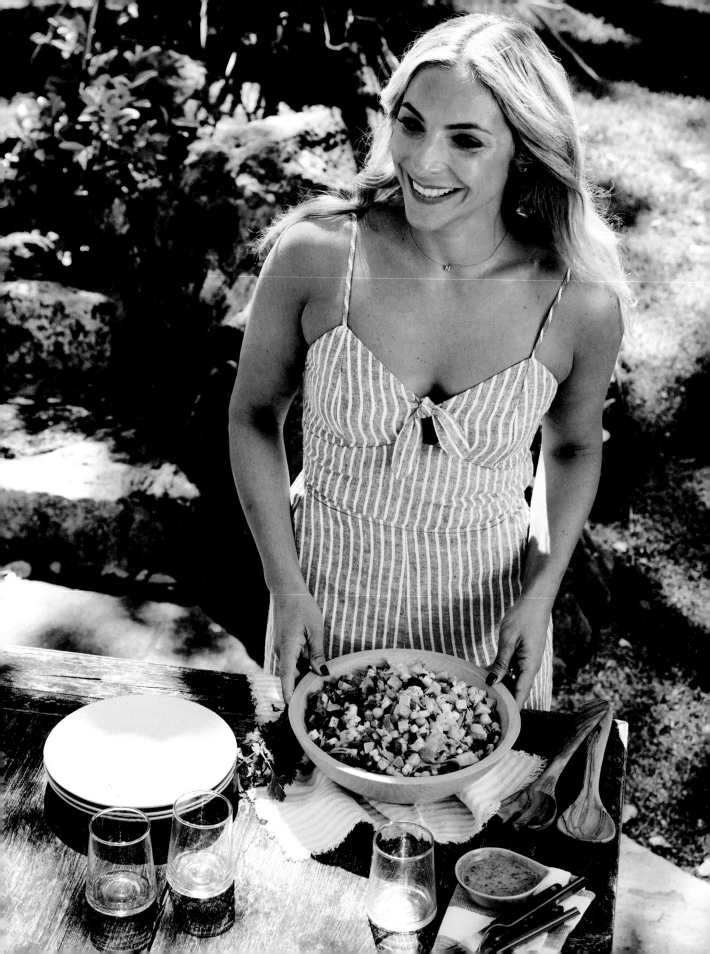

Chapter 5

SALADS AND DRESSINGS

I prepare a lot of elaborate dishes, but one of my favorite things to make and eat is salad. Apparently, my love of salad has made a lasting impression on my son. One summer when he was five, I was in Hong Kong, pregnant with my daughter Ayla, and he was vacationing with my parents in Montana. At the dinner table one night, just as the salad course came around, Ben started to cry. When my mother asked him what was wrong, he wistfully said, "We're eating salad. My mom's favorite food is salad. I miss my mom!"

Truth be told (and don't hate me for this, because it's the result of really hard work and many failed attempts—see page 186 on getting kids to eat veggies), my kids actually do eat salad. That's partly because it's what they see their dad and me eating at home (and when I serve it, I do so when the kids are famished). But more important, I make sure salads taste amazing. Forget about oil- and lemon-doused soggy lettuce. I'm talking tantalizing dressings and combos like Caesar salad with Parmesan crisps—it's the food you wanna eat for the way you wanna feel: hearty, delicious, light, and, ultimately, satisfying.

GIVE-ME-LIFE SALAD

STEPS: BLEND, ASSEMBLE, SERVE! / **Makes 6 servings**

When Hong Kong's iconic Life Café closed several years ago, I knew I needed to get their famed Life Salad back in my life—and get it to you. This salad ticks all the boxes of a covetable meal: satisfying, hearty, healthy, good-looking, and totally addicting. I remembered that my friend Carlos, the head chef and recipe creator, had one day scribbled notes with the salad's ingredients after I begged him to tell me how to make it. Miraculously, I dug up the crinkled handwritten list and used it as the basis for writing this recipe. Get ready for a new addiction, and go get a life... salad, that is.

Tools: Blender

DRESSING

2 cups assorted fresh green herb leaves (basil, parsley, oregano, thyme)

3 tablespoons lemon juice

2 tablespoons nutritional yeast, plus more for serving

1 tablespoon tahini

1 garlic clove

1 teaspoon Dijon mustard

½ teaspoon salt

⅓ cup extra-virgin olive oil

SALAD

6 cups mixed greens

1½ cups peeled, shredded carrots

1½ cups peeled, shredded beets

Alfalfa sprouts, for garnish

3 tablespoons chopped assorted nuts and seeds, for garnish

1½ cups Hummus Any Way Any Day (recipe page 274)

Store-bought crackers, for serving

1 To make the dressing: Blend the herbs, lemon juice, nutritional yeast, tahini, garlic, mustard, and salt. Then continue blending, slowly drizzling in the olive oil until the mixture is emulsified. If needed, add a touch of water to thin the dressing to your desired consistency, as it is quite thick.

2 To assemble the salad: Plate a handful of greens in individual bowls, or serve them all on a family-style platter. Drizzle some of the dressing on the greens. Mound carrots, beets, and alfalfa sprouts on top. Sprinkle with nuts, seeds, and nutritional yeast, and then drizzle more dressing on top. Scoop a large spoonful of hummus per person onto the salad (I like to use an ice cream scoop). Serve with crackers.

3 The dressing keeps in the refrigerator, covered, for 2 days. The salad, once dressed, should be eaten immediately so the greens stay crisp.

» *flip it*

Use the dressing on anything!

Vary your veggies. Eliminate the hummus if you want.

Nutritional yeast gives this dressing a cheesy, rich flavor without the cheese. But, hey, substitute Parmesan if you prefer.

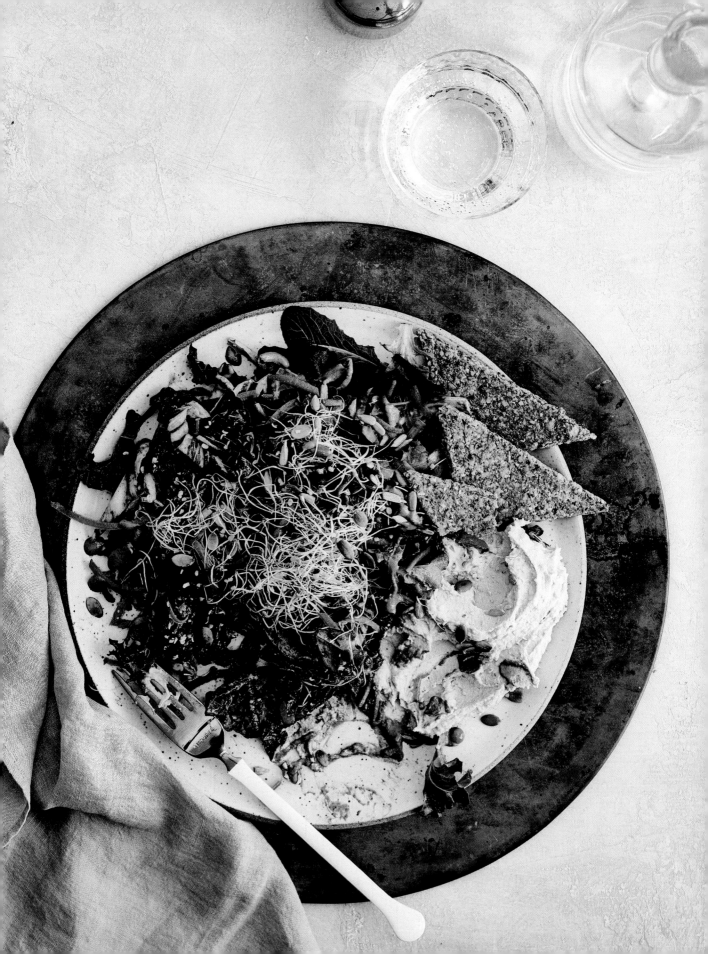

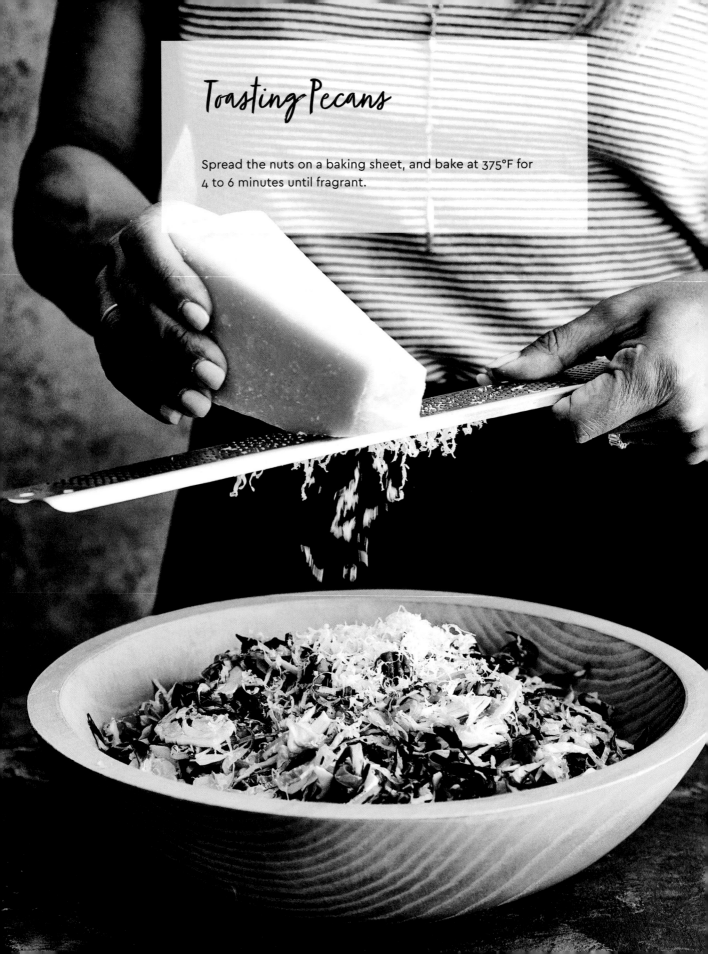

Toasting Pecans

Spread the nuts on a baking sheet, and bake at 375°F for
4 to 6 minutes until fragrant.

GROWN-UP COLESLAW

STEPS: SLICE, WHISK, TOSS! / **Makes 4 servings**

Brussels sprouts often get a bad rap, but they're one of the most nutritious veggies on the planet, and when prepared right they are scrumptious—yes, even raw! This shaved Brussels slaw bursts with a surprisingly varied texture and big flavor (thanks to the radicchio and Parmesan). Top the salad off with your favorite protein.

Tools: Mandolin (optional)

SALAD

1 pound Brussels sprouts
(4 cups shredded)

1 small head radicchio
(2 cups shredded)

1 cup thinly sliced green
onion

⅓ cup chopped pecans,
toasted (see sidebar)

DRESSING

2 tablespoons lemon juice

1 teaspoon Dijon mustard

2 small garlic cloves,
minced

2 teaspoons maple syrup

⅛ teaspoon salt

Freshly ground black
pepper, to taste

⅓ cup extra-virgin
olive oil

Grated Parmesan cheese,
for serving (optional)

1 Prepare the vegetables: Slice the Brussels sprouts very thinly lengthwise, using a mandolin if possible. Then thinly slice the radicchio. Place the shredded veggies in a large bowl. Stir in the green onions and pecans, and set aside.

2 Make the dressing: In a medium-size bowl, whisk together the lemon juice, mustard, garlic, maple syrup, salt, and pepper. Slowly pour in the olive oil, whisking constantly, until the mixture is emulsified.

3 Coat the slaw with as much dressing as you prefer, and top with a sprinkle of Parmesan cheese, if desired. Reseason with salt, as needed.

4 May be made up to 30 minutes before serving to marinate. While waiting, place in the refrigerator to chill.

> *nail this*

Top the slaw with grilled chicken, salmon, or sliced steak for the perfect lunch.

Serve the slaw as a side dish—it goes well with BBQ!

>> *flip it*

Feeling sweet? Grab a bag of glazed pecans or walnuts from the supermarket. Or chop in some Rosemary Party Nut Trail Mix instead (page 261).

Eliminate the Parmesan completely if you wish; serve with any dressing you love.

No Brussels? No problem. Use cabbage!

Save some shaved raw Brussels sprouts, and pan-fry them with butter or olive oil, salt, and pepper—adding any other veggies you have on hand. Serve as a side dish or for breakfast with eggs.

KALE SALAD WITH CREAMY CASHEW DRESSING

STEPS: BLEND, TOSS! / **Makes 6 to 8 servings**

Can kale really be that interesting? Yup, especially if you smother it with this addictive dressing. When I serve versions of this salad to friends, they always ask, "What's in this that makes it so good?" The cashew-based dressing is creamy and Caesar-like, but so delightful and different from almost any other dressing you'll try. Not convinced yet? Pop the dressing ingredients into a blender, and wait for the compliments from your diners to flow.

Tools: Blender

DRESSING

½ cup raw cashews, soaked for 10 minutes, then drained

⅓ cup rice vinegar

¼ cup extra-virgin olive oil

2 tablespoons minced shallot

2 tablespoons tamari or soy sauce

1½ teaspoons coconut sugar or maple syrup

1 garlic clove

½ teaspoon salt

Freshly ground black pepper, to taste

SALAD

6 cups kale, ribs removed, leaves rolled and sliced into ribbons

2 cups bite-sized raw cauliflower florets

1 cup Sweet and Salty Chickpeas (page 262)

¾ cup dried cherries

1 Make the dressing: In a blender, combine the soaked cashews, vinegar, olive oil, shallot, tamari, sugar, garlic, salt, and pepper. Blend until creamy. If you make ahead and chill, you might need to dilute the mixture ever so slightly with water, as it will thicken in the fridge.

2 To assemble: In a large bowl, toss the kale and cauliflower with just enough dressing to coat (save the rest of the dressing for the next day). Unlike other tossed salads that benefit from the lightest coating of dressing, the kale needs to be massaged with the dressing for about a minute to soften the leaves. Use your hands (with or without gloves) to toss.

3 Transfer the mixture to a serving bowl, sprinkle the top with chickpeas and cherries, and serve immediately. Or refrigerate for 30 minutes for the kale to soften further.

> *nail this*

Ensure that the kale is chopped into small pieces or sliced into small ribbons, because there's nothing worse than gnawing on a larger-than-your-mouth piece of kale. Alternatively, use baby kale.

>> *flip it*

Use the dressing as a marinade for chicken or veggies.

Substitute romaine, spinach, or another firm lettuce for the kale.

Make homemade kale chips: Spread any extra kale on a baking sheet, and top with a smattering of oil, salt, and pepper. Bake at 350°F until crisp, about 15 minutes. Stay vigilant, watch for crisping, and beware of burning. Remove when a sample makes your taste buds happy.

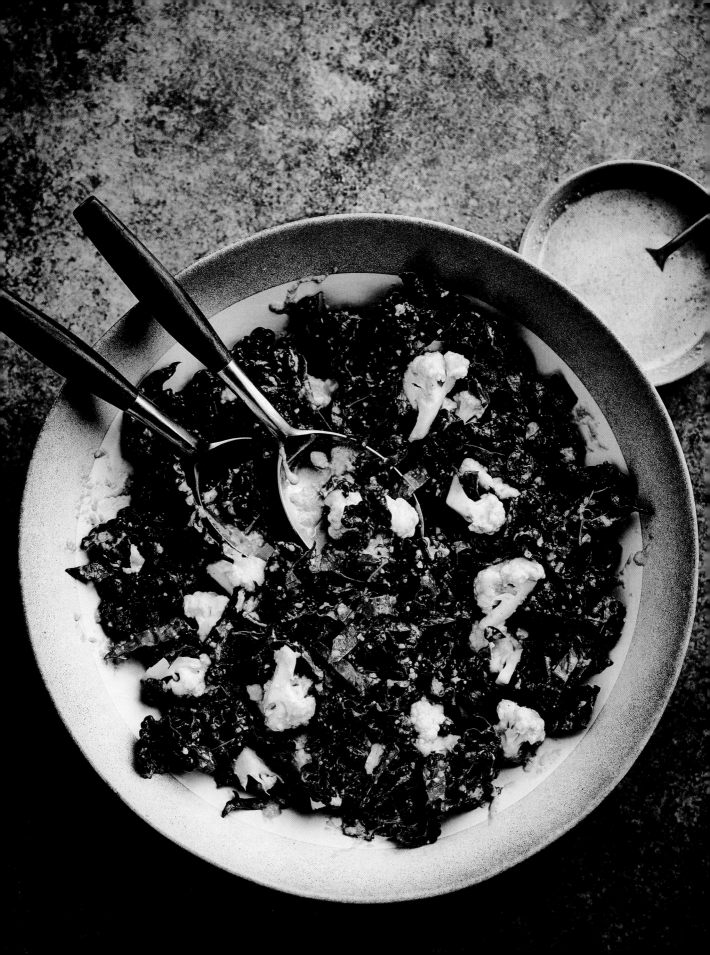

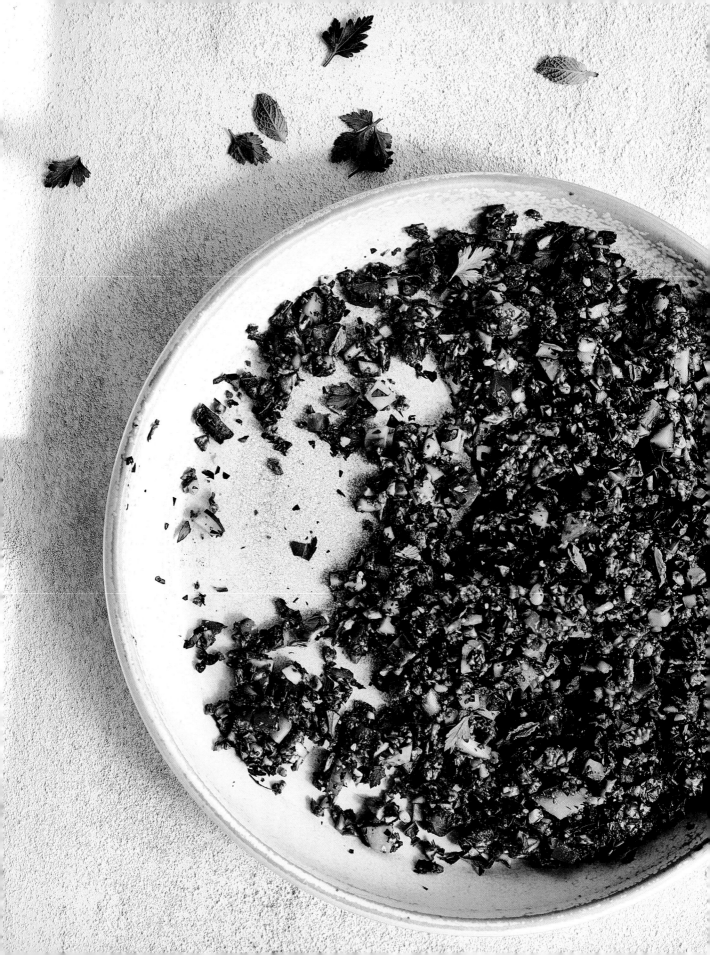

CAULIFLOWER-CRUNCH TABOULI

STEPS: CHOP, TOSS! / **Serves 6**

There's nothing ordinary about this stunning herb-specked, grain-free tabouli. Raw cauliflower and pine nuts take center stage and combine to add an unexpected and essential nuttiness and color that elevate the dish. This recipe takes just minutes to whip up and seconds to devour. It's crunchy, fresh, and the very definition of craveable clean food that makes you want more.
I really shouldn't play favorites, but this salad may well be my favorite!

Tools: Food processor (optional)

½ head purple or white cauliflower, core removed

3 Persian cucumbers, chopped

2 medium tomatoes, chopped

1 cup loosely packed fresh mint leaves, chopped

1 cup loosely packed fresh parsley leaves, chopped

2 tablespoons finely diced red onion

3 tablespoons extra-virgin olive oil

3 tablespoons fresh lemon juice

1 garlic clove, pressed (optional)

Salt, to taste

Freshly ground black pepper, to taste

½ cup chopped pine nuts, toasted

1 In a food processor, chop the cauliflower into ¼-inch pieces. Do not overprocess. Alternatively, chop it by hand.

2 In a large bowl, stir together the cauliflower, cucumber, tomato, mint, parsley, and red onion.

3 Toss the vegetables with the olive oil, lemon juice, and garlic (if desired). Season with salt and pepper to taste. Top with pine nuts just before serving.

4 Serve immediately, or it may be made an hour ahead. If making in advance, toss the pine nuts in right before serving so they stay crunchy.

> *nail this*

Because the fresh, raw ingredients are the centerpiece here, only make this recipe when you have access to the freshest herbs and cauliflower.

Nuts are crucial. They add an essential flavor and crunch that are unexpected and should be included.

>> *flip it*

Use any color cauliflower you can find.

Substitute another nut for the pine nuts. Toasted would be yummiest.

Add chopped anything! Red bell peppers and olives are favorite flavor profiles.

LIGHTENED-UP CURRIED CHICKEN SALAD

STEPS: BLEND, TOSS, SERVE! / **Makes 4 to 6 servings**

This dish is inspired by my favorite classic curried chicken salad from Ina Garten. I reduce the mayonnaise significantly by including an avocado, and the goldenberries add a sweet but tart punch (although they may not make it into the salad after you devour them). This salad is a great way to use up leftover chicken, is fun served as an accompaniment to a salad bar, and is an easy to-go lunch layered on a bed of greens with a light dressing.

Tools: Blender (optional)

DRESSING

⅓ cup mayonnaise
(I use an olive oil–based, "healthier" mayo)

1 avocado, peeled, pitted, and smashed

2 tablespoons fresh lime juice

2 tablespoons mango chutney

1 tablespoon extra-virgin olive oil

1 tablespoon curry powder

½ teaspoon salt

¼ teaspoon freshly ground black pepper

SALAD

4 cups diced, cooked chicken (preferably grilled or broiled; see sidebar)

½ cup finely chopped red onion

½ cup diced celery

¼ cup chopped cashews, toasted

4 teaspoons dried goldenberries

1 tablespoon chopped fresh cilantro leaves, plus more for garnish

1 Make the dressing: Combine all the dressing ingredients in the blender, and pulse until smooth. Or to prepare by hand, make sure the avocado and the chutney's mango pieces are smashed smooth (you can use a fork to do this), then whisk all of the dressing ingredients together in a medium bowl. Taste the dressing and adjust the seasoning to your liking.

2 In a serving bowl, stir together the chicken, red onion, celery, cashews, goldenberries, and cilantro. Toss with just enough dressing to coat. Taste and add more if necessary.

3 Garnish with extra cilantro to serve. May be made an hour ahead of serving and refrigerated to chill.

» *flip it*

Goldenberries add a surprising twist, but you can use regular or golden raisins, dried cranberries, or dried cherries instead—or omit.

If you have dressing left over, add a touch of oil and vinegar to dilute it, and season with salt and pepper. Drizzle over greens, and place a mound of chicken salad on top.

Leftover dressing is also great as a marinade for chicken or tofu prior to broiling or baking.

Roast some firm tofu and use it instead of chicken to make this dish vegetarian.

Marcona or toasted almonds are a great sub for the cashews.

Can't find mango chutney? Swap in 1 tablespoon apricot jam or orange marmalade.

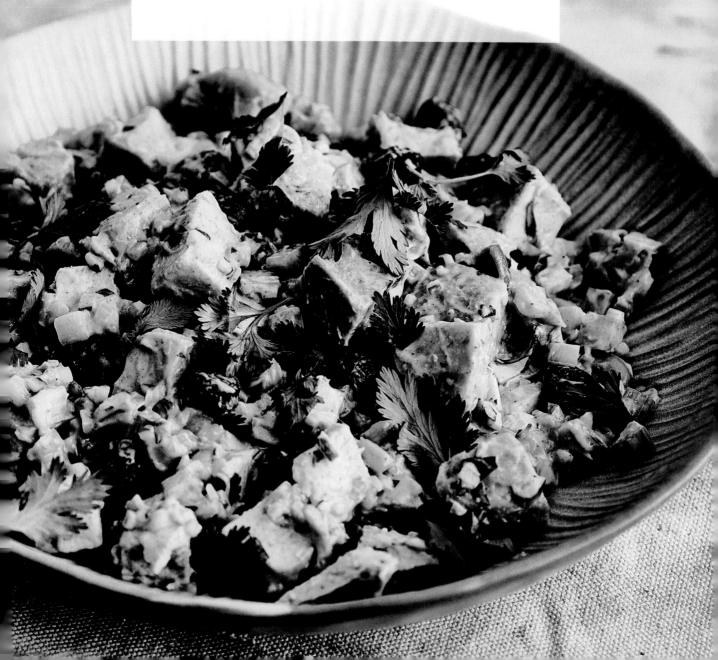

Easy Broiled Chicken in a Pinch

Arrange 8 boneless chicken thighs (about 1½ pounds) on a large sheet pan. Drizzle with olive oil, lemon juice, and a pinch of salt and pepper. Broil the chicken for a total of 12 to 18 minutes, or until cooked through. Set aside to chill before dicing.

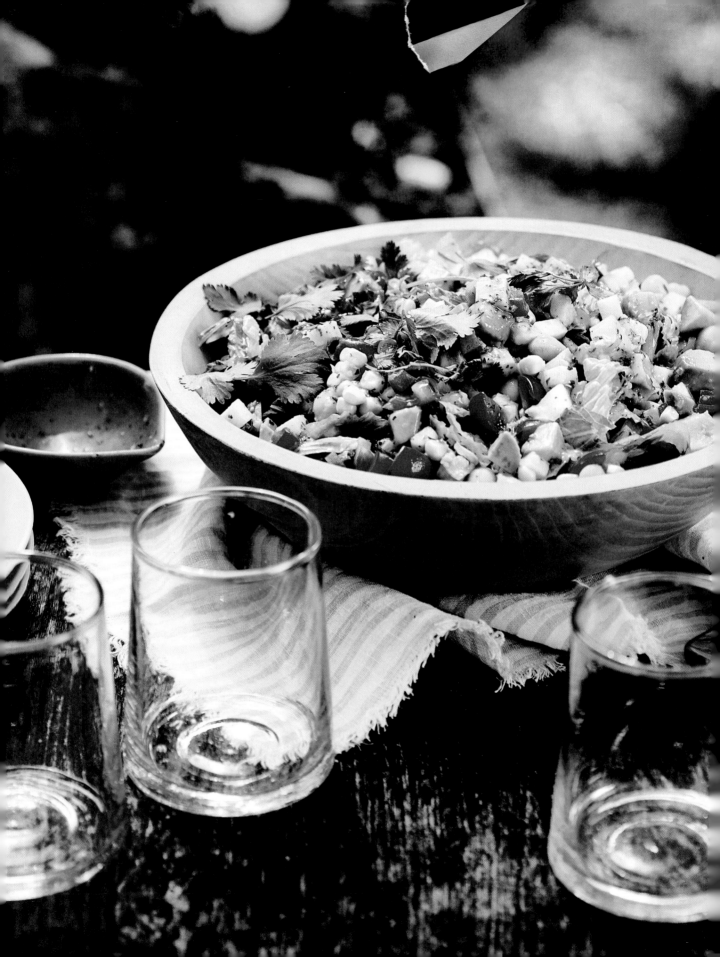

CHOPPED AND LOADED MEXICAN-ISH SALAD

STEPS: BLEND, TOSS! / **Makes 8 to 10 servings**

Here's my semi-Mexican take on a chopped and loaded salad. It's the kind of dish to whip up to go alongside a simple grilled fish or chicken, or as a one-bowl lunch when a hearty salad craving hits. I've even eaten leftovers for breakfast (weird but true). You'll love the crunchy mix of veggies, but it's the thick and creamy cilantro dressing that pulls them all together and makes this salad pop with fresh flavors.

Tools: Blender

CREAMY CILANTRO
DRESSING

½ cup chopped fresh
cilantro (leaves and stems)

⅓ cup chopped red onion

⅓ cup fresh lime juice

1 tablespoon raw honey

1 to 2 garlic cloves

1 teaspoon salt

1 teaspoon cumin

Pinch of cayenne pepper

Freshly ground black
pepper, to taste

1 cup extra-virgin olive oil

SALAD

3 ears fresh corn, husked
and cleaned (omit if not
in season)

1 medium head romaine
lettuce, thinly sliced
crosswise

1 medium red bell
pepper, cored and diced

2 small Persian
cucumbers, diced

½ medium jicama, peeled
and diced

1 cup diced cherry
tomatoes

2 avocados, pitted and
diced

1 cup canned chickpeas,
rinsed and drained

Cilantro leaves, for garnish

1 Make the dressing: In a blender, mix all the ingredients except olive oil until smooth. Continue blending, drizzling the oil in slowly to emulsify. The dressing can be made a day in advance.

2 Taste your corn. Is it sweet? If so, use it raw. If not, cook it until crisp-tender: Bring a saucepan of water to a boil over high heat, add the corn, and cook for 5 minutes. Drain and let cool. Use a sharp knife to cut the kernels off the cob.

3 Mix all the salad ingredients in a large bowl. Stir to combine. Toss with just enough dressing to coat. Taste, and add more dressing and salt and pepper, if needed. Garnish with cilantro leaves and serve immediately. Leftovers are a tad soggy but taste divine.

> nail this

The dressing will only achieve true creaminess if you blend it in a blender. You could use a hand blender or a food processor in a pinch, but it will be chunkier.

>> flip it

Use any sweetener in place of honey in the dressing.

Customize salad however you feel fit—omit or add what suits your palate.

ROASTED-CAULIFLOWER SALAD WITH ARUGULA AND CRISPY ONIONS

STEPS: ROAST, TOSS, SERVE! / **Makes 6 servings**

Whether mashed, roasted, "riced," puréed, steamed, or raw, cauliflower rules the cruciferous vegetable world in my book. It's low in calories and carbs, but off the charts in flexibility and nutrition. In this salad it shines, served warm on a bed of greens, topped with a tangy dressing, and delivering a whole lot of crunch. I had the hardest time sitting down to write out the recipe because it's the sort of dish that happens better when you just sprinkle a bit of this or that into it. Once you've mastered the gist of this salad, go get sprinkling and don't overthink it.

Tools: Rubber gloves, large baking sheet

Tangy Mustard Vinaigrette (page 122), or your favorite

1 large head cauliflower, cut into bite-sized florets (about 5 heaping cups)

¼ cup olive oil

½ teaspoon salt

¼ teaspoon turmeric

¼ teaspoon cumin

¼ teaspoon paprika

¼ teaspoon garlic powder

Freshly ground black pepper, to taste

SALAD

4 cups arugula

⅓ cup roasted almonds, chopped

⅓ cup Crispy Onions (see recipe page 269)

Handful of parsley leaves, for garnish

1 Preheat the oven to 425°F.

2 Make the vinaigrette (or pull out one you have already).

3 Prepare the cauliflower: Spread the florets on a large baking sheet in one layer. Use two pans if needed. Mix the oil, salt, turmeric, cumin, paprika, garlic powder, and pepper in a small bowl, then spread over the cauliflower. Toss to coat the cauliflower. (Wear gloves if you use your hands for this step.)

4 Roast the cauliflower for 30 minutes or until lightly browned on the edges. Remove from the oven and set aside.

5 To assemble: Toss the arugula with your preferred amount of vinaigrette, then mound it at the base of a shallow serving bowl or on a large platter. Top the arugula with the cauliflower, almonds, crispy onions, and parsley. The salad can be made and dressed up to 15 minutes before serving. If dressing ahead of time, add the onions just before serving so they don't get soggy.

› *nail this*

Using gloves or tongs to toss the cauliflower is essential unless you like turmeric-orange stained nails!

›› *flip it*

Serve the flavorful roasted cauliflower on its own as a side dish.

Substitute the Outrageous Lemon Caper Dressing (page 124) with this recipe—yum!

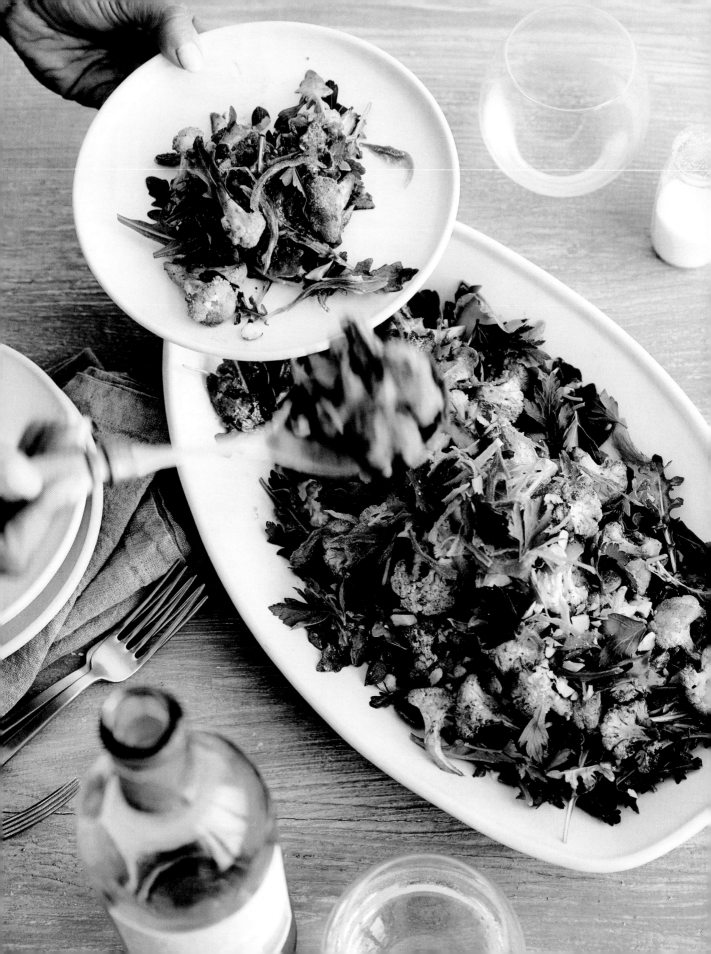

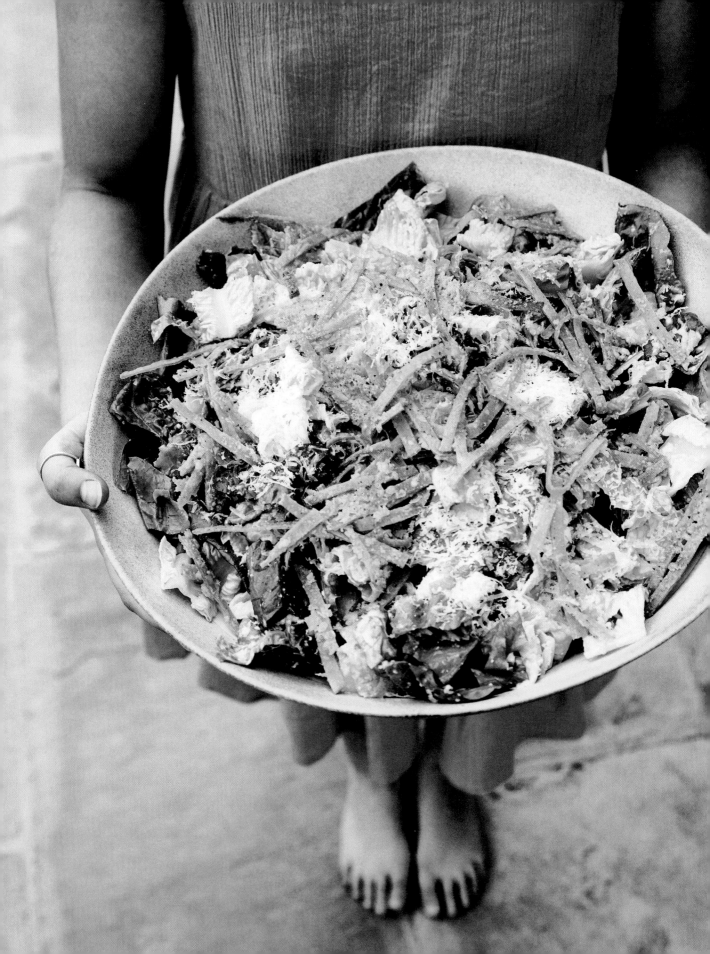

CAESAR SALAD WITH PARMESAN TORTILLA CRISPS

STEPS: BOIL, BLEND, BAKE, TOSS! / **Makes 10 servings**

Most Caesar salads use only raw egg yolks, which add creamy richness to the dressing—but it means you miss out on all that good extra protein from the whites. So, I got to thinking: Why does the egg have to be raw? Turns out, it doesn't. If you boil the egg for just a few minutes, the whites are semicooked, and you maintain the awesome Caesar experience. Even better? Parmesan Tortilla Crisps stand in for croutons. You're welcome.

Tools: Blender, pastry brush

DRESSING

2 large eggs

¼ cup fresh lemon juice

5 to 6 anchovies

2 garlic cloves

1 teaspoon Dijon mustard

¼ teaspoon Worcestershire sauce

¼ teaspoon salt

Freshly ground black pepper, to taste

½ cup extra-virgin olive oil

½ cup grated Parmesan cheese, for topping

PARMESAN TORTILLA CRISPS

4 6-inch corn tortillas

1 tablespoon plus 1½ teaspoons garlic-infused olive oil (see sidebar)

½ teaspoon salt

½ cup grated Parmesan cheese

2 heads romaine lettuce, chopped

1 Preheat the oven to 400°F.

2 Prep the eggs: Boil water in a medium saucepan over high heat. Add the whole eggs, and boil for 4½ minutes. The whites will be almost firm, and the yolks will still be runny. Cut off the top shell of each egg, and scoop out the whites and yolks (as if you were serving a soft-boiled egg).

3 Put the eggs in a blender, and add the lemon juice, anchovies, garlic, mustard, and Worcestershire, and season with salt and pepper. Blend to combine, then drizzle in the oil, still blending, until emulsified. Chill the dressing in the fridge—it will be warm from the cooked eggs.

4 Make the crisps: Brush the tortillas with garlic oil, and season with salt. Stack the tortillas on a cutting board, and cut them in half. Then cut each stack of halves crosswise into ¼-inch strips.

5 Transfer the tortilla strips to a sheet pan. Sprinkle them with Parmesan, and bake until light golden-brown and crisp, 10 to 15 minutes, flipping every 5 minutes. Set aside to cool.

6 Toss the romaine in a bowl with just enough dressing to coat, and top it with Parmesan cheese before serving. Garnish with the tortilla crisps, and serve at once to avoid soggy lettuce.

CONTINUED

› nail this

Be careful not to overcook the eggs; you want the yolks soft and runny.

You could attempt whisking the dressing by hand (first, finely mince the anchovies and garlic), although you'll have a chunky dressing from the cooked egg. A blender is essential to achieve creaminess.

» flip it

For a dairy-free version, omit the cheese, but add an extra clove of garlic and another anchovy to the dressing to intensify the flavor. Make the tortilla crisps without the Parmesan. And adjust the salt—if you omit Parmesan, the dressing could use a pinch more.

Toss the dressing over raw kale and top with a poached egg for a kale Caesar breakfast.

Make Your Own Garlic Oil

Crush a few cloves of garlic, and submerge them in a few tablespoons of extra-virgin olive oil.

Let sit, covered, for an hour (or up to a whole day), to allow the garlic to infuse the oil.

Strain the garlic out using a mesh strainer so you're left with the flavored oil. Store, covered, in the refrigerator for up to 1 month.

Wow Your Friends with an Extravagant Salad Bar

Salad bars are the easiest and most gorgeous spread to create for a fun meal at home. The chopping and prepping are annoyingly time-consuming but are still far easier than cooking a whole meal. Build your own salad, and you're free to run with your innovative ideas to balance flavor, texture, nutrition, and more.

SALAD BAR COMPONENTS

Vegetable base: Romaine, mixed greens, spinach, kale, and/or cabbage.

Vegetable add-ins: Chopped anything, but consider color and crunch—carrots, cucumbers, colored peppers, jicama, cooked and cubed beetroot are great options.

Proteins: Shredded beef or chicken, cooked or canned salmon and tuna, roasted tofu, edamame.

Toppings: Chopped nuts, olives, seaweed crisps, flax meal, dried cranberries.

Dressings: Serve with any dressing you love. I save wine bottles or other good-looking jars, rinse off the labels, and repurpose them to serve dressings—gorgeous! See my dressing recipes on pages 122 to 127, or concoct your own.

Assorted dips: Add decorative bowls of tahini, hummus, tapenades, or other dips to the spread for flavor infusions. Sometimes you'll just be tempted to sweep some hummus up with a slice of romaine.

DRESSED-UP QUINOA SALAD

STEPS: STEAM, MIX, MARINATE! / **Makes 4 to 6 servings**

Humble quinoa marries creamy chickpeas, crunchy veggies, and a sweetish zippy dressing to balance this earthy and satisfying salad. Cook the quinoa a day in advance, and chop up your veggies right before serving so that prep is fast. This salad is equally delicious the next day too, so save your leftovers in a container, and pack them for lunch!

2 cups cooked red quinoa (see cooking instructions page 38)

1 15.5-ounce can chickpeas, drained and rinsed

½ cup chopped green onion, green and white parts

1 red bell pepper, chopped

½ medium jicama, peeled and finely chopped (about 1½ cups)

⅓ cup extra-virgin olive oil

½ cup dried cherries or dried cranberries (optional)

¼ cup chopped fresh cilantro leaves, plus more for garnish

2 tablespoons plus 2½ teaspoons lemon juice

1 teaspoon curry powder

1 tablespoon maple syrup

¾ teaspoon salt

½ teaspoon freshly ground black pepper

½ teaspoon cumin

¼ teaspoon allspice

1 In a large bowl, stir together all the ingredients. It's best to marinate the mixture, covered in the refrigerator, for at least 4 hours before serving.

2 To serve, mound the salad into serving dishes; garnish with fresh cilantro.

» flip it

Red quinoa is pretty, but use white if that's what you have in your pantry.

What else to do with quinoa? Alone it's bland, so steam it and serve it with something saucy for it to cling to, like the Island-Style Chicken Adobo (page 149) or Simply Succulent Beef Stew (page 159). Or substitute it for the cauliflower "rice" in the Cauliflower Fried Rice (page 176).

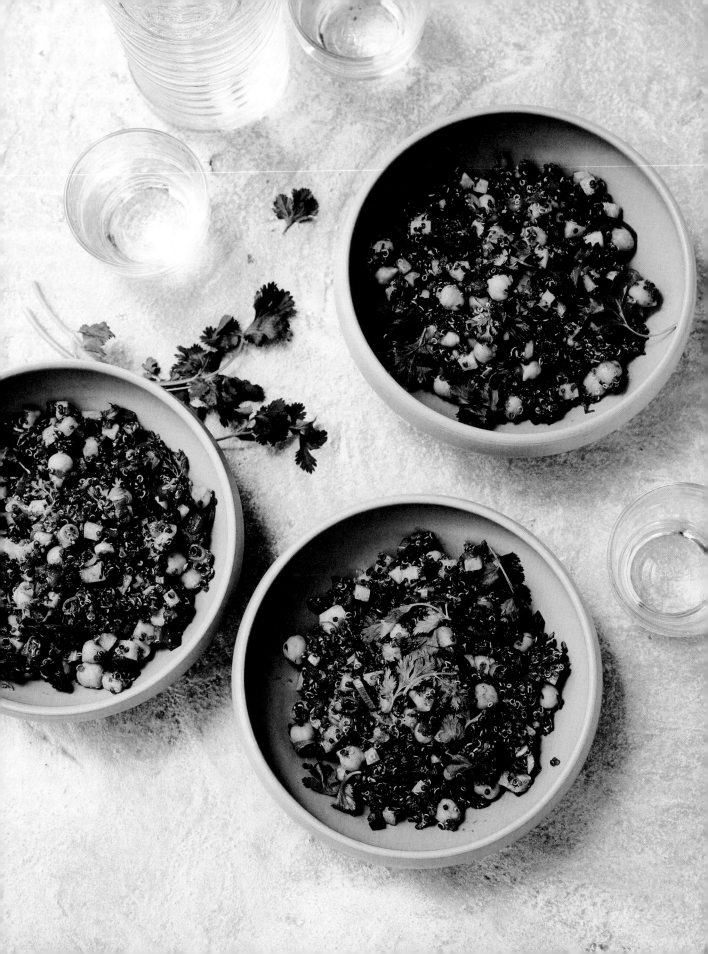

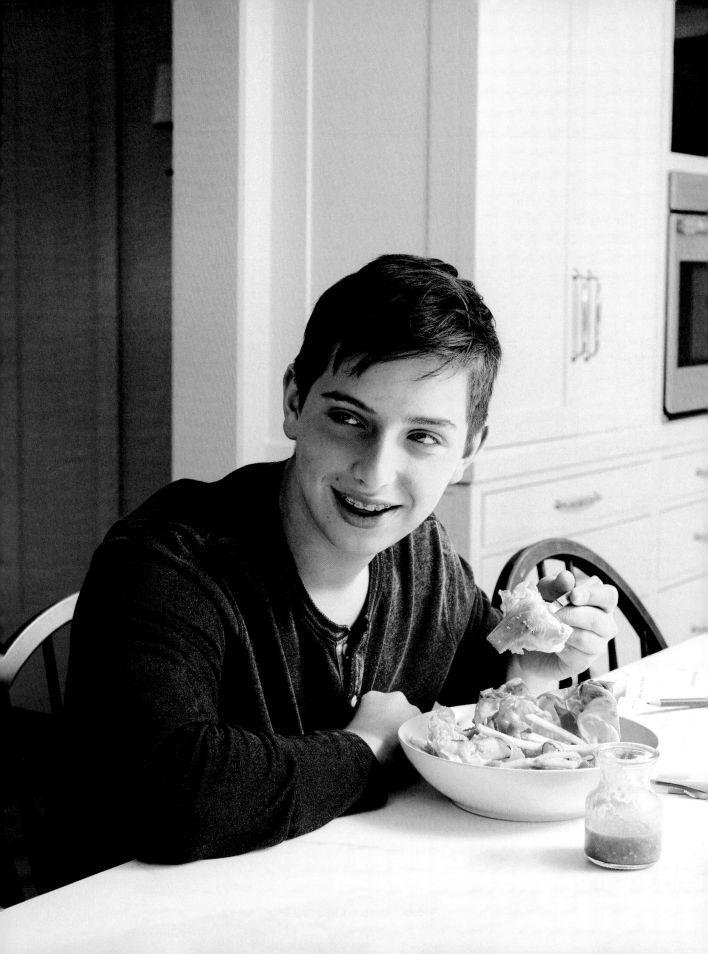

EITAN'S FAVORITE JAPANESE SALAD

STEPS: BLEND, SLICE, TOSS! / **Makes enough for 4 hungry kids**

One night, when my son Eitan was just four years old, we found ourselves famished after a long ski day in Japan. The first thing we ordered was a Japanese salad, served dressed in a creamy onion vinaigrette. To our surprise, Eitan gobbled the tossed lettuce and asked for more. I figured either he was ravenous or that dressing was miraculous. To cover my bases, I began to feed my kids salads on empty, grumbly tummies to increase the chances that they'd eat fresh greens—and I make my version of Japan's wonder dressing to this day, tossed with kid-friendly veggies: sweet butter lettuce, crunchy cucumber, jicama, and carrot.

Tools: Blender, vegetable peeler or mandolin

CREAMY ONION DRESSING

¼ cup rice vinegar

¼ small yellow onion, roughly chopped

2 tablespoons tamari

2 tablespoons sesame seeds

2 teaspoons maple syrup (or to taste)

½ cup plus 2 tablespoons extra-virgin olive oil

Freshly ground black pepper, to taste

SALAD

2 Persian cucumbers

1 large carrot

Leaves from 2 heads butter lettuce

1 cup julienned (or matchstick-cut) jicama

1 To make the dressing: Place the vinegar, onion, tamari, sesame seeds, and maple syrup in a blender, and blend until smooth. Continue blending, adding the oil in a slow stream to emulsify. Add black pepper to taste. Keeps for 4 days, refrigerated.

2 Slice the cucumber and carrot into ribbons using a vegetable peeler or mandolin.

3 In a large bowl, combine the lettuce, jicama, cucumbers, and carrots.

4 Toss the vegetables with the desired amount of dressing, and serve.

 » flip it

Make it by hand. It will be a different dressing, but you could crush the sesame seeds in a mortar or in a Ziploc bag. The onions can be grated. Whisk the ingredients together, adding the oil last to emulsify.

Use the dressing as a marinade for crispy roasted tofu or grilled vegetables. It's also great on roasted cauliflower.

TANGY MUSTARD VINAIGRETTE

STEPS: MIX, WHISK! / **Makes about 1 cup**

The test of a great recipe is if it's one that you keep coming back to over and over again. In my household, this dressing is our fallback. You can prepare it either by hand or in a blender, which makes it easy to whip up in minutes. Keep a jar of this vinaigrette in your fridge, and you'll have no excuse not to assemble a quick salad for lunch.

2 tablespoons plus
1½ teaspoons honey
mustard

2 tablespoons red wine
vinegar

1 tablespoon minced
fresh chives

1 teaspoon finely grated
peeled fresh ginger

1 teaspoon soy sauce

1 garlic clove, minced

¼ teaspoon salt

½ cup extra-virgin
olive oil

1 In a blender or a medium bowl, mix together honey mustard, vinegar, chives, ginger, soy sauce, garlic, and salt.

2 Slowly blend or whisk in the oil to emulsify.

3 Keeps, refrigerated, up to 4 days.

» *flip it*

Use this to marinate Unfried Chicken Schnitzel (page 152).

Stocking Your Fridge with Dressings

- Choose airtight containers, and label and date the dressing. As I always say, a salad is only a second away if you have a dressing ready-made.

- Most dressings stay fresh for 4 to 5 days in the fridge. Stock up!

- Always taste your dressing on a small piece of lettuce, and then adjust the seasonings to taste.

- Dressings presented in pretty jars are killer hostess gifts.

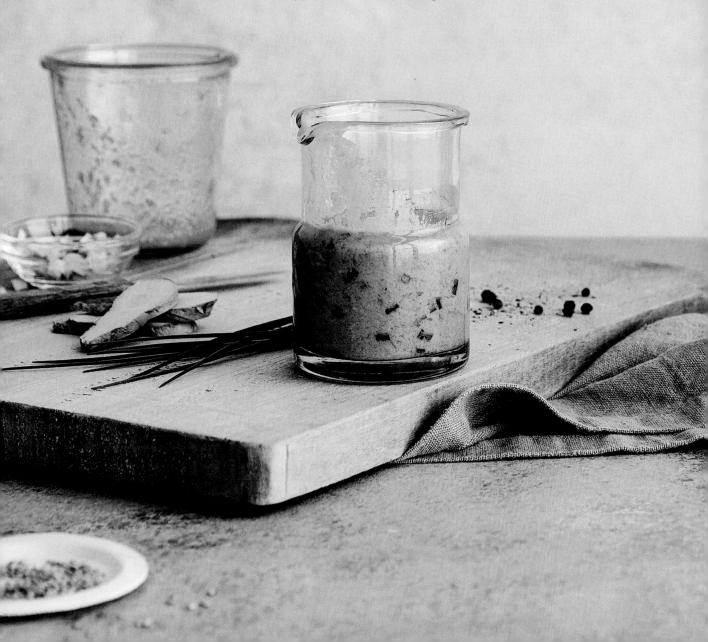

OUTRAGEOUS LEMON CAPER DRESSING

STEPS: WHISK OR BLEND! / **Makes about 2 cups**

Can I just say—my salad life has been transformed by this flavorful dressing. It's inspired by a vinaigrette created by Chef April Bloomfield, and I literally cannot get enough. You can make this recipe two ways: Whisk it by hand to produce a dressing with texture from the capers and shallots, or make it smoothly divine in a blender. Whip up a double batch, and try it both ways. It'll last in a jar in the fridge all week, but I doubt you'll have leftovers that long.

Tools: Whisk or blender

6 tablespoons lemon juice (from about 2 lemons)

⅓ cup diced shallot

¼ cup minced fresh chives

¼ cup drained capers, minced

¼ cup Dijon mustard

1 tablespoon orange juice

1 teaspoon sea salt

1 teaspoon granulated sugar

½ teaspoon freshly ground black pepper

⅔ cup extra-virgin olive oil

1 In a medium bowl, mix together lemon juice, shallot, chives, capers, mustard, orange juice, salt, sugar, and pepper.

2 While whisking, slowly pour the olive oil into the mixture to emulsify the dressing.

3 Alternatively, place all the ingredients except the oil in a blender, and purée until smooth. Continue blending, and add the oil in a drizzle until it's emulsified.

DATE-NIGHT VINAIGRETTE

STEPS: BLEND! / **Makes about 1 cup**

Who doesn't love a great date? In a salad, that is. Dates lend both sweetness and tanginess to this thick and creamy dressing. It's best when made in a blender so that the shallots, garlic, mustard, and dates can emulsify into magic, but if you only have a hand blender, keep reading for a tip on how to "Nail This." Nothing says "I love you" more than feeding your loved ones delicious and nourishing foods, so serve this up with any of your favorite salads.

Tools: Blender

⅓ cup red wine vinegar

2 Medjool dates

2 tablespoons minced shallot

1 garlic clove

1 teaspoon Dijon mustard

1 teaspoon salt

¼ teaspoon freshly ground black pepper

¾ cup extra-virgin olive oil

1 Mix the vinegar, dates, shallot, garlic, mustard, salt, and pepper in a blender until smooth.

2 Continue blending, adding the oil in a stream. Do not overblend once the mixture has emulsified.

3 Keeps for 4 days, refrigerated.

› *nail this*

You need a powerful, high-speed blender to blitz the dates into a smooth paste. If you only have a regular blender or an immersion blender, pour boiling water over the dates and soak them for 30 minutes to soften. Drain and finely chop before blending.

If the dressing solidifies in the fridge, bring it to room temperature before serving, or splash in a little hot water and shake it to bring it back to liquid form.

›› *flip it*

If you really can't get yourself a date, then sweeten this dressing with a tablespoon of maple syrup or honey.

The sweet and pungent flavors of this vinaigrette lend themselves well to a marinade. Marinate chicken or veggies in this mixture for a few hours and grill!

All Dressed Up: Presenting the Perfect Salad

The secret to serving salads that your guests will rave about and that you will crave is dressing them properly. Too little dressing leaves your salad bland, and too much drowns your veggies.

1 Dress your salad in a large bowl, not the one you serve it in. You want some space to coat your ingredients properly.

2 Toss lighter leaves like mesclun, baby spinach, or butter lettuce with your hands (if you have a manicure, wear gloves). Hands are your best tool—you can really feel and disperse the ingredients better than you can with tongs.

3 *Do not* pour the entire quantity of dressing over your salad at once! Add small drizzles at a time, and toss. Stop once the veggies are evenly coated but not overly so.

4 Taste the salad to determine if it needs anything more. More lettuces, vegetables, or dressing? Salt and pepper? A squeeze of lemon? A drizzle of oil?

5 Time your dressing. Some salads benefit from marinating, while others must be dressed right before serving so they don't get soggy. For fragile veggie bases (soft lettuces and spinach) that tend to wilt, wait. Heartier greens like cabbage and kale benefit when marinated for a short time in the dressing.

ORANGE BALSAMIC DRESSING

STEPS: BLEND! / **Makes about 1⅓ cups**

A solid balsamic dressing is a staple we all ought to keep in our arsenal and pull out when appropriate. I drizzle this creamy vinaigrette over a hot mushroom salad, and I keep it in the fridge for when I'm in the mood for a more strongly flavored dressing. The orange mellows the balsamic, and the aromatic herbs add an unexpected twist.

Tools: Blender

¼ cup balsamic vinegar

2 tablespoons orange juice

1 tablespoon plus 1½ teaspoons tamari

2 teaspoons Dijon mustard

2 teaspoons maple syrup

1 garlic clove

¼ teaspoon dried thyme

¼ teaspoon dried rosemary

¾ cup extra-virgin olive oil

Salt and freshly ground black pepper, to taste

1 Mix all the ingredients except the oil in a blender until smooth. Continue blending, and add the oil in a stream to emulsify. Season with salt and pepper.

2 Alternatively, whisk by hand, drizzling the oil in last.

3 Keeps for 4 days, refrigerated.

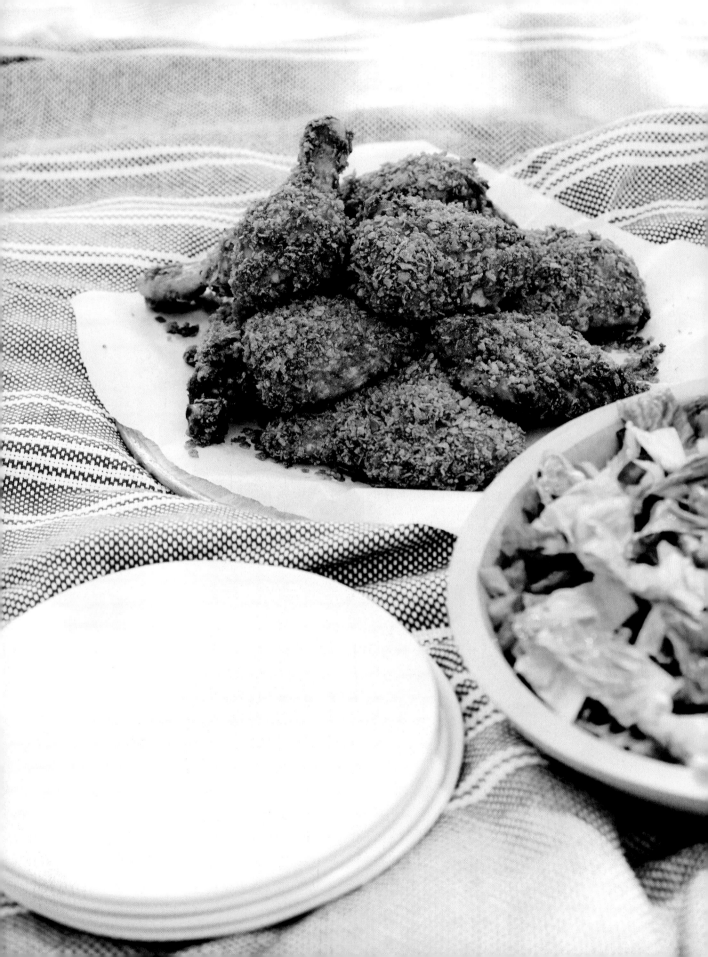

Chapter 6

FISH, POULTRY, AND MEAT

I didn't eat chicken or red meat for twenty years. In those less-educated days, my primary reasoning was "It's bad for me." But one night during my last pregnancy, I was preparing a beef roast for my family and I, guiltily, snuck a taste. Oh, it was so good! I thought my body would go into paroxysms when I fed it meat for the first time in so long. No such thing. Coincidentally, I had a doctor's appointment shortly afterward and discovered that my iron levels were dangerously low. No wonder I craved beef. Moderate amounts of beef have been a part of my diet ever since. It's amazing how well we fare when we finally cave in to listening to our bodies.

If you crave steak, eat it. If you want to avoid meat altogether, honor the impulse. What's right for you might be wrong for me. Whenever possible, choose the best-quality seafood, poultry, and meat you can find and afford. Seek out wild-caught seafood, antibiotic-free or organic chicken, and grass-fed beef, but don't freak out on the occasion when you can't find them.

In each main dish in this chapter, I've offered you a variety of swaps and suggestions, so the chicken oven stir-fry can easily become a red meat dish, or the chicken adobo can always be made with tofu (yes, please, borrow ideas from this chapter for vegetarians). Dig deep to use recipes as a springboard of ideas for you to customize. Flexibility is always the magic word. With a few minor tweaks, you can make each dinner idea work for you.

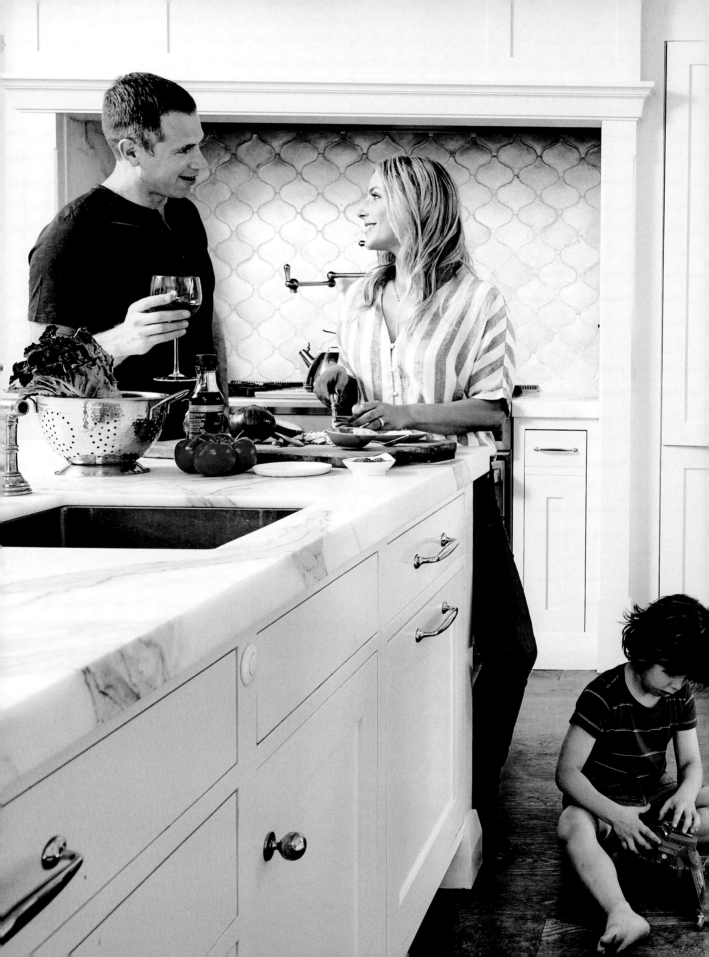

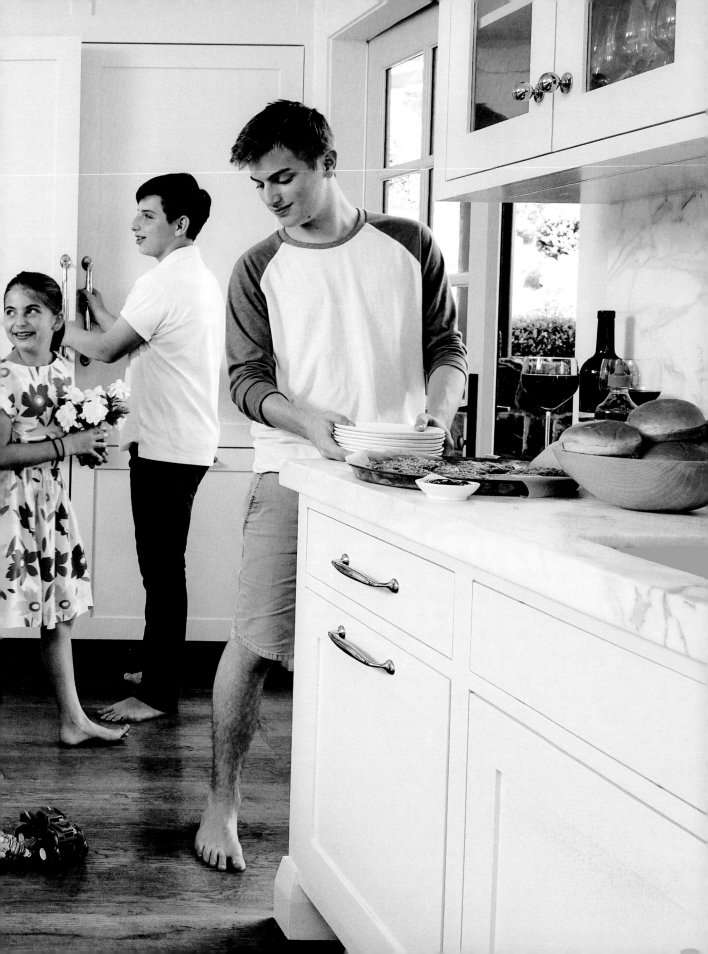

What the Heck Is for Dinner Tonight?

(IN TEN MINUTES OR LESS)

I don't know about you, but some nights, despite my best-laid plans, six p.m. arrives and I wonder "What the heck should I serve for dinner?" The kids are starving, I'm exhausted, and the last thing I want to do is cook. There are the odd nights when we just order in or eat out, but I prefer to turn to my emergency stash. This is when stocking your pantry (page 12) and keeping foods in the freezer (page 12) are your lifelines. My criteria for whipping up these last-minute dinners is that they take ten minutes or less—because any longer and my kids will just pour themselves a bowl of granola.

Soup using last night's leftovers: Sauté onions, carrots, and any veggie you have in the fridge and add broth. Or make a corn soup using a sautéed veggie base and canned or frozen corn. Purée with an immersion blender or leave chunky.

Quickie Bolognese: Sauté onions, mushrooms, and peppers with ground beef, turkey, or chicken. Crumbled tofu works, too. Add defrosted marinara sauce or your favorite jarred sauce, and season with fresh herbs, salt, and pepper.

Cheesy noodles to the rescue: Boil gluten-free pasta, and jazz it up with marinara sauce and cheese. For a grain-free option, swap steamed cauliflower for pasta, and mix it in a frying pan to melt the cheese.

Easy niçoise salad: Make tuna salad, add romaine, olives, green beans, or whatever veggies you want to chop in. Or just pop open a can of tuna and serve with sliced bread, avocado, and a green salad with whatever vinaigrette you have on hand.

Breakfast for dinner! Make an omelet or a "kitchen sink" scramble with a salad and toast.

Fried quinoa "rice": Steam quinoa (it cooks in half the time as rice), and stir in sautéed veggies. Top each portion with a fried or sunny-side-up egg.

Quick tacos: Toast corn tortillas, and whip out a can of black beans or chickpeas. Fry the beans with taco seasoning or just cumin and chili powder. Serve with a bowl of shredded Cheddar or Jack cheese, chopped avocado, chopped tomatoes, jalapeño, and sliced romaine lettuce.

Avocado toast any way: Top toasted bread with smashed avocado and the toppings of your choice.

Curried chickpeas: Fry an onion. Add a generous amount of curry powder and a can of rinsed and drained chickpeas. Serve over steamed rice (if you have the time to cook rice) and/or a steamed or sautéed green veggie. It's great served with yogurt.

Poke bowl: If you have any leftover cooked fish or sushi-grade fish you can defrost, serve it sliced on a bed of chopped veggies with a drizzle of your favorite vinaigrette. Or use canned tuna, sardines, or salmon.

Express chicken: Forget preheating your oven, just season a chicken fillet with salt and pepper and sear in a skillet. Or sear salmon and drizzle both with lemon.

SHOWSTOPPING HERB-CRUSTED SALMON

STEPS: COAT, BAKE! / **Makes 10 servings**

This is one of the more stunning ways to serve a whole salmon fillet. You'll crave the crispy browned edges as they blend with the succulent, herby, nutty topping. I love having friends over for casual weekend lunch buffets, when I serve this fish accompanied by a bountiful display of salads. After lunch, we all go for a hike, topping off a day made in healthy heaven.

Tools: Large baking sheet

SALMON

2 tablespoons olive oil

3-pound side of salmon, whole, skin on

3 tablespoons Dijon mustard

1 tablespoon honey

Salt and freshly ground black pepper, to taste

COATING

⅔ cup Gluten-Free Cracker Crumbs (page 276)

⅔ cup almond flour

4 tablespoons butter, melted

Handful of roughly chopped fresh basil

1 teaspoon dried or fresh rosemary

Pinch of salt (see note below)

¼ teaspoon freshly ground black pepper

1 Preheat the oven to 400°F. Brush the olive oil over a large baking sheet.

2 Place the salmon on the baking sheet, skin side down, and spread the mustard and honey over the flesh. Season with salt and pepper.

3 In a separate bowl, combine all the coating ingredients. Use your hands for easy mixing (but wear gloves if you have a fresh manicure).

4 Sprinkle the coating over the top of the salmon, making sure you have an even layer that covers all or most of the flesh.

5 Bake for 20 to 30 minutes or until the edges are browned and a knife inserted in the center reveals that the salmon is opaque and cooked through.

> *nail this*

You're looking for the salmon skin to bubble and the topping to crisp up, forming a deliciously buttery, flavorful crust.

If you're using (already salty) cracker crumbs, add only a pinch of salt to the coating. If you're using almond flour only, or in combo with breadcrumbs, increase the amount of salt to 1 teaspoon. Adjust to taste.

If your salmon is larger, make extra mustard and honey and double the coating if you need more.

>> *flip it*

Use gluten-free breadcrumbs instead of cracker crumbs, or use all almond flour. Crackers really add the best crisp, but these options will do if necessary.

Get a skinless fillet if you prefer to go "naked," or use precut salmon pieces instead of a whole side of fish.

Make salmon burgers with the leftovers. Crumble the salmon, and follow instructions for Tuna and Veggie Cakes (page 139).

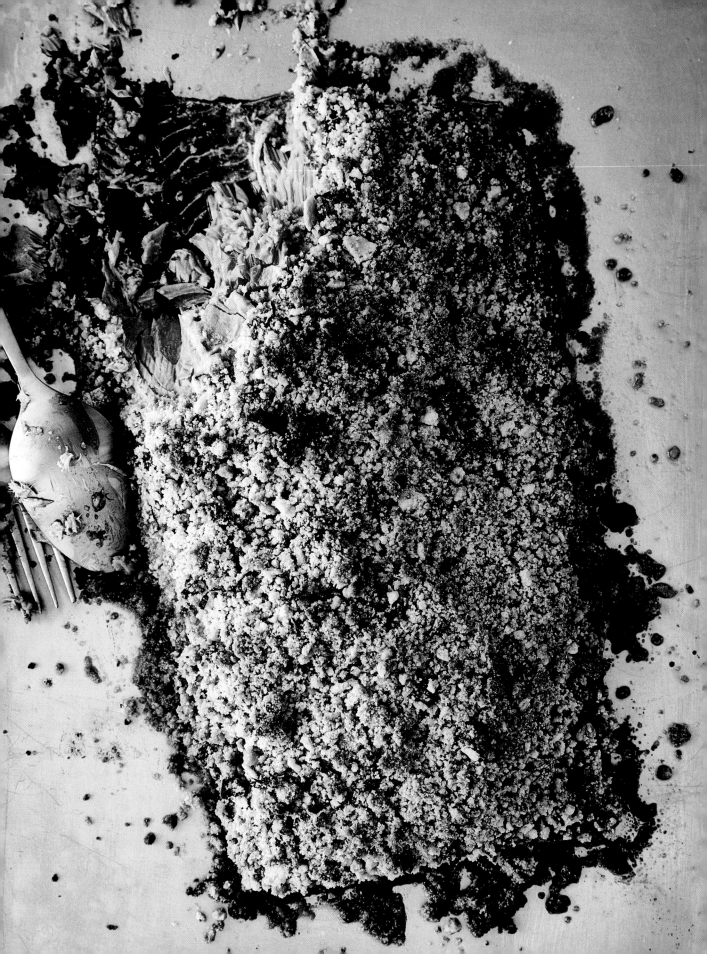

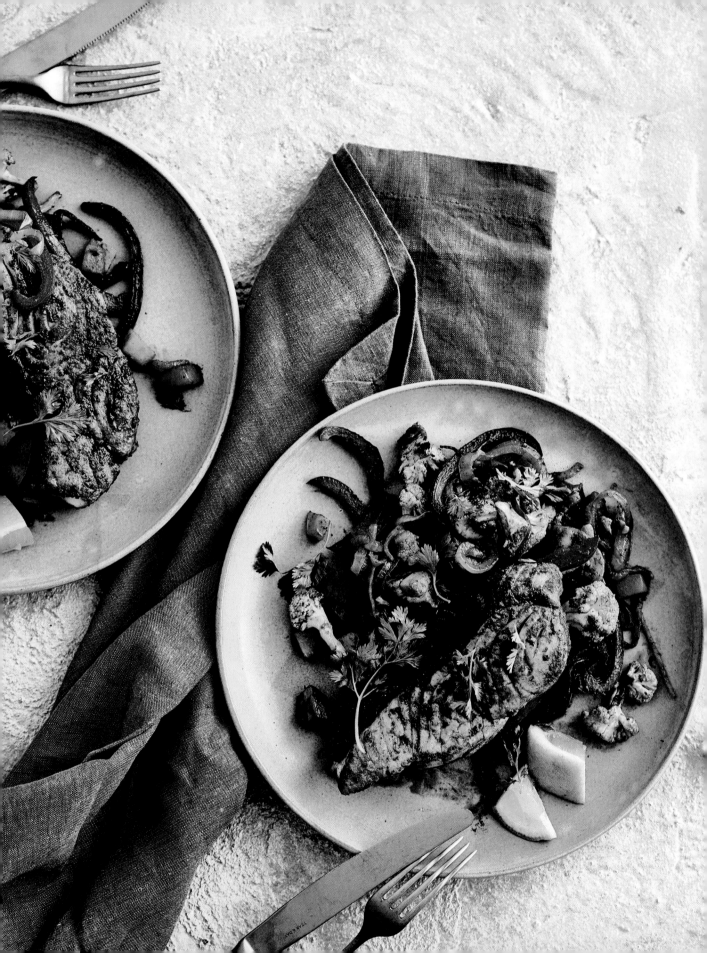

MELT-IN-YOUR-MOUTH MOROCCAN HALIBUT

STEPS: MIX, DREDGE, SAUTÉ, SERVE! / **Makes 8 servings**

Seth can always tell when I've cooked this fish because I smell like a Middle Eastern market afterward. It does—it really does—melt in your mouth, and the result is worth having to wear rags while cooking and shower later. The flavor combo is divine, and the ease of adapting this dish to serve picky eaters ("Spice? Yuck," says my five-year-old) or vegetarian diners makes this dish a flexible winner.

Tools: Large nonstick frying pan

SPICE RUB

3 teaspoons cumin

2 teaspoons turmeric

2 teaspoons paprika

2 teaspoons salt

1½ teaspoons ground coriander

1 teaspoon freshly ground black pepper

HALIBUT

8 6-ounce pieces halibut

Juice of 2 lemons, plus wedges, to serve

Salt and freshly ground black pepper

4 tablespoons olive oil

1 yellow onion, thinly sliced

2 cups quartered mushrooms (white button or your favorite)

2-inch piece fresh ginger, peeled and julienned

1 cup chopped pumpkin

2 cups small cauliflower florets

½ red bell pepper, cored and thinly sliced

½ green bell pepper, cored and thinly sliced

Fresh cilantro, for garnish

1 To make the spice rub: In a shallow bowl, combine all the ingredients for the rub. Set aside 2 teaspoons.

2 Sprinkle the fish with the lemon juice, salt, and pepper, and toss to coat. Dredge the fish in the spice mixture, using about 1 to 1½ teaspoons of mixture per fillet to lightly coat.

3 Warm a few tablespoons of oil in a large skillet over medium heat. Working in batches, pan sear the fish on both sides until almost cooked through, about 4 minutes total; the timing will depend on the thickness of the fillets. (Don't worry too much because you finish cooking it later.) Transfer the fish to a plate.

4 In the same skillet over medium heat, heat a bit more oil if needed. Cook the onion until translucent, about 5 minutes. Add the mushrooms and ginger and cook, stirring frequently, until the mushrooms release some juice, about 7 more minutes.

5 Stir in the reserved 2 teaspoons spice rub. Add the pumpkin and cauliflower and cook, stirring, until the pumpkin and cauliflower are almost fully cooked but still firm, about 7 minutes. Stir continuously to fry the vegetables uniformly and to avoid burning. Add the peppers and cook for an additional minute. Taste the veggies, and adjust the salt and pepper, if needed.

6 Arrange the halibut fillets on top of the almost-done vegetables. Continue to cook until the fish is cooked through, 5 to 8 minutes.

7 Serve with fresh cilantro leaves.

CONTINUED

> *nail this*

In any recipe that calls for a variety of vegetables, always start with the onions (if called for) and fragrant additions like ginger to layer your flavors. Next, add the veggies that require the longest cooking times, and finish with the faster-cooking ones.

If you are working with a small pan, cook in batches. You want the fish to rest in a single layer on a low pile of vegetables.

Warning: If your nails are painted, wear gloves, because turmeric stains!

>> *flip it*

Sea bass or cod makes a great substitution for the halibut. Salmon always works, too.

Use any colorful veggies you like. Consider carrots or pumpkin, toss in some fennel for flavor and crunch, or use zucchini or kohlrabi.

Oven method: If you want to make this dish in advance and reheat it later, cook the fish and vegetables as described above through step 5. Transfer the vegetables to a large casserole, and arrange the fish fillets on top. Finalize the cooking of the fish and vegetables together in the oven, uncovered, at 400°F.

For picky eaters, reserve the fish to grill separately with some butter and fresh herbs. For vegetarians, make the spiced vegetables only, and add some chickpeas or tofu. Or skip the veggies, and just pan-fry or grill the halibut for a simple Moroccan-spiced, blackened fish!

TUNA AND VEGGIE CAKES

STEPS: SAUTÉ, SEAR, BAKE! / **Makes 20 cakes**

Dinner doesn't get easier than this—just open a can of tuna and whip up the best tuna burgers, period. The key to this dish's success is using flavorful tuna packed in olive oil. The sneaky addition of sautéed vegetables guarantees flavor, moistness, and nutrition. Bonus: No breadcrumbs or carbs are involved here, just good, real ingredients. Truth: On some desperate nights, you might just ditch the burgers and serve a can of tuna with a salad.

4 tablespoons olive oil, divided

1 whole yellow onion, finely chopped

1 cup chopped button mushrooms

1 cup grated carrots

1 cup grated zucchini

2 garlic cloves, minced

4 5-ounce cans olive oil–packed tuna, drained

Salt and freshly ground black pepper

5 large eggs, beaten

2 teaspoons Dijon mustard

1 In a large skillet, heat 3 tablespoons olive oil over medium heat. Add the onions and cook, stirring, until translucent, about 5 minutes.

2 Add the mushrooms and cook until their juices are released, about 5 minutes.

3 Add the carrots, zucchini, and garlic, and cook, stirring frequently, until the veggies are crisp-tender and have released their juices, about 5 minutes more. Transfer the veggies to a bowl. Allow to cool.

4 Stir in the tuna. Season the mixture with salt and pepper. Stir in the eggs and mustard.

5 Preheat the oven to 350°F. Line a baking sheet with parchment paper, or oil it well.

6 Shape the tuna into 2½-inch patties (the mixture will be fairly wet), and arrange them on the prepared baking sheet.

7 Heat a large frying pan over medium heat with the remaining tablespoon of oil, and fry up your tuna cakes just to crisp, about 2 minutes on each side (they will finish cooking in the oven).

8 Transfer the cakes back to the baking sheet, and finish them in the oven until browned, cooked, and firm, about 10 to 15 minutes.

>> flip it

Don't need 20 burgers? Freeze any leftovers they reheat beautifully.

If you limit your tuna consumption due to its mercury levels, substitute canned salmon.

Use any combo of veggies that you wanna sneak in!

Skip the pan-fry part and place the patties directly in the oven. They won't have the same depth of flavor, but you will save time and mess.

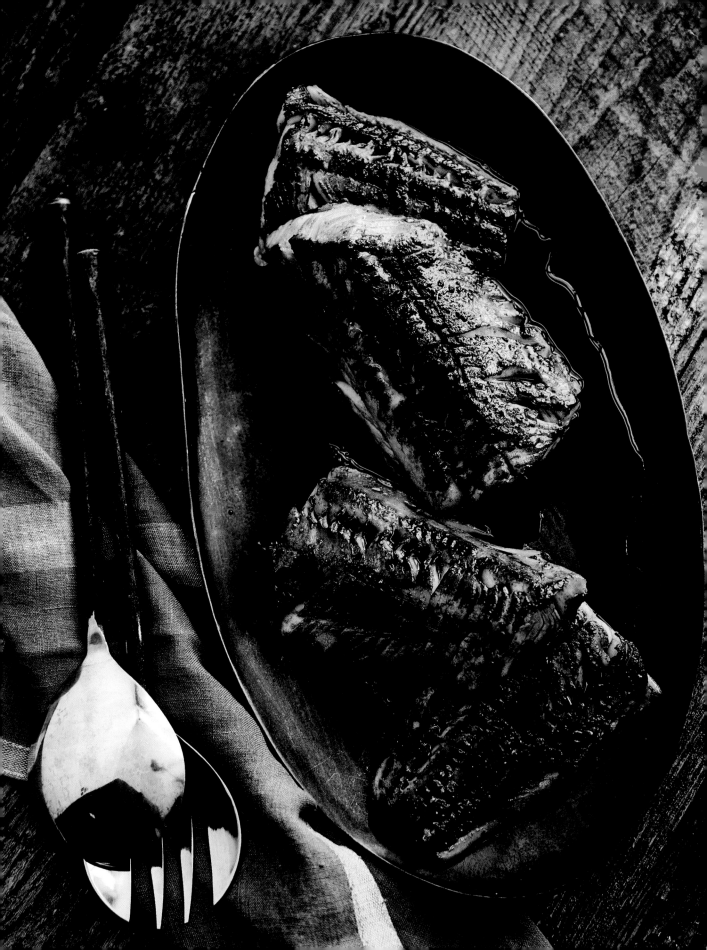

CRISPY MISO BLACK COD

STEPS: MARINATE, SAUTÉ, BROIL, SERVE! / **Makes 6 servings**

Chef and restaurateur Nobu Matsuhisa's iconic black cod is delectable, and versions of it are now served in Japanese restaurants around the world. In his original recipe, he cooks the sauce to evaporate the alcohol from the sake and then marinates the cod for three days. When I'm truly craving this dish, I never have the patience to cook, cool, and marinate. So I've devised a version that skimps on time but certainly not on taste. The result is a full-flavored, flaky, decadent cod that you'll find familiar and comforting—minus the kitchen time! Serve on a bed of smashed sweet potatoes or cauliflower rice, or with a scoop of rice and roasted broccoli.

MISO MARINADE

¾ cup dry sake

¼ cup plus 2 tablespoons white miso

¼ cup maple syrup

COD

2 tablespoons olive oil, or enough to coat the pan

6 6-ounce black cod fillets

1 In a large baking pan or bowl, mix the marinade ingredients. Marinate the cod in the sauce, covered in the refrigerator, for 24 to 48 hours— or as long as you have. The longer the better, but just a few hours is good enough in a pinch. Turn the fillets every few hours to make sure all sides are exposed to the marinade.

2 Preheat the broiler.

3 Heat the oil in a large sauté pan over medium-high heat. Remove the cod fillets from the marinade, and, working in batches if necessary (depending on the size of your pan), sear them until well browned, about 2 minutes on each side. (The fish won't be cooked through yet.)

4 Transfer the cod to a lightly oiled baking sheet (or keep it in the sauté pan if it is oven safe), and broil the fish until it is cooked through, 2 to 3 minutes on each side. (Test to see if the fish is fully cooked after flipping once.) When done, the fish flesh will be opaque and start to separate or flake, just slightly. Remove from the broiler and serve.

> *nail this*

Note that black cod is different from regular cod. It's actually sablefish and is very oily, much like salmon (which you can sub). If you can only find regular cod, don't flip it when it's in the oven; just let the broiler do its thing. Regular cod's lower oil content means it doesn't blacken as quickly; thus it has no problem cooking through without being turned.

» *flip it*

Vegetarian option: Choose a meaty-textured veg like mushrooms or eggplant, and skewer your veggies on a stick for a fun presentation.

Make-Ahead Recipes

RECIPES TO PREPARE AHEAD AND DEFROST FOR DINNER:

- Tuna and Veggie Cakes (page 139). Or salmon burgers.
- My Mom's Comforting Chicken Soup (page 74). Or use the base as stock for Asian Hot and Sour Soup (page 78).
- Velvety Carrot Soup (page 71).
- Thai Green Curry Chicken (page 143). Freeze leftover sauce to use as a base for fresh veggies and chicken.

- Simply Succulent Beef Stew (page 159).
- Sneakily Good-for-You Beef Burgers (page 160).
- Maple-Brined Turkey (page 155). These leftovers reheat well, so make a double batch.

FOUNDATIONS FOR EASY MEALS:

- Turkey gravy or Island-Style Chicken Adobo gravy (pages 155 and 149). Make extra, or freeze leftovers to jazz up rice, etc.
- Herbed Everyday Bread (page 62). Great to freeze in slices for morning toast and quick sandwiches.

- Muffins and quick breads (pages 41–65). Frozen individually, these quick breads live up to their name for breakfast, brunch, or snacking.
- Veggie-Full Marinara (page 282). Defrost for instant pasta, lasagna, or noodleless lasagna.

GREAT TO HAVE ON HAND:

- Quick Chicken Stock (page 75).
- Gluten-Free Cracker Crumbs (page 276).
- Ice Cube Infusions (page 266). For smoothies and drinks.
- Flexible Green Pesto (page 272) and Family Secret Red Spread (page 271). Freeze in cubes or small bags.
- Crispy Onions (page 269).
- Roasted nuts for making desserts or for snacks, such as Rosemary Party Nut Trail Mix (page 261).

- Chocolate Chip Cookies (page 233) or other cookies.
- Decadent Frozen Almond Brownie Pie (page 213).
- Pie crust (page 227).
- Riced cauliflower. Why buy it packaged? Process fresh cauliflower, freeze it, and have it on hand for a quick stir-fry with veggies and protein.

THAI GREEN CURRY CHICKEN

STEPS: BLEND, BROIL, SIMMER! / **Makes 10 servings**

Years ago, I took cooking classes at the Blue Elephant cooking school in Bangkok. The locals made their dishes look so simple, but I was timid about re-creating Thailand in my own kitchen. With the application of smart technique, quality ingredients, and a spoonful of confidence, it turns out that I can cook Thai, and so can you! It's all about the curry: The paste is the recipe's foundation. I love this curry so much I've even woken up with a craving and eaten it for breakfast after a long run. There's never a leftover, other than some sauce perhaps, which you should spoon over fresh steamed veggies to avoid wasting a drop.

Tools: Mortar and pestle or food processor, wok or big pot

CURRY PASTE

2 bunches cilantro (roots, stems, and leaves)

2 stalks lemongrass, tough outer leaves removed

4 to 5 mini spicy jalapeño peppers (the spiciest), or to taste

3-inch piece galangal (see note below)

2 shallots

3 garlic cloves

6 kaffir or makrut lime leaves

Juice and zest of 1 lime

1 teaspoon ground cumin

1 tablespoon coconut oil, if using blender

CHICKEN

8 boneless, skinless chicken thighs, cut into thirds

3 tablespoons curry paste

1 to 2 tablespoons olive oil

½ teaspoon salt

1 Make the curry paste: Place all the paste ingredients (except the coconut oil) in a mortar, and combine using a pestle. Alternatively, place all the paste ingredients in a food processor (with the coconut oil), and blend. If you prefer less spice, use fewer hot peppers.

2 Prep the chicken: Unless you already have cooked chicken (lucky you), mix 3 tablespoons of the prepared curry paste with the raw chicken thighs. Drizzle the chicken with olive oil, and season with salt. Broil the chicken on high for 7 minutes on each side, or until the thighs are cooked through (but not overcooked) and browned on the edges. Set the chicken aside.

3 Make the sauce: In a large saucepan over medium heat, warm 1 tablespoon olive oil and cook the shallots, stirring, until fragrant, about 2 minutes. Add 2 to 4 tablespoons of the curry paste (use less if you want a milder curry, and more if you like a moderately spicy curry; you can always add more later) and cook, stirring, until fragrant, about 2 more minutes. Add the coconut milk gradually, ½ can at a time, to allow it to absorb the flavors. Simmer for a few minutes.

4 Stir in the lemongrass, galangal, kaffir lime leaves, brown sugar, salt, and pepper. Bring to a boil, then lower the heat to a simmer. Taste for flavor in case you need more curry paste.

5 Add the baby eggplants, and cook until moderately softened, about 5 to 7 minutes.

6 Stir in the broccoli, chicken, and Thai basil, and cook until heated through. Finish by stirring in the coconut cream just before serving.

CONTINUED

CURRY

1 tablespoon olive oil

3 shallots, sliced

2 to 4 tablespoons curry paste, or to taste

2 13.5-ounce cans full-fat coconut milk

2 stalks lemongrass, tough outer leaves removed, smashed to release aroma

2-inch piece galangal, smashed to release aroma

4 kaffir or makrut lime leaves

1 tablespoon dark brown sugar

1 teaspoon salt

Pinch of freshly ground black pepper

10 baby eggplants, cut lengthwise in half (see note below)

2 cups broccoli florets

Handful of Thai basil leaves

Solids from 1 6.8-ounce chilled can coconut cream, to finish (optional)

› nail this

The secret is the combo of the curry paste and the coconut milk. Don't forget to taste the sauce to determine if it needs more curry paste or seasoning.

Newsflash: Thai basil is not the same as basil. If you can't find Thai basil, omit it.

Galangal root, found in Asian stores and many supermarkets' produce sections, is not the same as ginger. Could you use ginger? Sure. It will taste slightly different. If you're cool with that, I am.

Kaffir (aka makrut) lime leaves can be found in specialty Asian grocers, often in the freezer section. They impart a gorgeous fragrance to the curry so they are worth seeking out, but the dish will still be delicious without them.

» flip it

Swap tofu for chicken: Marinate sliced tofu in curry paste, salt, and olive oil. Oven-roast the marinated tofu until crispy and golden (see page 88 for tofu method). Or eliminate the chicken completely and just do a vegetable curry, adding carrots, cauliflower, and whatever else you love.

Adjust the spiciness by adding more or fewer jalapeño peppers. You can also reduce the spiciness by seeding the jalapeños before using.

Make the curry paste and chicken up to a day ahead. Assembly is then only 10 minutes.

Freeze the curry paste in ice cube trays to always have some on hand (page 266).

Swap any eggplant, peeled and chopped, for the baby eggplants, or substitute a different vegetable entirely.

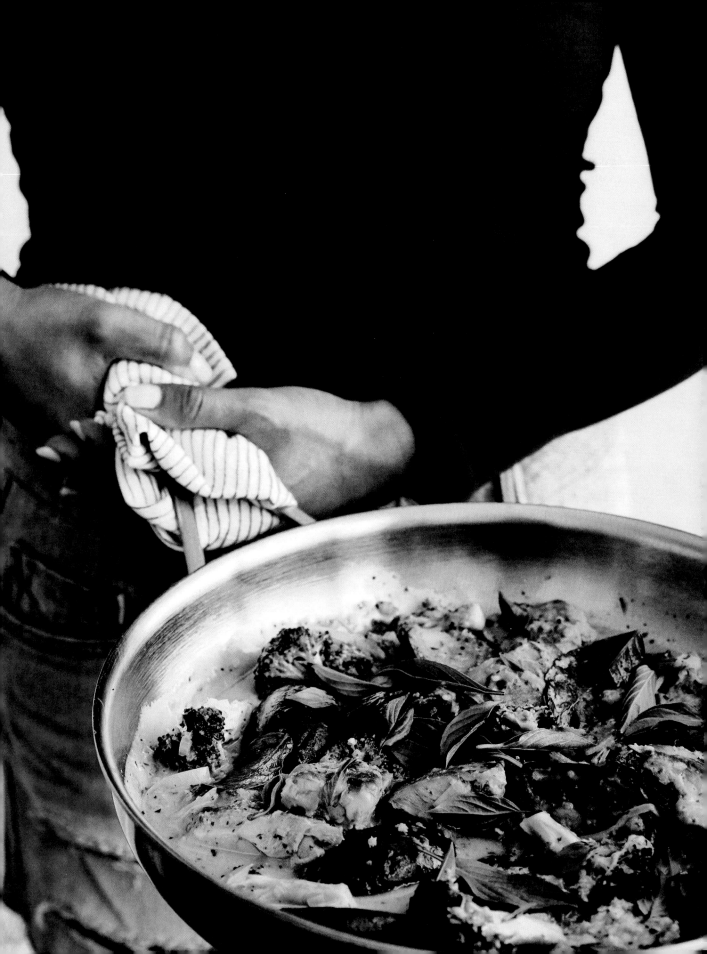

MIRACLE CHICKEN AND VEGETABLE STIR-FRY

STEPS: TOSS, BAKE! / **Makes 4 to 6 servings**

Some of the best recipes are born from a flop, a mishap, or a problem that you're forced to solve. Enter: Making a stir-fry without stir-frying at all. Say what? One day when we were craving Chinese comfort food, my stovetop broke down (great timing, huh?)—so I improvised. I baked this baby in about forty minutes, and it turned out better than Chinese takeout! Ditch the idea of standing at a wok and frying your next Chinese meal. This one-pan wonder makes prep and cleanup a breeze.

Tools: Rubber gloves (for mixing), large baking sheet(s)

CHICKEN

2½ pounds boneless, skinless chicken breast or thighs, cubed or cut in strips

2 tablespoons cornstarch

1 teaspoon salt

½ teaspoon freshly ground black pepper

SAUCE AND VEGETABLES

6 cups chopped assorted vegetables, such as broccoli, red bell pepper, mushrooms, and cauliflower

1 yellow onion, thinly sliced

½ cup unsalted chicken stock or water

⅓ cup olive oil

⅓ cup tamari

1 tablespoon plus 1½ teaspoons maple syrup

4 garlic cloves, minced

2-inch piece peeled fresh ginger, minced

2 teaspoons hot chile oil

1 Preheat the oven to 425°F.

2 Coat the chicken with cornstarch, salt, and pepper (either shake it in a Ziploc bag or toss it in a bowl). Set aside.

3 Spread the mixed vegetables and onion on a large sheet pan in a single layer. If they are piled too high, use two pans.

4 Toss the chicken stock, olive oil, tamari, maple syrup, garlic, ginger, and chile oil with the veggies (I like to do this with gloved hands to ensure even spreading).

5 Add the chicken to the pan, and gently toss it with the sauce, coating evenly.

6 Bake, uncovered, for 35 to 40 minutes or until the chicken is cooked through and the vegetables are tender and slightly browning on the edges. Check every now and again, and toss to ensure even cooking.

> **nail this**

If you want to use snow peas or other quick-cooking vegetables, toss them in for the last 10 minutes of cooking to ensure that they don't get overdone.

If broccoli wilts quickly, remove it and continue cooking the chicken.

>> **flip it**

Like it saucy? Double the sauce ingredients. This recipe can expand or shrink to fit your crowd.

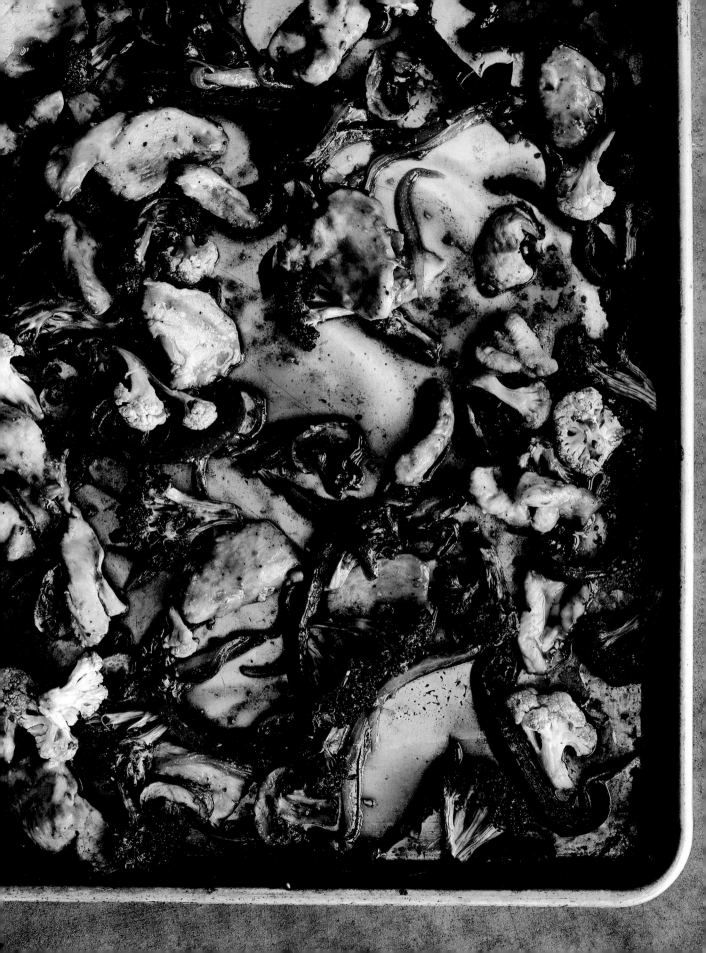

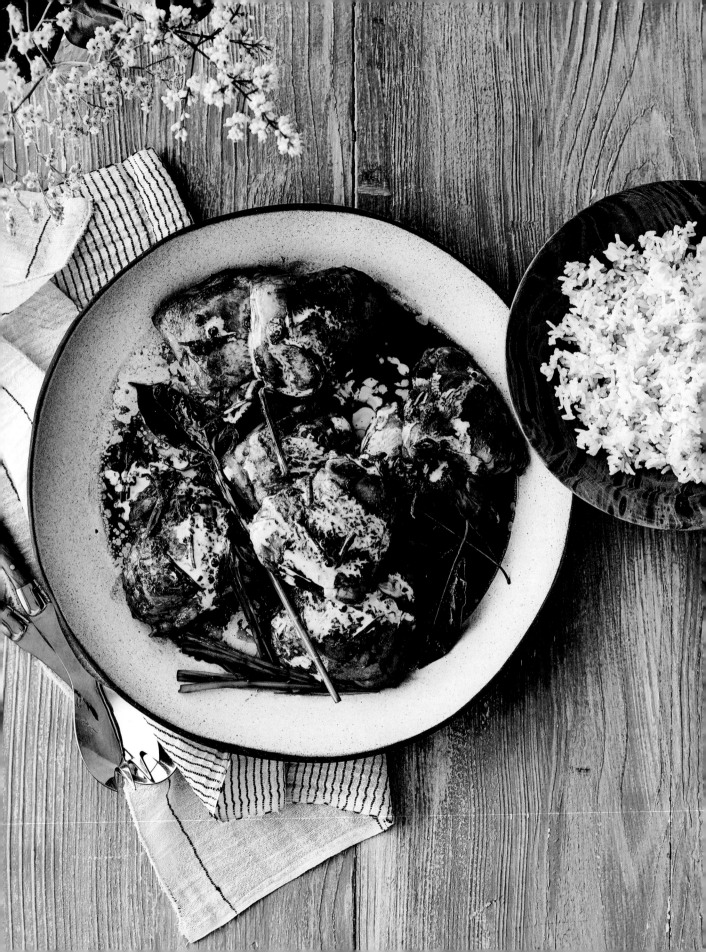

ISLAND-STYLE CHICKEN ADOBO

STEPS: MARINATE, BROWN, BRAISE! / *Makes 4 to 6 servings*

I've been making a home-style chicken adobo since I was young, and have refined it over the course of a decade while living in Asia. This popular Filipino dish is simple to make, it relies on inexpensive ingredients, and its lip-smacking sticky glaze sets it apart. On a recent trip to a resort in the Philippines, executive chef Erwin shared his mom's secrets for an adobo upgrade: Infuse the dish with ginger and lemongrass, then finish it with coconut milk. His island-style twist adds an unparalleled complexity and richness. Trust me, you'll be licking your plate once you're through.

Tools: Large skillet with cover

8 bone-in, skin-on chicken thighs

½ cup white vinegar

½ cup tamari or soy sauce

1 tablespoon olive oil

1½ to 2½ cups chicken stock or water, divided

3 stalks lemongrass, tough outer leaves removed

8 garlic cloves, crushed

2-inch slice fresh ginger, peeled and thinly sliced

4 bay leaves

1 teaspoon peppercorns or ground black pepper

½ cup full-fat coconut milk

Cooked rice, for serving (optional)

1 Place the chicken, vinegar, and tamari in a large Ziploc bag, and marinate in the refrigerator overnight, for at least 12 or up to 24 hours.

2 Remove the chicken from the marinade, reserving the marinade. In a large skillet over medium-high heat, heat the oil. Brown the chicken pieces on both sides, 4 to 6 minutes total.

3 Add the reserved marinade to the pan. Add about 1½ cups of stock, the lemongrass, garlic, ginger, bay leaves, and peppercorns. Bring the liquid to a boil, then lower the heat to a simmer and cover the pan.

4 After about 10 minutes, uncover the pan to allow the sauce to thicken. If the chicken looks cooked enough to be safe, taste the sauce. If it's way too salty, add more stock or water. Flip the chicken frequently to ensure an even coating of the sauce. If the sauce feels too thick, cover the pan to retain more juice; if it feels too thin, uncover the pan to reduce the sauce. Continue to simmer until the chicken is completely cooked, about 20 more minutes.

5 Remove the chicken from the pan, bring the sauce to a boil, and cook to reduce it until it's slightly thickened—this can happen really quickly or can take up to 10 minutes. Remove the lemongrass if you don't want to serve it, and finish by stirring in the coconut milk (use less than ½ cup if you prefer). Return the chicken to the pan.

6 Serve immediately, or set it aside and reheat it just before serving. Serve with rice, if desired.

CONTINUED

› nail this

Don't leave the dish alone. Keep turning the chicken and playing with the sauce, whether the pan is covered or uncovered, to get the right texture and taste. The secret lies in deglazing the pan to maximize the flavor.

Marinating the night before adds a ton of extra flavor, so it's best not to skip this step. But if you skip it you'll survive—with chicken that's just a tad less robust in flavor.

›› flip it

Slow-cooker method: Cook approximately 1 hour on high or 5 to 6 hours on low—or until the chicken is cooked through. Do not add more than 1 cup of broth or water. Transfer the sauce to a saucepan, and simmer until it's reduced, then strain. Pour the reduced sauce over the chicken and serve.

Use a whole chicken, cut up, or boneless thighs if that's what you have.

If you have leftover pan gravy from the chicken, a few tablespoons added to rice pilaf or Cauliflower Fried Rice (page 176) will kick their flavor up a notch.

Cut up leftover chicken for a stir-fry— or even better, use it in the Miracle Chicken and Vegetable Stir-Fry (page 146), adding some of the adobo sauce to the stir-fry gravy.

Cheats and Time-Savers

There are days when, frankly, I'd rather be doing something else than smelling like fried onions, and cooking is not at the top of my list. Alas, life demands we show up even when we don't feel like it. Sigh. Enter: The Cheats. Times like these call on us to be creative and sometimes cheat a little.

Recycle leftovers

Burgers can transform into a Bolognese sauce; noodleless lasagna can become a cheesy pasta sauce; turkey, chicken, or beef can get tossed into a stir-fry; and cauliflower rice (page 176) can get a makeover in pancake form.

Play up store-bought, ready-made foods

Buy rotisserie chicken and add it to spring rolls, a stir-fry, salads, and so much more. Buy hummus and tapenade or other ready-made dips for quick snacks. Or buy the main dish and cook up the sides and salads.

Buy veggies prewashed and chopped

There's an abundance of choice today in the ready-chopped produce department. But these items usually spoil faster, so only buy what you think you need. They also tend to be more expensive—just saying.

Take advantage of ready-made cookie dough

I love buying this stuff; even gluten-free versions can be found in the refrigerated section of the store. Roll the dough into cookies or bars, or press it into a pie crust.

Plan your menu for the week

Ironically, a menu takes time to prepare now but saves you time later. Consider planning leftovers into your weekly menu. For instance, if you're making succulent grilled chicken thighs and roasted potatoes, the next night you might plan a chicken stir-fry and potato pancakes. You'll save on grocery store trips too!

Double up and freeze

Double recipes and freeze the extra for later. See page 142 for a list of suggested recipes that freeze well, plus page 142 for more make-ahead and freeze ideas.

Boxed mixes: Cheat your way to a great muffin

You don't need to apologize for using boxed mixes. In fact, be proud and flexible! Don't just follow the directions on the back of the box, though. See page 00 for ideas.

UNFRIED CHICKEN SCHNITZEL

STEPS: MARINATE, COAT, BAKE! / **Makes 4 to 6 servings**

The kicker to this recipe is to marinate the chicken overnight in a honey mustard dressing. Instead of discarding the marinade, you savor it like gold and keep every last drop in the bottom of the pan while the chicken cooks. The crumbs melt into the mustard sauce, making this dish sing. Complexity can be overrated—many of the best simple recipes, like this one, are the most requested.

1 whole 4½-pound chicken, cut into 8 pieces

Tangy Mustard Vinaigrette (page 122)

3 cups cornflake crumbs (store-bought or crushed cereal)

Pinch of salt and freshly ground black pepper

1 Marinate the chicken in the vinaigrette directly in the baking dish, refrigerated, overnight or up to 24 hours. Alternatively, to save space in the fridge, marinate it in a Ziploc bag—but don't discard the marinade; you'll pour it into the pan with the chicken before roasting.

2 Preheat the oven to 400°F.

3 Season the cornflake crumbs with salt and pepper.

4 Place about 1 cup of the crumbs in a shallow bowl or plate. Coat the chicken pieces in the crumbs, then return them to the pan with the marinade. Replenish the crumbs as needed. Make sure each chicken piece is well covered.

5 Bake the chicken for 40 to 50 minutes. Start checking at the 35-minute mark: Prick the chicken to see if the juices run clear and it's cooked through.

6 This dish can be made a day in advance and reheated, uncovered, just before serving. If making in advance, underbake the chicken by a few minutes so that it remains moist after reheating the next day.

> *nail this*

Don't skimp on the flavor infusion achieved by marinating the chicken overnight.

You can either buy a box of Kellogg's cornflake crumbs or (what I usually do because I often can't find ready-made crumbs) crush a box of cornflakes in a food processor or by hand—just put them in a Ziploc bag and crush away. A rolling pin is a good tool for this task. This is a great way to involve your kids in meal prep. Don't forget to season the crumbs to taste.

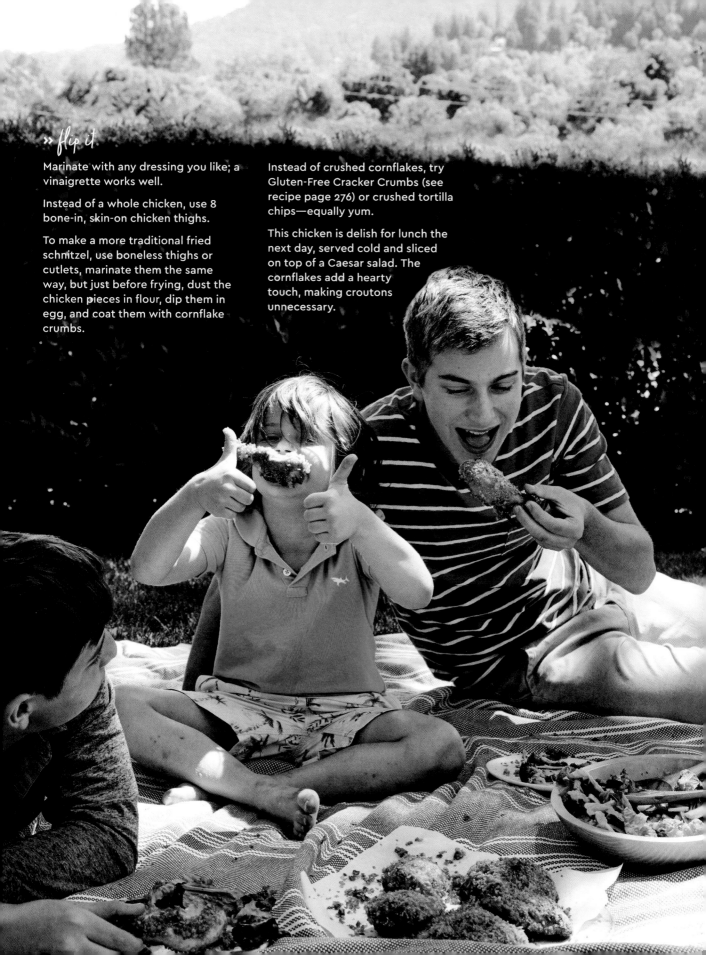

» flip it

Marinate with any dressing you like; a vinaigrette works well.

Instead of a whole chicken, use 8 bone-in, skin-on chicken thighs.

To make a more traditional fried schnitzel, use boneless thighs or cutlets, marinate them the same way, but just before frying, dust the chicken pieces in flour, dip them in egg, and coat them with cornflake crumbs.

Instead of crushed cornflakes, try Gluten-Free Cracker Crumbs (see recipe page 276) or crushed tortilla chips—equally yum.

This chicken is delish for lunch the next day, served cold and sliced on top of a Caesar salad. The cornflakes add a hearty touch, making croutons unnecessary.

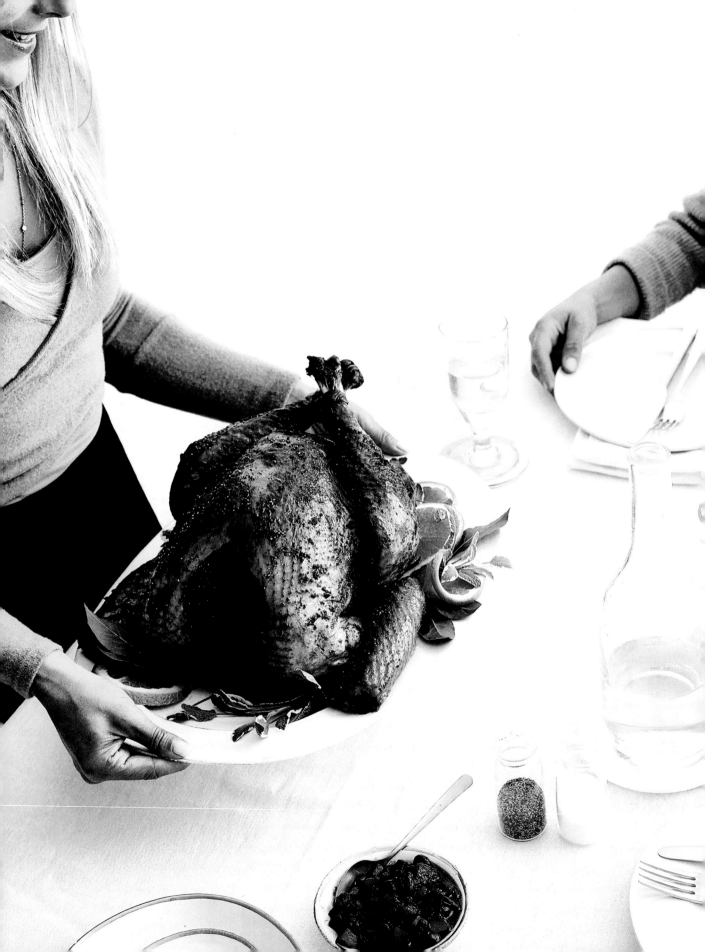

MAPLE-BRINED TURKEY WITH APPLE CRANBERRY SAUCE

STEPS: BRINE, RUB, ROAST, BASTE, SLICE! / **Serves 10**

Best. Turkey. Ever. Said every human who has tried it. (Even my labradoodle sneakily devoured a platter one day—don't ask.) Unlike many turkey recipes that easily dry out, this version just falls off the fork and melts into your mouth. Any dream turkey, however, doesn't just magically cook itself. It requires a great deal of attention, determination, and TLC. So, yes, you'll have to plan your movements around getting the turkey on the table, but once you've mastered the challenge, cooking this bird will get easier, and as with all challenges, you'll get better.

Tools: Large stockpot for brine, bag for brining (you can buy special turkey-brining bags, or use a clear garbage bag or a jumbo Ziploc), large roasting pan (or large disposable aluminum pan), meat thermometer

BRINE

1½ cups maple syrup

1 cup kosher salt

1 cup sugar

6 fresh sage leaves

4 fresh thyme sprigs

3 bay leaves

8 cloves

1 tablespoon allspice

1 teaspoon dried juniper berries, crushed

1 teaspoon black peppercorns, crushed

4 cups ice cubes

15½ pound turkey, giblets removed

1 In a large stockpot, prepare the brine by combining 8 cups of water with all the brine ingredients (except the ice cubes). Bring to a boil over high heat, and cook for about 3 minutes. Remove the pot from the heat, and add the ice cubes. Set aside to cool to room temperature.

2 Once the brine has cooled, transfer it to a large plastic bag. Add the turkey to the bag. Seal the bag, and refrigerate it for at least 2 days and up to 3 days.

3 Preheat the oven to 350°F.

4 In a small bowl, combine all the rub ingredients.

5 Remove the turkey from the brining liquid. Pat the skin dry, then coat it with the rub, applying it both under and on top of the skin.

6 Place the turkey in the roasting pan breast-side up, and stuff the cavity with onion, carrots, fresh thyme, and bay leaves. Pour ½ cup of the orange juice over the top.

7 One hour into cooking, baste the turkey with the remaining ½ cup orange juice and 1 cup white wine. Tent the turkey with aluminum foil if and when the skin starts to brown during roasting.

CONTINUED

TURKEY RUB

2 tablespoons olive oil

1 tablespoon paprika

1 tablespoon onion powder

1 teaspoon salt

1 teaspoon freshly ground black pepper

FOR ROASTING

1 whole onion, roughly chopped

2 carrots, roughly chopped

1 bunch fresh thyme

3 bay leaves

1 cup orange juice, divided

1 cup dry white wine, plus 1 cup for gravy (optional)

TO SERVE

Apple Cranberry Sauce (recipe follows)

8 Throughout the roasting process, baste the turkey about every 20 minutes. Test for doneness with an instant-read thermometer inserted into the center of the breast, making sure it does not touch bone. The turkey is done when it reaches 165°F in the center, but keep in mind the temperature will rise several degrees while it rests. Roast the turkey for roughly 15 minutes per pound for bone-in brined; I start checking the temperature after 2½ hours, to be super safe.

9 Remove the turkey from the oven, and transfer it to a serving platter. Rest the turkey, tented with foil, for 10 to 15 minutes before carving.

10 Make the gravy: If you have the time, reduce the turkey pan drippings, along with a second cup of wine, the onions, and the thyme (both retrieved from the cavity of the turkey), in a saucepan over medium-high heat until reduced by a third, about 20 minutes. Pour the reduced sauce over the sliced turkey. Serve with Apple Cranberry Sauce.

❯ nail this

Never leave your turkey alone. Once it goes in the oven, plan to stick around to baste, tent, and check. It's a labor of love!

Use a meat thermometer to get the turkey out at the right moment; otherwise it's a guessing game. You can carve the white meat and return the remaining dark pieces (whole, to preserve their juices) to the oven to fully cook, if need be. Or try using a remote-read thermometer with dual sensors so you can gauge the heat in two places at once without opening the oven—takes the guesswork away!

❯❯ flip it

To prepare a boneless turkey breast, simply adjust the roasting time to 30 or 45 minutes, or until it reaches 160°F, then let it rest before slicing.

Try brining a chicken! The brine imparts a flavor that's hard to replicate. Roast the bird with a spice rub and simple veggies, and it's a divine dinner anytime.

These turkey leftovers are to die for heated up in their gravy the next day, tossed into a quick stir-fry, sliced into Asian Hot and Sour Soup (page 78), diced as a protein topping for a lunch salad, or frozen for later.

Can't find fresh or frozen cranberries? Swap in 2 cans of whole cranberry sauce, use 3 apples, and omit the maple syrup. Proceed with the recipe, using a 10-minute-shorter cooking time.

CONTINUED

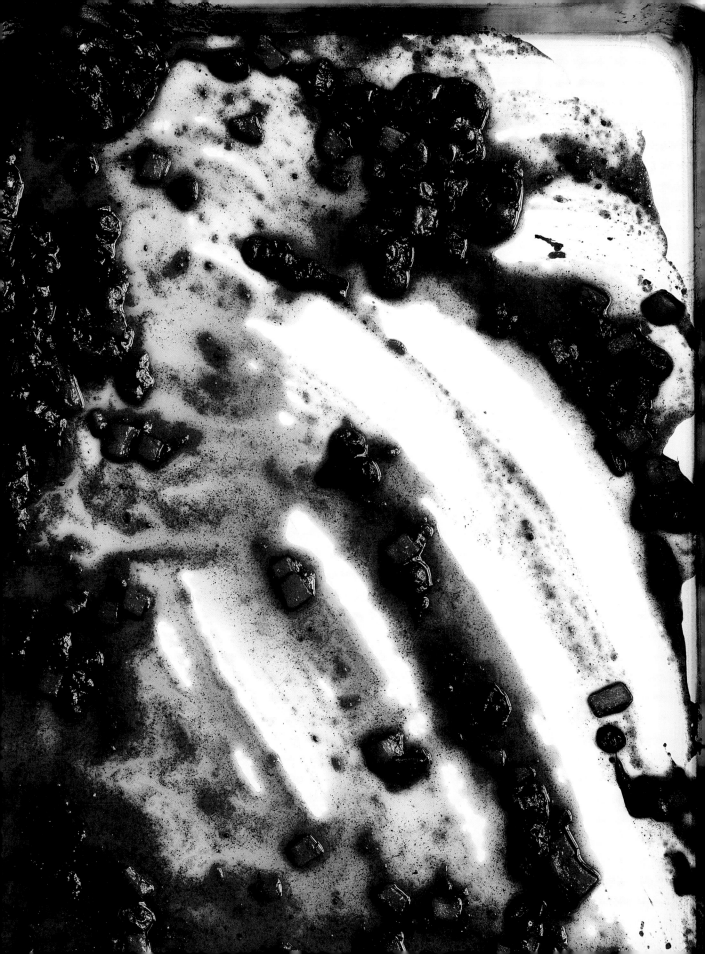

APPLE CRANBERRY SAUCE

Makes about 4 cups

4 cups fresh or frozen cranberries

2 cups peeled and diced Granny Smith apples (about 2 apples)

¾ cup maple syrup

1 teaspoon ground cinnamon

1 teaspoon vanilla extract

Pinch of salt

Zest of ½ orange (optional)

I love a good cranberry sauce, but not one that's loaded with sugar or cornstarch. I've added apples to balance out the texture here. This recipe is just so easy and fun to serve alongside turkey, or try it with chicken or brisket—or even with zucchini or potato latkes! I always make this a day ahead of serving, so when company comes it's one less thing to worry about.

1 In a medium saucepan over high heat, mix together ¾ cup water with the cranberries, apples, maple syrup, cinnamon, vanilla, and salt. Bring the mixture to a boil, then lower the heat to a simmer. Cook, uncovered, until the cranberries pop, 20 to 25 minutes. The cranberries will start to break apart, the apples will be cooked, and the mixture will be runny.

2 Stir in the orange zest. Set the pan aside, and allow the sauce to cool and thicken. Refrigerate it to chill (and to thicken some more) before serving.

SIMPLY SUCCULENT BEEF STEW

STEPS: BROWN, SAUTÉ, SIMMER! / **Makes 10 servings**

One-pot meals are hard to beat and almost impossible to flop. If you choose the right cut of beef, this slow-cooked, melt-in-your-mouth stew is a crowd pleaser. You could try this with osso buco, beef shank, beef ribs, short ribs, or another slow-cooking cut, and add whatever veggies you love. Serve it in bowls with some cauliflower rice or steamed rice.

Tools: Large Dutch oven (or see the slow-cooker flip)

2 to 3 tablespoons olive oil, divided

4 pounds beef shoulder, cut into 1- to 2-inch cubes

2 large yellow onions, chopped

5 garlic cloves, smashed

¼ cup soy sauce or tamari

3 bay leaves

1 teaspoon dried thyme

1 teaspoon paprika

½ teaspoon cayenne pepper

½ teaspoon coarsely ground black pepper

1 cup dry red wine

2 cups tomato sauce

1 cup pineapple juice

4 medium carrots, chopped

2 red bell peppers, cored and chopped

½ cup 1-inch-cubed pumpkin or any firm squash (such as kabocha)

Salt and freshly ground black pepper, to taste

1 Heat 2 tablespoons of the oil in a large Dutch oven or other pot over medium-high heat. Working in batches, add the beef, and cook until browned on all sides, about 4 minutes per batch. Remove the beef from the pot with a slotted spoon and set aside.

2 Add the onion and garlic to the pot, with a bit more oil if necessary, and cook them in the beef juices, stirring frequently, until lightly browned, about 8 minutes.

3 Return the beef to the pot and add the soy sauce, bay leaves, thyme, paprika, cayenne, and coarsely ground black pepper. Cook, stirring well, to allow the beef to absorb the flavors, for 1 minute. Add the wine, and bring to a boil. Boil until the alcohol evaporates, about 5 minutes.

4 Reduce the heat to low, and stir in the tomato sauce and pineapple juice. Cover and simmer until the beef is fork tender, about 2 hours.

5 Add the carrots, bell pepper, and pumpkin, and cook, covered, until soft, about 45 minutes. Season to taste with salt and pepper.

> *nail this*

Use high-quality beef!

Searing the beef and browning the onions and garlic add depth of flavor, so don't skip these steps.

» *flip it*

Slow-cooker option: Brown the beef and onions, then cook all the ingredients in the slow cooker for 1 hour on high and then 6 hours on low.

If you want a heartier dish, add cubed potatoes 15 minutes before the other vegetables. Or swap out any veggies with others that you love.

Add beef bones to intensify the flavor.

SNEAKILY GOOD-FOR-YOU BEEF BURGERS

STEPS: MIX, SHAPE, BROIL! / **Makes 8 burgers**

After transitioning from vegetarian to once-in-a-while carnivore, I realized I had to work a little harder to ensure sufficient veggie intake. Enter these sneaky beef burgers. The flavor boost from the veggies enhances the beef more than just nutritionally—they make the patties irresistibly tasty and moist. Dare I say these are the best burgers ever?

Tools: Food processor (optional)

1 tablespoon olive oil

1 cup finely chopped mixed vegetables (e.g., combo of garlic, mushrooms, carrot, zucchini)

2 pounds lean or grass-fed ground beef

½ medium yellow onion, grated or finely diced (use the food processor if you wish)

2 large eggs

2 teaspoons tamari or soy sauce

1 teaspoon sriracha sauce

1 teaspoon Dijon mustard

½ teaspoon salt

¼ teaspoon freshly ground black pepper

Oil spray, for pan or grill

Burger buns or lettuce leaves, Spicy Sriracha Mayo (page 277), sliced red onion, sliced tomatoes, and ketchup, for serving

1 Preheat an outdoor grill or indoor broiler.

2 Caramelize the vegetables: Heat the olive oil in a large skillet over medium heat. Add the chopped veggies, starting with the firmer ones first and adding the softer ones 5 or 6 minutes later. Cook, stirring frequently, until they are a rich brown in color and soft in texture, 10 to 15 minutes total. Allow to cool slightly.

3 In a large bowl mix the beef, vegetables, onion, eggs, tamari, sriracha, mustard, salt, and pepper.

4 Divide the mixture into 8 round patties, and flatten them just slightly.

5 Arrange the burgers on the grill grate or in a greased broiler pan, and cook until lightly browned on the first side, 7 to 9 minutes. Flip the patties and cook for 4 to 6 minutes more, or until cooked to medium (with a light pink center).

6 Serve, if desired, on buns or lettuce leaves, with Sriracha Mayo, red onion, tomatoes, and, yup, ketchup, if you like.

> nail this

If you make your burgers in the oven they will release a ton of yummy juice. Don't you dare dump that liquid gold. Drizzle it atop your burgers before serving, or reserve (even freeze) it for later, and stir it into rice or veggies.

The key to the moistness of these burgers is the sautéed vegetables. Don't be tempted to eliminate them!

>> flip it

Bake your veggies at 350°F instead of sautéing them: Toss them with olive oil and salt, spread them on a baking sheet, and slide them into a preheated oven until they're cooked and lightly brown, 15 to 20 minutes. Pop them in the food processor, or finely chop before adding.

Leftovers? Chop up a burger for your lunch salad.

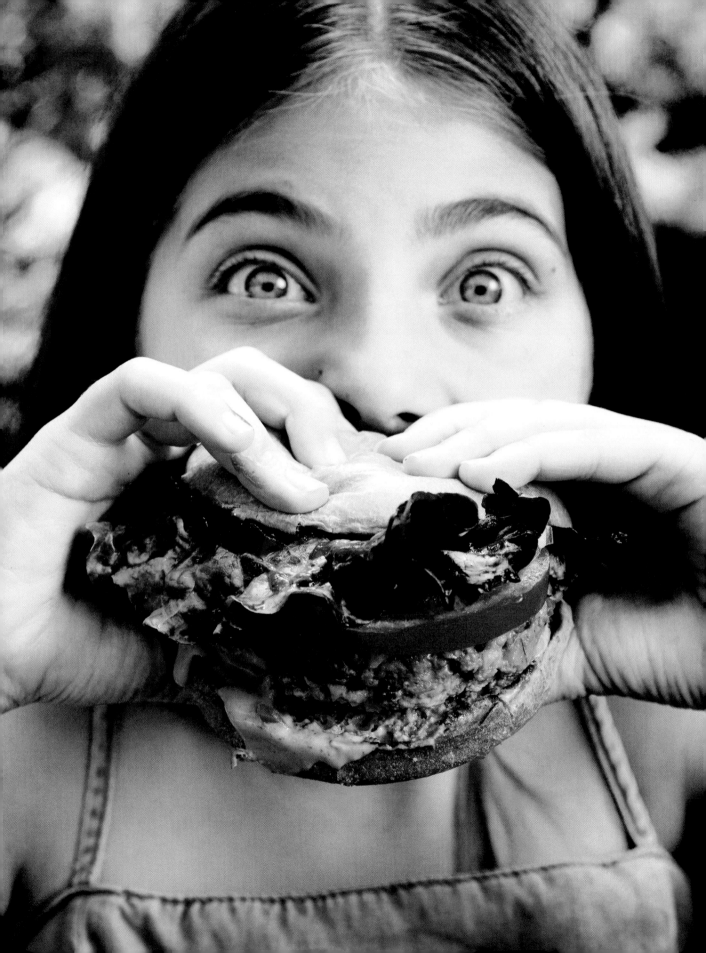

KNOCK-YOUR-SOCKS-OFF CHILI

STEPS: SEAR, SAUTÉ, BRAISE! / **Makes 6 to 8 servings**

This chili represents winter comfort food at its best. I used to include red kidney beans. Although it tasted good, it didn't agree with any of our stomachs (enough said). This one is bean-free (but if you have an iron stomach, get liberal with your beans). My kids love the addition of corn, which is, of course, totally optional. I make this overnight in a slow cooker, but you can certainly cook it on the stovetop if you prefer. Don't skip the step of browning your beef first, which keeps it flavorful. Play around with the spice and the heat to suit your diners' tastes—the chipotles are spicy!

Tools: Slow cooker

4½ pounds short ribs (or chuck or round), cut into 1- to 2-inch cubes

2 tablespoons olive oil

1 large or two small yellow onions, chopped

3 tomatoes, finely chopped

3 carrots, cut into 1-inch chunks

2 stalks celery, cut into 1-inch chunks

1 small red bell pepper, cored and chopped into 1-inch chunks

1 small green bell pepper, cored and chopped into 1-inch chunks

1 14.5-ounce can diced tomatoes with juice

1 6-ounce can tomato paste

1 3.5-ounce can chipotles in adobo sauce, chopped (or use less according to your heat preference)

½ whole head of garlic, outer peel removed but head kept whole

1 Pat the beef dry so it won't splatter in the oil. Heat the olive oil in a large skillet over medium-high heat, and, working in batches, brown the meat on all sides, approximately 4 minutes per batch. Transfer the beef to the slow cooker. Add the onions to the skillet and cook them, stirring, until translucent, about 4 minutes. Transfer the onions and all the pan juices to the slow cooker.

2 Add all the remaining ingredients except the corn to the slow cooker.

3 Cook for 2 hours on high, then reduce the heat to low and cook for 5 hours more. Or if you want to cook it overnight or before you leave home for the day, cook on high for 1 hour, then on low for an additional 8 hours.

4 About 1 hour before serving, once the beef has cooked through but before the chili is ready, check the seasoning and adjust the salt and pepper. About 30 minutes before serving, add the corn, if using.

5 To serve, spoon the chili into bowls. Serve alongside avocado, lime wedges, and tortillas. Garnish with cilantro or parsley.

CONTINUED

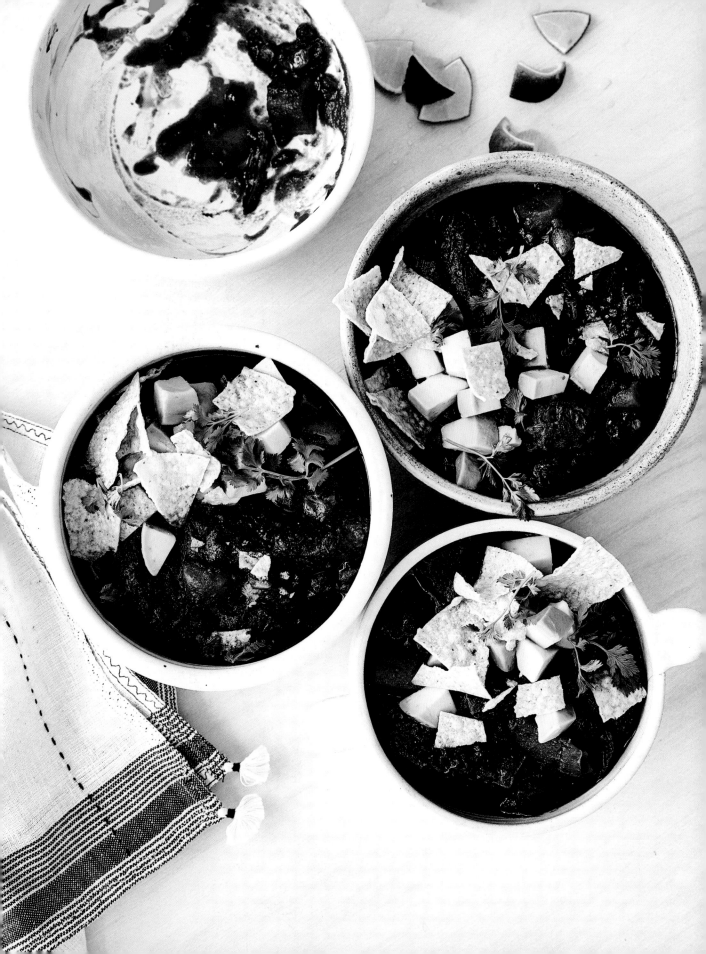

2 tablespoons dark
brown sugar

1 tablespoon plus
1½ teaspoons cumin

1 tablespoon chili powder

2½ teaspoons salt

2 teaspoons freshly
ground black pepper

½ 14-ounce bag (about
1½ cups) frozen corn
(optional)

TO SERVE

Peeled and diced
avocado

Fresh lime wedges

Corn tortillas or
tortilla chips

Fresh cilantro or parsley
leaves

› nail this

Add a few turkey necks or beef bones
for flavor before you turn the slow
cooker on.

Plan ahead—make this in the morning
for dinnertime, or cook overnight
for the next day. To speed up the
cooking, keep the slow cooker on
high for longer. To cook it for longer,
keep the setting at low.

The garlic infuses this chili with great
flavor, but remove the intact head
before serving.

» flip it

Stovetop method: Follow the
instructions through step 3, but
simmer in a medium-sized pot or
Dutch oven for approximately 3 hours
over medium-low heat, or until the
beef is soft.

If your fresh tomatoes are off-season
or mealy, omit them and use a
24-ounce can of tomatoes in place of
the fresh tomatoes (and in addition to
the 14.5-ounce can). Likewise, if corn
is in season, use fresh kernels.

Chipotle chiles add a distinct,
smoky, and delicious flavor. If you
can't find them, the dish will still
be delectable—just add heat in
another form (e.g., red pepper flakes,
chopped spicy fresh red peppers,
jalapeños).

Repurpose leftovers into tacos; serve
with chopped tomato, avocado, and
cilantro.

SARAH'S MELTAWAY BRISKET

STEPS: SEAR, SOFTEN, SIMMER, SLICE! / **Makes 10 to 12 servings, depending on the size of the brisket**

I wasn't your typical Jewish mom, mostly because for years I couldn't cook a killer brisket. My friend Sarah's brisket (which I later discovered was pioneered by noted NYC culinary bookstore owner Nach Waxman) melts in your mouth, as brisket should. She slices the brisket midway through the cooking process. I was initially mortified upon hearing this. It breaks all brisket rules! All the juices will run out! But it works, I promise. Sarah and I worked and reworked this recipe so many times that I had enough test briskets in my freezer to feed my family for a year (thankfully, brisket freezes beautifully). In the end, I officially feel like a good Jewish mother serving this—aside from the bourbon, which I snuck in to kick the sauce (and the cooking experience) up a notch.

Note: Brisket cook time is over 4 hours.

Tools: Large, deep skillet or frying pan with cover (big enough to fit brisket), tongs

SAUCE

¾ cup BBQ sauce

¼ cup bourbon

3 tablespoons soy sauce

3 tablespoons hoisin sauce

3 tablespoons dark brown sugar

1 tablespoon Dijon mustard

4 garlic cloves, pressed

2 teaspoons paprika

1½ teaspoons cumin

½ teaspoon salt

¼ teaspoon freshly ground black pepper

¼ teaspoon cayenne (optional)

1 Make the sauce (this step can be done in advance): Whisk together all of the sauce ingredients. Set aside.

2 Sear the brisket: Season the beef with salt and pepper. In a large, deep skillet that is big enough for your brisket to lie flat, warm the oil over high heat. Sear the meat on all sides just until lightly browned, about 1 to 2 minutes on each side. This helps prevent the meat from drying out while it cooks for several hours. Remove the brisket from the heat, and transfer it to a separate pan or large plate to rest while you cook the veggies.

3 Add the onions to the skillet (pouring in a touch more oil if necessary), and cook over medium heat until fragrant and softened, about 5 minutes. Stir in the mushrooms and garlic.

4 Return the meat to the skillet, fat side up, and pour the prepared sauce over the brisket. Move the onions and sauce around so that both surround the meat on all sides. Bring the mixture to a boil; add the carrots. Reduce the heat to a gentle simmer and cook, covered, on the stovetop until the brisket is fork tender, 3 to 3½ hours.

5 Using tongs, transfer the brisket to a cutting board. Allow it to cool enough to slice. Cutting against the grain of the meat, slice the brisket into long, very thin (⅛-inch-thick) slices.

CONTINUED

BRISKET AND VEGETABLES

1 6- to 7-pound brisket, first cut (also called the flat), trimmed, with a ¼-inch-thick layer of fat remaining

1 teaspoon salt

1 teaspoon freshly ground black pepper

¼ cup olive oil

2 large yellow onions, finely chopped

3 cups sliced mushrooms

4 garlic cloves, smashed

3 carrots, peeled and sliced into 1-inch chunks

6 Return the sliced brisket to the skillet and gently simmer, covered, until further softened, 30 minutes or longer. Keep testing the meat, as the cook time will vary. Cook as long as it needs to soften.

7 Remove the pan from the heat, and allow the meat to cool. If you plan to serve it later, transfer it to a heatproof baking dish, pour the sauce and vegetables on top, refrigerate, and reheat before serving.

› nail this

Check your flame and ensure that it's at the correct, low level, so that the brisket is simmering but not bubbling—but also make sure the flame isn't so low that it will blow out (this has happened to me!).

Choose the right brisket to ensure softness. Get your meat from a reputable butcher, and avoid very lean cuts (they don't melt in your mouth).

Leftovers are even better (the longer the brisket sits the tastier it gets), but I usually freeze or discard it after 3 days in the fridge.

»› flip it

Oven option: Bake at 350°F for the same cook time. Once you've seared the meat and cooked the onions, arrange it all in an ovenproof dish. Keep tightly covered. Removing and slicing is more of a hassle, so just cook for 3 hours and then slice, and let it sit as long as possible in the gravy.

Got tough meat? Heat the slices and sauce in a pot, simmering more aggressively; don't panic, it will eventually become tender.

Adjust the size of your brisket depending on the crowd you're feeding; for a main course, consider ½ pound per person.

Use the sauce for chicken wings and chicken marinade!

Use your favorite BBQ sauce. If hoisin isn't available, substitute more BBQ sauce.

Make the same recipe using short ribs or beef stew meat.

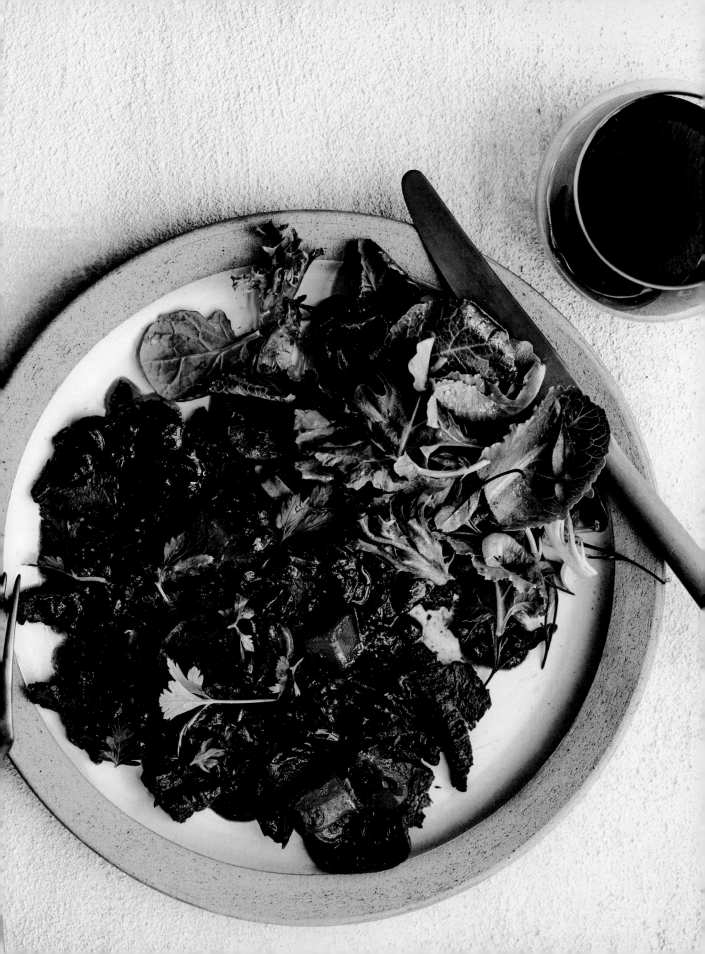

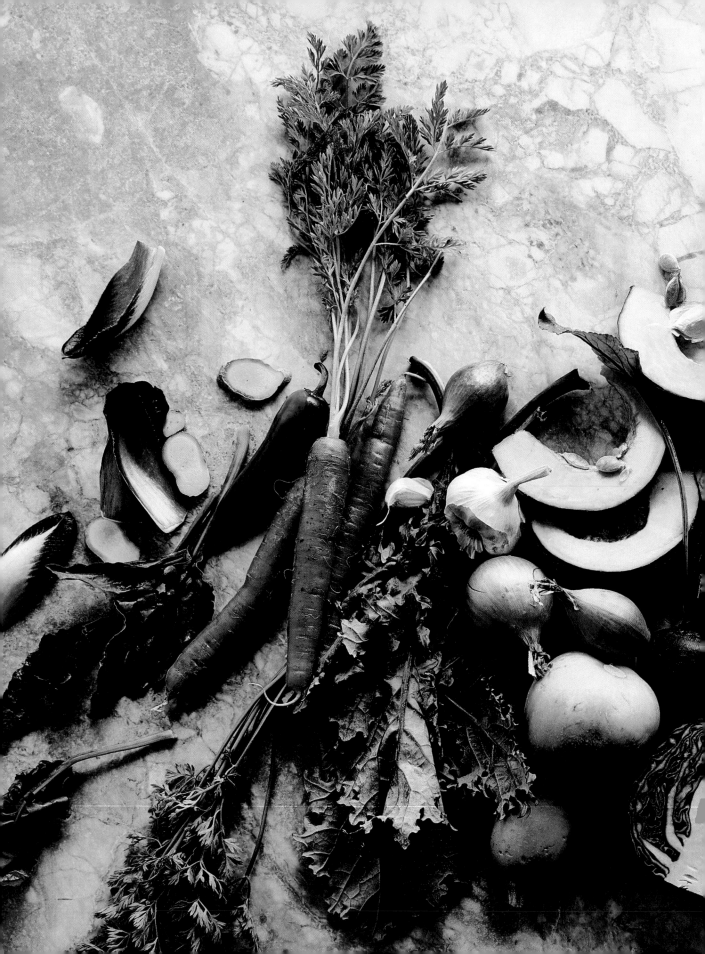

Chapter 7

VEGGIES ANYTIME

Side dishes are like a really great friend—supportive but never invasive. They shouldn't steal the show, only enhance it! In this chapter, the spotlight's on vegetables. You'll discover how to broil, sauté, and bake fresh ingredients so they have maximum flavor and flair. Learn to whip up other grain-free favorites, like Cauliflower Fried Rice (yum!) (page 176) and Sheet-Pan Tofu Medley (page 183) with mushrooms and onions. Enhance the recipes in this chapter to act as vegetarian main courses, and mix and match them with your meal plans.

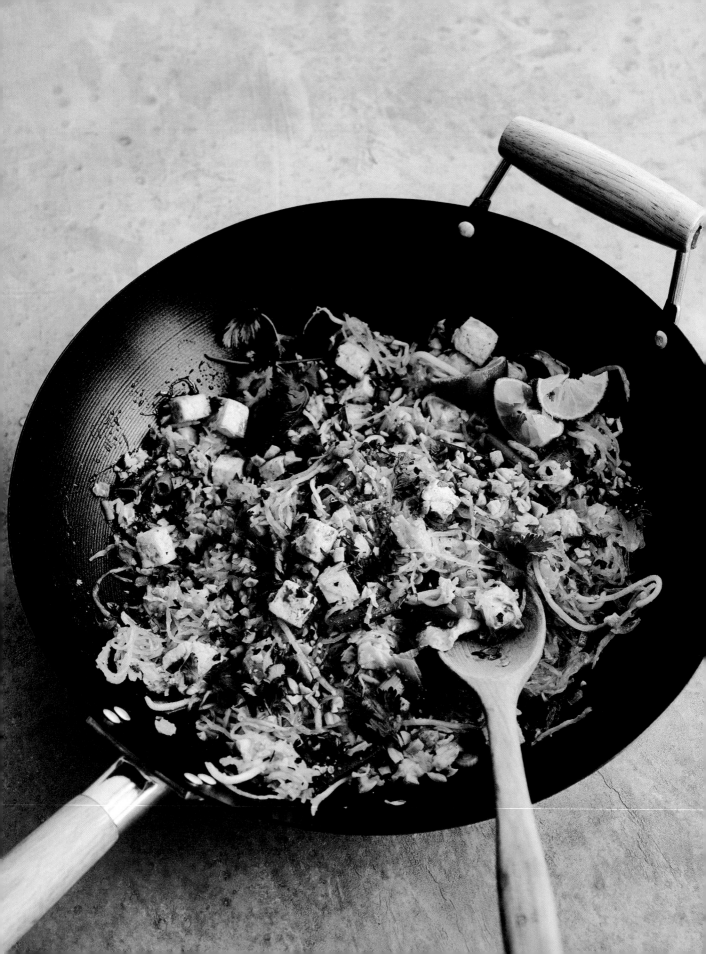

SPAGHETTI SQUASH PAD THAI

STEPS: BAKE, SAUTÉ, STIR-FRY! / **Makes 4 servings**

When I was pregnant with my oldest son seventeen years ago, I had an insatiable lust for spaghetti squash (so random). I searched every market in NYC, called every local farmer, and finally found a provider. This dish is my ode to the spaghetti squash. Plus, this healthified take on a classic Thai dish tastes almost identical to the carb-filled rice noodle version minus the belly bloat you get after a bowlful of noodles. Not interested in going on my pregnant-woman wild-goose chase for squash? Check out the zucchini noodle flip, which is equally irresistible and faster; use it in a pinch.

Tools: Wok

PAD THAI

8 ounces firm tofu, cut into ½-inch cubes

3 tablespoons peanut oil or olive oil, divided

¼ teaspoon salt

¼ teaspoon freshly ground black pepper

1 medium (3-pound) spaghetti squash

1 cup chopped yellow onion

4 large eggs, beaten

4 garlic cloves, minced

8 scallions, greens cut into 1-inch pieces, whites chopped

2 cups mung bean sprouts

PAD THAI SAUCE

2 tablespoons rice vinegar

2 tablespoons fish sauce

2 tablespoons dark brown sugar or raw honey

½ teaspoon salt

¼ teaspoon freshly ground black pepper

1 Preheat the oven to 400°F. Grease 2 large baking sheets.

2 Arrange the tofu on a prepared baking sheet, and season it generously with a tablespoon of oil, salt, and pepper. Set aside.

3 Slice the squash lengthwise in half; use a sharp knife and use caution, as the squash is hard to cut through. Place the halves flesh-side down on a prepared baking sheet.

4 Slide the tofu and the squash in the oven. Remove the tofu after 20 minutes, or when it is firm, crispy, and lightly browned on the edges. Set aside. Bake the squash for 10 to 15 minutes more, for a total cook time of 30 to 35 minutes, or until it is tender and separates into strands. Do not overbake or it will be mushy. Remove the seeds from the center. (Seeds are way easier to remove once the squash is cooked rather than attempting it raw.)

5 Whisk all the sauce ingredients together in a small bowl with 2 tablespoons of water. Set aside.

6 Heat the remaining 2 tablespoons of oil in a large wok over medium heat. Add the onion and cook, stirring frequently, until softened, about 5 minutes.

7 While the onion is cooking, scramble the eggs in a separate small frying pan coated with oil over medium heat until cooked, about 4 minutes. Set aside.

CONTINUED

TO FINISH

1 cup chopped fresh cilantro leaves

¼ cup chopped roasted, salted peanuts

3 teaspoons hot chile oil

1 lime, sliced into wedges

Red pepper flakes, to garnish

8 Raise the heat to medium-high. Add the cooked tofu, spaghetti squash, and garlic to the wok with the onions, stirring to combine. Stir in the sauce, and cook until incorporated, 2 to 3 minutes. Stir in the cooked eggs, scallions, and bean sprouts, just to heat through. This whole cooking process should take only minutes on a medium-high flame. Taste and season with salt and pepper.

9 To serve, garnish with cilantro, peanuts, and drizzles of chile oil and lime juice. Sprinkle with red pepper flakes for more spice, if you like. Arrange lime wedges on the side. Eat immediately!

› nail this

Prep and measure all of your ingredients before beginning, as you will need to move quickly once everything is in the wok to avoid overcooking the squash.

›› flip it

Use zucchini noodles: Spiralize 3 to 4 zucchini, enough to make 4 cups. Squeeze out excess water with a cheesecloth before adding them in step 8. This is vital or it will be mushy—trust me, I made it without squeezing, and it turned into pad thai soup!

TANDOORI-SPIKED VEGETABLE SKEWERS

STEPS: PARBOIL, MARINATE, ROAST! / **Makes 10 skewers**

I'm in love with skewered anything, especially when spiced with this flavorful and luscious Indian-inspired tandoori marinade. While traditional Indian marinades usually call for yogurt, you can easily swap in coconut cream as a dairy-free alternative. Set aside time to soak your skewers and marinate the veggies; the rest gets assembled in minutes. Here, I use cauliflower and broccoli with red bell peppers and onions, but skewer whatever you love.

Tools: 10 bamboo skewers (about 9 inches long, but any will do), sheet pan

MARINADE

½ cup plain yogurt or coconut cream

5 garlic cloves, minced

5 tablespoons olive oil

1 tablespoon chickpea or rice flour

1 tablespoon lemon juice

1 tablespoon minced fresh ginger

½ teaspoon paprika

½ teaspoon turmeric powder

½ teaspoon cumin

½ teaspoon coriander powder

½ teaspoon salt

¼ teaspoon cardamom

¼ teaspoon freshly ground black pepper

1 Soak the bamboo skewers in water for 1 hour to prevent them from burning in the oven. Grease a large sheet pan and set aside. Bring several inches of water to a boil in a medium pot for blanching vegetables.

2 Make the marinade: In a large bowl, mix together all the marinade ingredients. Set aside.

3 Plunge the broccoli and cauliflower florets into the boiling water for 60 seconds. They should only be parboiled and still hard.

4 Drain the vegetables in a colander, then immediately rinse them under very cold water to stop the cooking—or plunge them into a bowl of ice and water. Pat the vegetables dry, and add them to the bowl with the marinade (or in a Ziploc bag). Using gloved hands, massage the marinade into the veggies. Chill them in the refrigerator for 1 hour.

5 Preheat the oven to 400°F.

6 Thread the pieces of broccoli, cauliflower, pepper, and onion onto skewers, and arrange them on the greased sheet pan.

7 Bake the skewers until lightly browned on the first side, about 15 minutes, then flip and cook until the edges are browned and the vegetables' centers are cooked through, about 10 more minutes.

CONTINUED

VEGETABLES

1 medium head broccoli, cut into florets

1 medium head cauliflower, cut into florets

1 small red onion, cut into 4 wedges, layers separated

1 large red bell pepper, cut into wedges

Oil spray, for greasing pan

› nail this

You must soak the skewers in advance or they will burn. For added insurance, wrap the exposed bamboo sticks in foil to avoid charring the wood.

» flip it

For something quicker, you could grill the skewered vegetables without the tandoori marinade. Season with oil, salt, and pepper.

Skip the skewers, and bake the veggies with the tandoori sauce on a large baking sheet until crisp. Same timing applies.

Make this a full vegetarian meal by adding other vegetables to the skewers, such as white button mushrooms, cherry tomatoes, or eggplant, or proteins like tofu, paneer, or haloumi cheese.

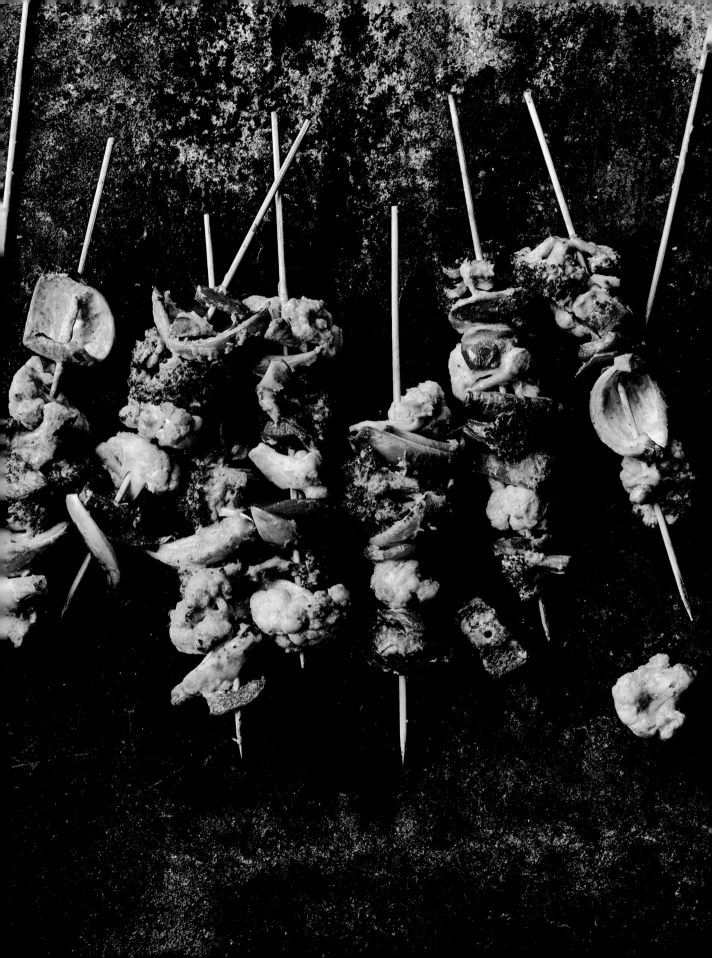

CAULIFLOWER FRIED RICE

STEPS: CHOP, SAUTÉ, SEASON, DEVOUR! / **Makes 6 servings**

Traditional fried rice has become a staple in our home in Hong Kong. But some days call for a lighter, grainless alternative that delivers that same taste-of-Asia succulent party in your mouth. This dish looks like rice and tastes just like fried rice, but it's nothing more than spiced-up vegetables. Simply toss your cauliflower into a food processor, and stir-fry the rice-like crumbles with a few veggies and spices. Mix in some soy sauce and a fried egg to complete the Chinese flavor. Make more than you think you need because leftovers are never wasted. You'll feel healthier just cooking this.

Tools: Large wok or heavy frying pan, food processor (optional)

¼ cup olive oil

1 medium yellow onion, finely chopped

2 large heads cauliflower

1 large or 2 small carrots, diced

1 cup chopped white button mushrooms

2 garlic cloves, chopped

½ cup frozen green peas

Kernels from 1 small ear fresh corn, or ½ cup frozen corn

Salt and freshly ground black pepper

2 large eggs, beaten

1 tablespoon tamari or soy sauce (or to taste)

Sriracha sauce, to taste

2 tablespoons chicken or beef gravy, if on hand (optional)

1 In a wok or frying pan over medium heat, heat the oil. Sauté the onions for 8 to 10 minutes, or until golden. Check on the onions often to make sure they don't burn.

2 While the onions are cooking, cut each cauliflower into 4 chunks, and pulse, in batches if necessary, in the food processor until crumbly, but not mushy; don't overprocess. If necessary, chop by hand to achieve rice-sized crumbs. Set aside.

3 Add the carrots, mushrooms, and garlic to the browned onions, and cook over medium-high heat, stirring frequently, to caramelize the vegetables and allow the mushrooms to release their juices, about 10 minutes.

4 Stir in the cauliflower, then add the peas and corn. Cook, stirring constantly, for 6 to 8 minutes, or until the cauliflower is al dente. Season with salt and pepper and set aside.

5 In a separate, lightly oiled, nonstick frying pan over medium heat, cook the egg into a thin omelet, until set, about 2 minutes. (Or, to save some cleaning time, cook the egg in the same wok the veggies are in; just move them aside.)

6 On a cutting board, thinly slice the omelet, and add it to the veggies.

7 Season the cauliflower rice with tamari and sriracha (and stir in the gravy, if desired), and serve.

> nail this

Allow the veggies to caramelize long enough to accumulate flavor. Properly browned onions, carrots, and mushrooms serve as the base of the dish's flavor.

You do not want mushy or watery "rice." Working quickly at high heat in a large wok helps to crisp the cauliflower's edges and absorb the water.

Flavor injection is a real bonus: To nail an even better dish, use leftover gravy from the Island-Style Chicken Adobo (page 149) or Simply Succulent Beef Stew (page 159).

>> flip it

The corn and peas are added for color and texture. If you're avoiding starches, just eliminate them. Add other vegetables into the mix, like broccoli, kale, or diced red bell pepper. Swap the white mushrooms for shiitake.

Still craving rice? Add about 1 cup of cooked rice to the dish, and you'll get the best of both worlds.

Change it up! Omit the soy sauce and egg, and use the base to make rice pilaf or Mexican rice.

Leftovers? Add a few heaping tablespoons to your morning omelet. Or add a beaten egg or two, and turn the combo into sautéed cauliflower-rice pancakes. Those are good!

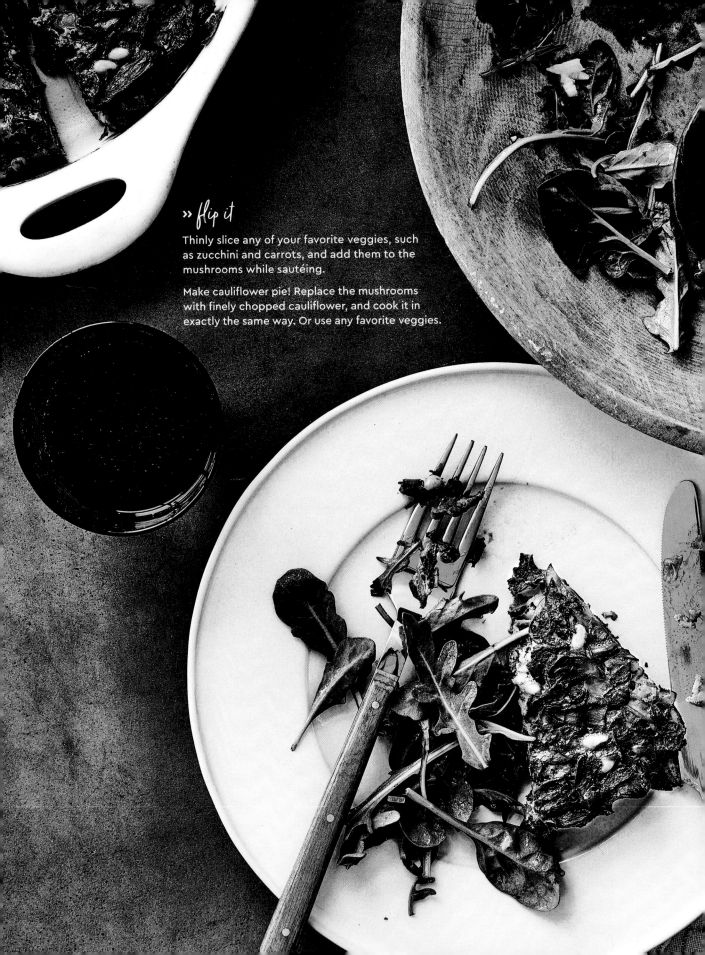

›› *flip it*

Thinly slice any of your favorite veggies, such as zucchini and carrots, and add them to the mushrooms while sautéing.

Make cauliflower pie! Replace the mushrooms with finely chopped cauliflower, and cook it in exactly the same way. Or use any favorite veggies.

CRUSTLESS MUSHROOM PIE

STEPS: SAUTÉ, MIX, BAKE! / **Makes 8 servings**

The other day I had a friend over for dinner who was watching her weight. When I offered her a slice of mushroom pie she politely declined. When she discovered that this pie was made of nothing more than mushrooms and eggs, she leapt out of her seat—and later asked for seconds. Meanwhile, my fourteen-year-old, who's on an all-you-can-eat diet, asked for thirds. Serve this crowd pleaser as a dinner side dish or a main course with a salad for lunch, and save some leftovers for breakfast.

Tools: 10-inch round glass or ceramic pie dish, or 11 × 7-inch baking dish

¼ cup plus 2 tablespoons olive oil, divided

2 medium yellow onions, finely chopped

8 cups thinly sliced white mushrooms (about 20 ounces)

6 heaping cups thinly sliced brown mushrooms (about 20 ounces)

1 cup julienned spinach

4 garlic cloves, minced

1 teaspoon salt, or to taste

½ teaspoon freshly ground black pepper, or to taste

4 large eggs, beaten

¼ cup pine nuts

2 cups shredded cheese, your favorite

1 Heat ¼ cup oil in a large skillet over medium heat. Add the onions and cook, stirring, until translucent, for about 5 minutes.

2 Add the mushrooms and cook until the juices are released, about 8 minutes.

3 Add the spinach, garlic, salt, and pepper and cook, stirring, until the mushrooms are cooked through, and the water is reduced to almost none, about 15 to 20 more minutes. Taste to adjust the seasoning. Cool the mushrooms completely, about 5 minutes, before continuing to the next step, to avoid having the eggs cook in the hot mushroom mixture.

4 While the mushrooms are cooling, preheat the oven to 350°F.

5 Add the eggs to the cooled mushroom mixture; stir in the pine nuts. Season again with salt and pepper, if desired, and cheese, if using.

6 Grease your pan with the remaining 2 tablespoons oil. Now here comes the trick to the best pie ever: Pop your oiled pan into the preheated oven until the oil is very hot, roughly 10 minutes. Be careful not to allow it to burn.

7 Remove the pan from the oven, and pour the mushroom mixture into the hot, oiled pan. This will create a sizzle effect, perfectly browning the outer edges of your pie.

8 Bake until the eggs are set, about 45 minutes. Slice and serve.

> nail this

The secret to this dish's awesomeness is preheating an oiled pan, so when the mushrooms go in, they sizzle and create the crispiest crust. Test whether your pan is hot enough by dropping a mushroom or flicking some water in it. It must sizzle.

NOODLELESS LASAGNA

STEPS: SLICE, LAYER, BAKE! / **Makes enough for 6 to 8 hungry people**

One bite of this lasagna and you'll wonder why lasagna has noodles to begin with. Zucchini strip "noodles" are layered with marinara sauce and cheese to produce drooly, cheesy, guiltless, deep-dish comfort food. I make this in a large baking pan, and it lasts for a few days. I even chop up the leftovers to make a pasta sauce and serve it on top of gluten-free spaghetti—and my family is tricked into a whole new dinner. *Shhhhh.*

Tools: 13 × 9-inch lasagna pan, mandolin (optional)

5 large zucchini (about 3½ pounds total)

1 teaspoon salt, plus more for seasoning

1 pound shredded mozzarella cheese

1 batch Veggie-Full Marinara (page 282)

¼ cup Parmesan cheese

1 Make the zucchini layers: Using a mandolin or a sharp chef's knife, slice the zucchini lengthwise into ⅛-inch-thick strips. Sprinkle the strips with salt and lay them on paper towels, with two more layers of towels on top to absorb the moisture they expel. Let them sit for 30 minutes, pressing down on the towels occasionally to squeeze out excess moisture.

2 Preheat the oven to 350°F.

3 Assemble: Line the bottom of the lasagna pan with a single layer of zucchini strips, overlapping the edges for complete coverage.

4 Top the zucchini with a thin layer of mozzarella cheese (about ¼ of the total mozzarella) followed by a layer of the marinara.

5 Repeat the layers—zucchini noodles, cheese, and then sauce—to make a total of 3 complete layers.

6 Top the final layer of marinara sauce with the remaining mozzarella and the Parmesan.

7 Bake, uncovered, for 40 minutes, or until the lasagna bubbles. During the last 10 minutes of cooking raise the oven temperature to 400°F to brown the cheese. Serve. Keeps for 2 days in the fridge.

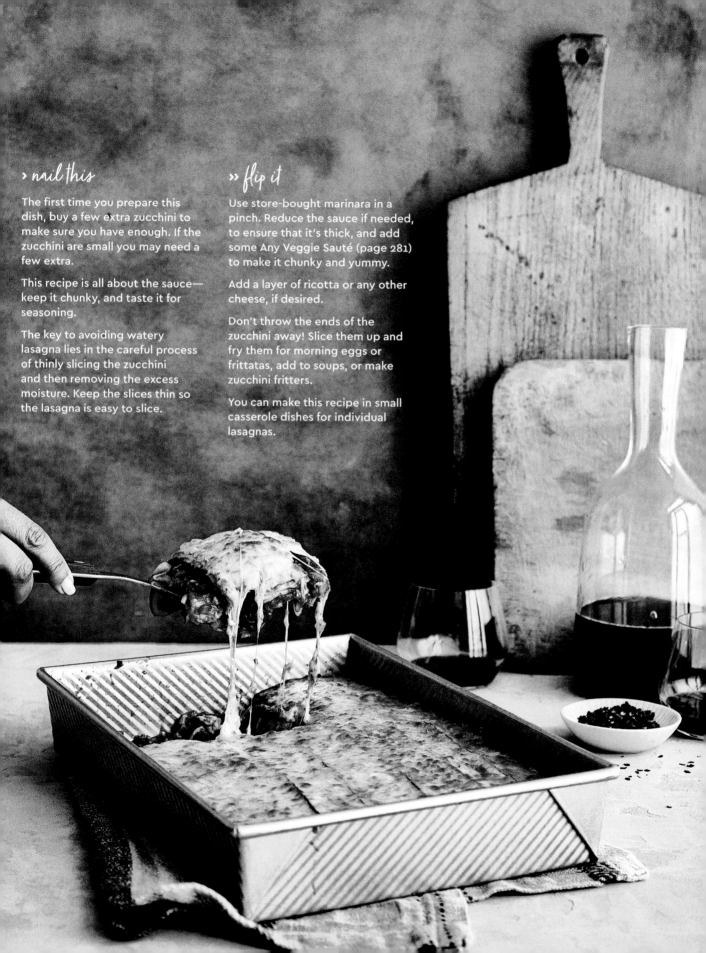

› nail this

The first time you prepare this dish, buy a few extra zucchini to make sure you have enough. If the zucchini are small you may need a few extra.

This recipe is all about the sauce—keep it chunky, and taste it for seasoning.

The key to avoiding watery lasagna lies in the careful process of thinly slicing the zucchini and then removing the excess moisture. Keep the slices thin so the lasagna is easy to slice.

›› flip it

Use store-bought marinara in a pinch. Reduce the sauce if needed, to ensure that it's thick, and add some Any Veggie Sauté (page 281) to make it chunky and yummy.

Add a layer of ricotta or any other cheese, if desired.

Don't throw the ends of the zucchini away! Slice them up and fry them for morning eggs or frittatas, add to soups, or make zucchini fritters.

You can make this recipe in small casserole dishes for individual lasagnas.

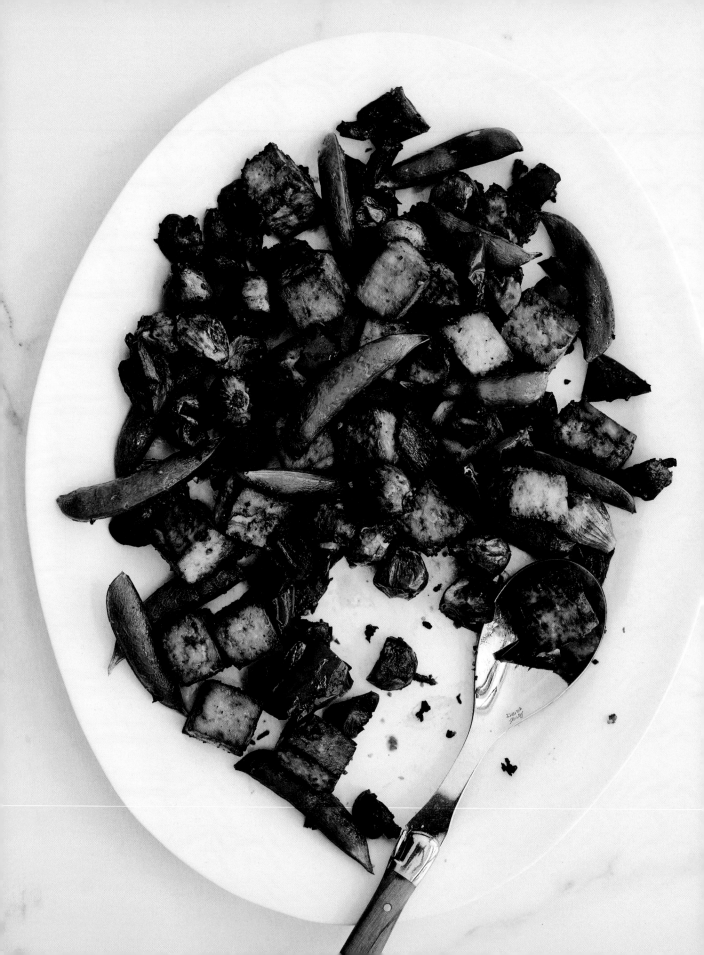

SHEET-PAN TOFU MEDLEY

STEPS: MARINATE, BAKE! / Makes 4 to 6 servings

I kid you not, this tofu might convert all you non–tofu eaters into tofu cravers. Tofu takes on the flavor of the marinade, and when you crisp the bites in the oven they caramelize on the corners and taste divine. Serve this one-pan meal with simple steamed rice, or roast the tofu on its own and serve it as a protein topper to salads. Or use it as a meat substitute in Thai Green Curry Chicken (page 143) or Make-Your-Own Beef Wraps (page 83). Experiment away.

2 8-ounce blocks of firm organic tofu, cut into 1-inch cubes

¼ cup tamari or soy sauce

¼ cup olive oil

2 tablespoons minced fresh ginger

3 garlic cloves, minced

1 tablespoon plus 1½ teaspoons maple syrup

1 teaspoon rice vinegar

½ teaspoon freshly ground black pepper

3 cups quartered white mushrooms

1 red bell pepper, cored and sliced in chunks

1 cup pearl onions, trimmed and outer skins left on

1 cup whole sugar snap peas

1 Spread the tofu on a greased baking sheet. Add the tamari or soy sauce, oil, ginger, garlic, maple syrup, vinegar, and black pepper, and toss to coat.

2 Marinate the tofu for at least 1 or up to 4 hours.

3 Preheat the oven to 425°F.

4 Add the mushrooms, red bell pepper, and onions to the tofu, and toss to combine. Put the baking sheet in the oven.

5 After 30 minutes, add the sugar snap peas. Bake for 10 to 15 minutes more, for a total cook time of 40 to 45 minutes, checking and flipping often to ensure even browning of the tofu and vegetables. Remove when the tofu and mushrooms are golden-brown and crispy.

> nail this

If you don't have the time to marinate, just omit that step. The flavor will be less intense, but your time will be spared.

» flip it

Roast tofu with any of your favorite veggies, such as cauliflower and broccoli instead of mushrooms and peppers. You can also swap thinly sliced red onion or shallots for the pearl onions.

Toss this into my Glass-Noodle Stir-Fry (page 184) or Oven-Roasted Secret Broccoli (page 195) to make it a main dish!

Want your tofu extra crispy? Follow the crispy-tofu instructions on page 88, in the Vietnamese Veggie Spring Rolls. Hint: Cornstarch is the secret.

GLASS-NOODLE STIR-FRY

STEPS: SOAK, FRY, SOFTEN, SERVE! / **Makes 8 servings**

This satisfying comfort food is always a big hit. Glass or cellophane noodles, often made from mung bean or sweet potato starch, are a totally underused, lighter noodle alternative. You can usually find them in the Asian aisle of the grocery store, but don't go on a wild-goose chase if you can't. If you must, use thin rice vermicelli noodles instead. This kid-friendly recipe is packed with hidden veggies that make it a winning family dish.

Tools: Wok or large frying pan

1 8.8-ounce package glass (cellophane) noodles

5 tablespoons olive oil

6 shallots, sliced (about 1 cup)

4-inch piece fresh ginger, peeled and sliced thin

1 head green cabbage, shredded

4 carrots, julienned

2 cups sliced mushrooms

4 garlic cloves, minced

4 cups diced choy sum or bok choy

2 tablespoons plus 1½ teaspoons tamari or gluten-free soy sauce

1 tablespoon maple syrup

1½ teaspoons chile oil (or red pepper flakes, to taste)

A few small red chiles, thinly sliced (optional)

Salt and freshly ground black pepper, to taste

Cilantro leaves and thinly sliced green onion, to garnish

1 Submerge the glass noodles in a bowl of warm water until soft, about 10 minutes. Drain and set aside.

2 Meanwhile, heat the olive oil in a wok over high heat. Cook the shallots, stirring frequently, until soft, about 3 minutes. Add the ginger and cook until fragrant, about 2 minutes. Add the cabbage, carrots, mushrooms, and garlic. Lower the heat to medium and cook, uncovered, until the vegetables are very soft, about 15 minutes. Every few minutes, check on them and stir.

3 Raise the heat to high, add the choy sum, and cook for a few more minutes to sweat the veggies. Stir in the drained noodles, and season with tamari, maple syrup, chile oil, and red chiles, if desired. Season with salt and pepper to taste. Remove from the heat immediately.

4 Serve the noodles garnished with cilantro and green onion.

> nail this

To avoid soggy noodles, always add them last, with the seasoning. And don't oversoak them; they will soften a bit more when you add them to the pan.

The noodles sometimes stick together. Grab your kitchen scissors and cut the noodles in half if they clump after cooking.

>> flip it

Add cooked beef or chicken to the final cooked meal. Or toss in my Sheet-Pan Tofu (page 183) for extra texture and flavor.

At some stage, give yourself the freedom to eyeball and experiment—to just throw your veggies in without measuring. Add any leftover veggies you have in the fridge; make sure you cook them long enough to caramelize them and build flavor.

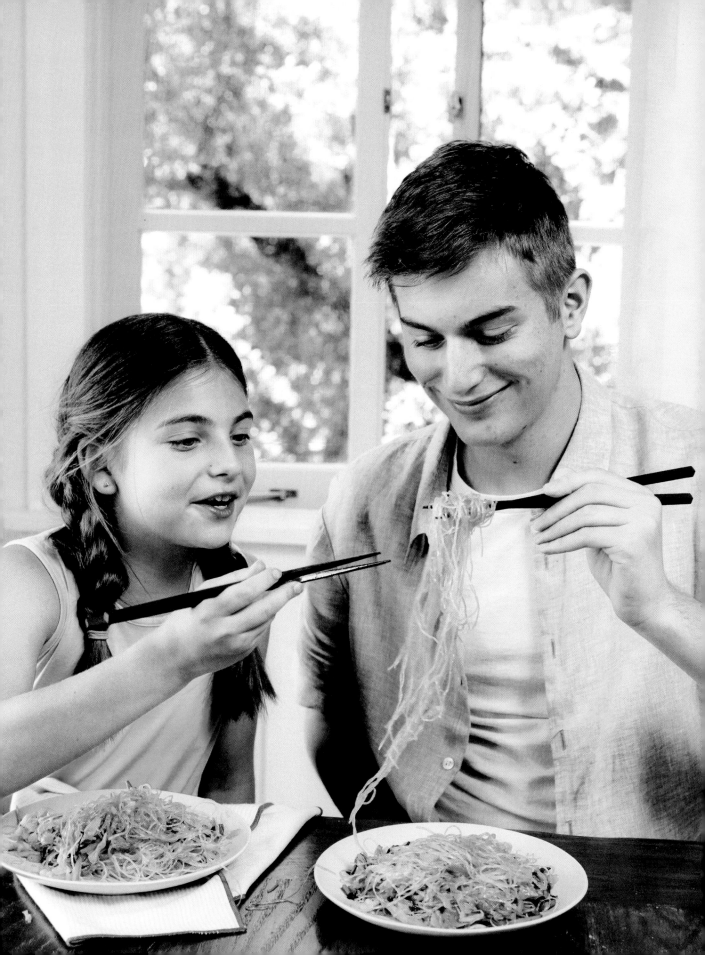

Help! Your Survival Guide for Picky Eaters

We all know one. The kid or the friend who just won't touch this or that, making meal planning a potential nightmare. I've been there.

MODEL

People will model how you behave more than they will follow what you tell them to do. Persistence, dedication, and modeling will encourage children to adopt good habits. Even if you aren't a parent, your friends might start to have what you're having when they see how good you look and feel.

STARVE THEM!

Yep, you read that right. Make sure the picky diners are actually hungry when they sit down to eat. This means no snacking after a certain time, which is a rule at our house. Put out the salad first—they'll be more inclined to fill their plates in order to fill their tummies. If I'm serving oven fries for dinner with burgers and a salad, I always serve the meat and salad first and bring the fries out once they've eaten some.

START THEM EARLY

I was never prepared to raise kids who only ate "kid" food. Start kids early on real foods, and you'll train their palates. After all, kids in China eat stir-fries, and kids in India eat curries!

HIDE OR ELIMINATE THE JUNK

Years ago, I helped my kids' school make their lunch buffet healthier. We reshuffled the buffet line so that instead of the bread, pasta, and rice being served first, the veggies and proteins were brought forward (and we eliminated some processed items altogether). Get rid of junk food at home that might readily be within reach or stored at eye level.

SNEAK VEGGIES IN EVERYWHERE

Think beyond the Green Smoothie Milkshake on page 20. Add greens to other smoothies. For a nongreen look try lettuce that can camouflage better than kale, like romaine; spinach, while bright green, is a great option because it has a very mild taste. Add finely shredded raw or cooked vegetables into baked goods. Hide white veggies like cauliflower or peeled zucchini in omelets, pastas, and quesadillas. Fold chopped spinach or any other veggies into beef, turkey, or fish burgers (page 281). Chop veggies superfine, and fold them into rice dishes. (If necessary, help the medicine go down with some extra cheese.)

TRAIN THEIR TASTE BUDS

Steer kids toward salads and other veggies by making them taste great. Put as much thought into preparing salads as you would into an entrée. Kids gravitate toward sweets. With slightly sweeter dressing options and colorful veggie medleys, salads can actually be tempting for kids.

THINK LONG-TERM

Trust me, I know—it's easier to give them what they want. I've given a wailing child a lollipop on an airplane (true, that's just survival parenting) or succumbed to boiling pasta when they refused everything else. It's easier to give them what they want in the short term because then they stop fussing. But it's wise to have a longer-term vision. You're giving them a healthy eating foundation that will last the rest of their lives. I ate salad at dinner and offered it to my children every night for a *full year* before Ben agreed to try it, and now he continues to be a salad fan. In time, your efforts will pay off. Stay persistent.

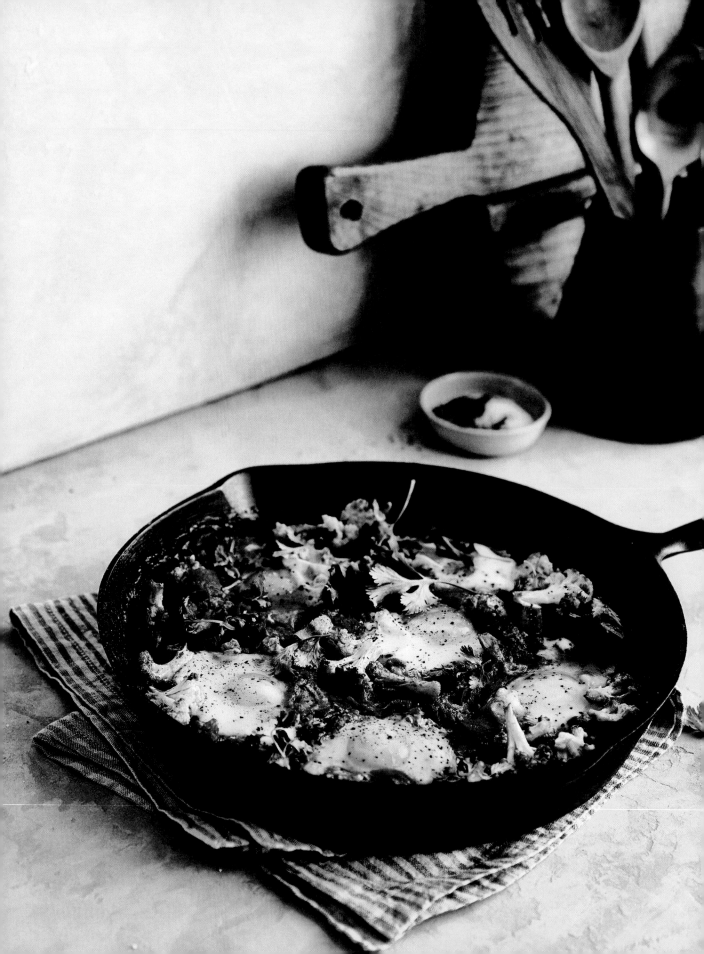

ROASTED-CAULIFLOWER SHAKSHUKA

STEPS: ROAST, SAUTÉ, SIMMER, BAKE! / Makes enough for 8 hungry people

I spent some years of my childhood in Israel eating "American"-style foods at home. It wasn't until I moved West (then East) that my yearning and appreciation for classic Israeli dishes returned. Shakshuka is a staple Israeli one-pan egg breakfast. Spiced tomato sauce is topped with cracked eggs and simmered until the whites are done and the yolks still run. Here, I add roasted cauliflower to the sauce (any excuse to incorporate my favorite veg), but you could add roasted just-about-anything. Or add nothing at all, and serve it up in the classic tomato style.

Tools: Large (12-inch) skillet or frying pan with a lid

1 head cauliflower, cut into bite-sized florets

Generous drizzle of olive oil

Salt and freshly ground black pepper

SAUCE

¼ cup olive oil

1 medium yellow onion, finely chopped

3 garlic cloves, minced

1½ teaspoons cumin

1 teaspoon paprika

½ teaspoon ground coriander

1 teaspoon crushed red pepper flakes

3 tablespoons tomato paste

1 28-ounce can diced tomatoes with juice

1 to 2 fresh, unpeeled medium tomatoes, diced

3 tablespoons Family Secret Red Spread (page 271; optional)

Salt and freshly ground black pepper, to taste

1 Preheat the oven to 400°F.

2 Spread the cauliflower florets on a baking sheet, drizzle with oil, and season with salt and pepper. Roast until the florets have softened and are slightly brown on the edges, about 30 minutes. Set aside. (Roast some extra to munch on!)

3 Prepare the sauce: In a large skillet over medium heat, heat the oil and cook the onion, stirring, until translucent, about 5 minutes. Add the garlic, cumin, paprika, coriander, and pepper flakes, and stir until fragrant, 1 or 2 minutes.

4 Add the tomato paste, ⅓ cup water, the canned and fresh tomatoes, and the Red Spread. Bring to a boil, then reduce the heat and simmer until the tomatoes are softened, about 20 minutes. Be patient—the longer the sauce cooks on low heat, the more robust the flavor.

5 Dot the shakshuka sauce with the cauliflower florets.

6 Crack the eggs carefully on top, making sure the yolks don't break. Season with salt and pepper.

7 Cook, checking every few minutes, until done, about 3 or 4 minutes— cover the pan only at the very end to set the whites. Garnish with fresh cilantro.

CONTINUED

TO ASSEMBLE

8 large eggs

Salt and freshly ground
black pepper

Leaves from 1 bunch fresh
cilantro, chopped, for
garnish

› nail this

Shakshuka seems simple, but
perfecting the sauce's texture and
the balance of spices is an art. Taste
as you go, and season accordingly.
Make this more than once to nail *your*
perfect shakshuka.

Once you've cracked the eggs on
top, watch carefully, and remove the
skillet from the heat while the yolks
are still runny.

» flip it

For a crowd: Pour the cooked sauce
into a 13 × 9-inch casserole, top it
with the cauliflower and then the
eggs, and bake it in the oven at 375°F
until the whites are set, 8 to
10 minutes.

Substitute the cauliflower with
roasted eggplant, pumpkin, or
mushrooms.

Use all fresh tomatoes—swap
4 additional whole, diced tomatoes
in place of the 28-ounce can.

Add olives or red bell pepper to your
sauce—yum.

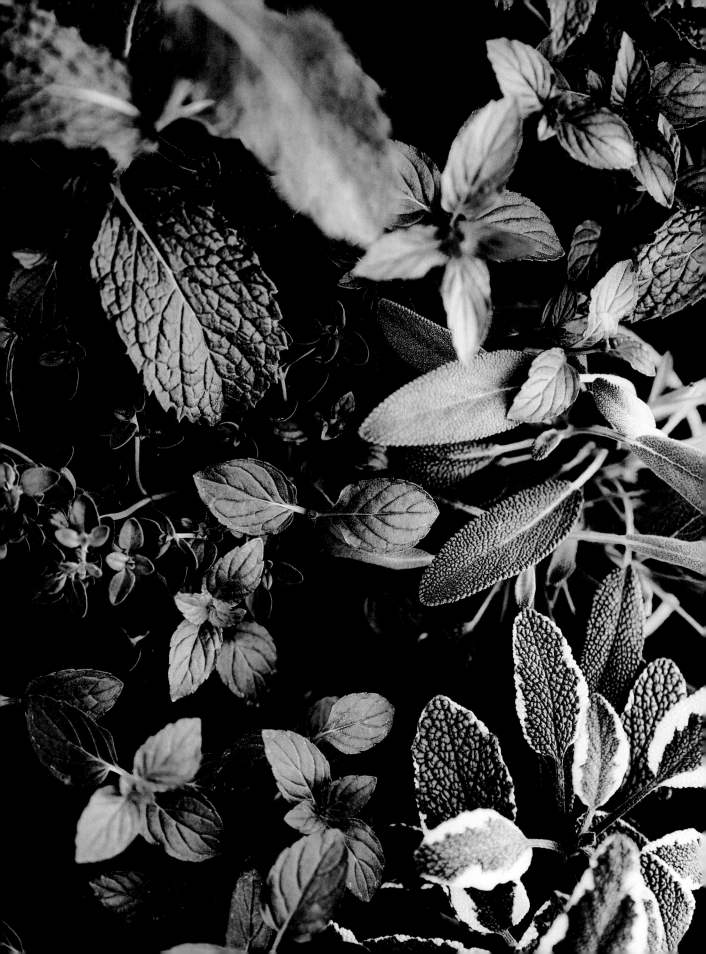

BETTER-THAN-FRIED FRENCH FRIES

STEPS: SLICE, SEASON, BAKE! / **Makes 8 servings**

These oven-baked fries are one of the most requested side dishes at my dinner table, and the simplest to make—double win! After years of making either mushy or dry baked fries that tasted more like roasted potatoes, I concocted this winning idea, together with our babysitter (and the amazing flexible chef), Marilyn. The secret is to blanch your potatoes before seasoning and baking them, delivering the perfectly crisp fry every time. After trying these you may never covet a fried fry again, but I must warn you it is quite hard to stop at just a few.

Tools: Large baking sheet

6 large Yukon gold potatoes

½ cup olive oil

2 teaspoons paprika

1 teaspoon onion powder

1 teaspoon garlic powder

¾ teaspoon salt

¼ teaspoon freshly ground black pepper

1 Preheat the oven to 425°F. Bring a pot of water to boil. Prepare a large bowl of ice water.

2 Cut the potatoes lengthwise into ¼- to ½-inch-thick slices, then cut each slice lengthwise into ¼- to ½-inch-thick fries.

3 Add the cut potatoes to the boiling water, and cook until the water returns to a boil, about 3 minutes. Drain the potatoes, and plunge them briefly in ice water to stop the cooking. (This step precooks the potatoes and helps them get crispy in the oven. They should be soft enough to bite into at this stage). Do not overboil.

4 Drain the potatoes again, and spread them in a single layer on one or two large baking sheets. Coat the potatoes with oil, and season them with the remaining ingredients. Use your hands to coat them evenly. Ensure that the fries do not overlap—it's essential to keep them in a single layer to ensure crispiness and reduce cooking time.

5 Bake for 30 minutes without turning—if you flip them too soon they fall apart. (But if the edges start burning, go ahead and flip them.) After 30 minutes, turn the fries, and continue to check and flip them every so often until they are crisped and browned on all sides, approximately another 15 to 20 minutes. Every now and again, rotate the pan in the oven to ensure even heat distribution.

> nail this

Don't overboil your potatoes or they will turn into mush. If they do become overly mushy, fix your flop and make mashed potatoes instead.

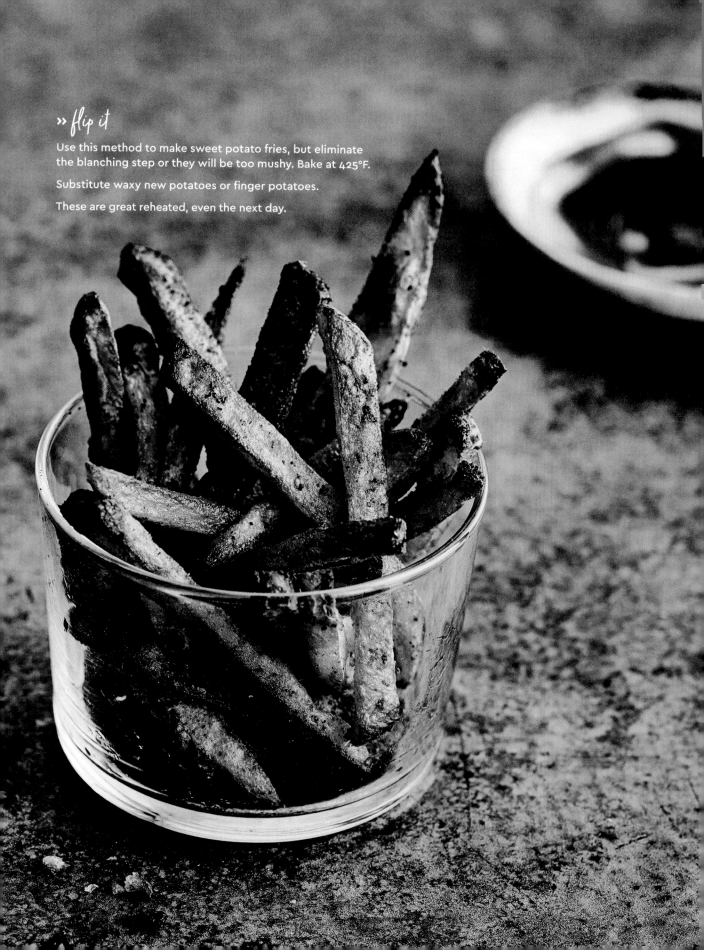

» flip it

Use this method to make sweet potato fries, but eliminate the blanching step or they will be too mushy. Bake at 425°F.

Substitute waxy new potatoes or finger potatoes.

These are great reheated, even the next day.

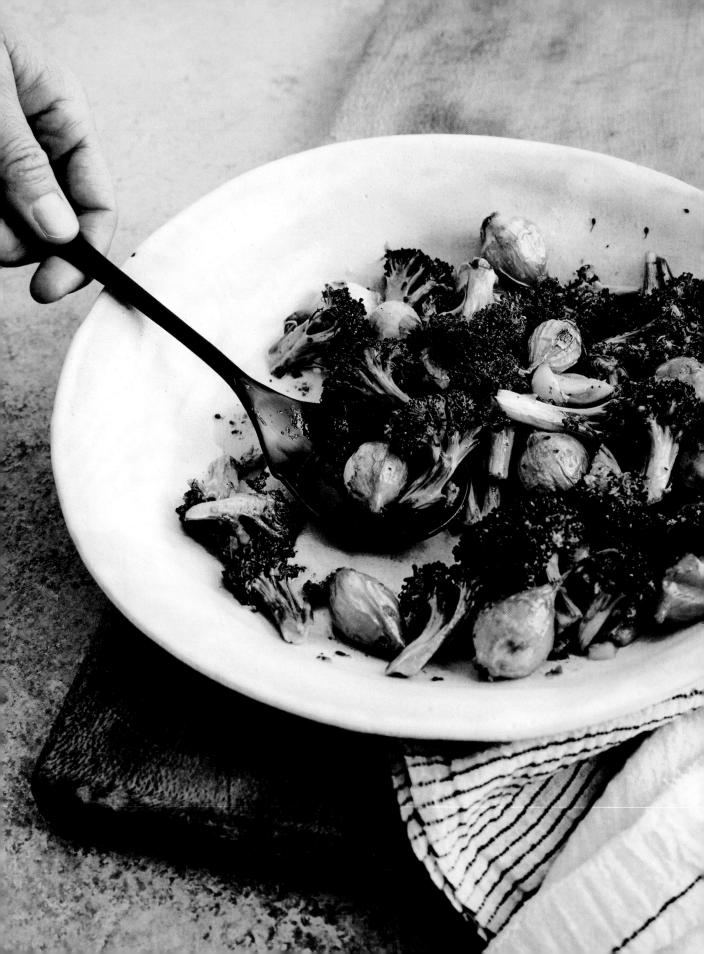

OVEN-ROASTED SECRET BROCCOLI

STEPS: ROAST, SERVE! / **Makes 6 servings**

I used to only steam, sauté, or stir-fry broccoli until I discovered the beauty of oven-roasting it with butter. And while this recipe may call for broccoli (because I'll do anything to get my kids to eat their greens), you should completely roast, like, uh, *every* veggie this way. Mushrooms, cauliflower, or even carrots and zucchini would be totally delish.

Tools: Rubber gloves (optional)

Olive oil or oil spray, to grease pan

2 heads broccoli, cut into florets (about 8 cups)

½ stick (4 tablespoons) unsalted butter, cubed, at room temperature

2 tablespoons white miso

2 garlic cloves, pressed

¼ teaspoon freshly ground black pepper

1 cup pearl onions, peeled

Salt to taste, if needed

1 Preheat the oven to 425°F. Lightly grease a large sheet pan. Bring a large pot of water to a boil, and prepare an ice bath.

2 Blanch the broccoli in the boiling water for 1 minute. Remove the broccoli from the water with a slotted spoon, and plunge it immediately into an ice bath for 1 to 2 minutes to stop the cooking. Drain and set aside.

3 In a small bowl, mix the softened butter with the miso, garlic, and pepper. Mash together with a fork.

4 Massage the miso butter into the broccoli (I use gloves—it's messy). Stir in the pearl onions, and spread the vegetables on the prepared baking sheet.

5 Place the baking sheet in the oven. Check after 5 to 10 minutes, and toss the vegetables with the melted miso butter. Roast for 15 to 20 minutes total, or until the broccoli is cooked and lightly charred but still crisp. Season with salt to taste, if needed.

» flip it

Stovetop method: Blanch and drain the broccoli. Melt the butter and miso and 2 tablespoons of olive oil in a skillet over medium-high heat. Stir in the garlic and broccoli and cook, stirring, until the sauce is bubbly and the broccoli cooked but still crunchy, 3 to 5 minutes. OMG.

Toss with my Sheet-Pan Tofu Medley (page 183) to make it a main!

Swap Brussels sprouts and cauliflower for broccoli.

Add Parmesan cheese.

Fold leftovers into salads, eggs, or anything else you can think of.

For dairy free, use olive oil.

Ten No-Recipe Side Dishes

1 **Rice or quinoa pilaf:** Steam rice or quinoa. Separately, sauté vegetables (see Any Veggie Sauté, page 281). Mix the veggies into the rice or quinoa. Add spices to amp the flavor, or cook the rice in coconut milk in place of water for coconut rice. Serve with a protein and a vegetable, or with anything that has a sauce.

2 **Sweet potato smash:** Bake a few large sweet potatoes. Allow to cool. Scoop the flesh out of the peel. Purée the flesh in a food processor, or mash with a potato smasher. Add milk or coconut milk, butter or coconut oil, salt and pepper. Add a touch of cinnamon or vanilla, if desired, plus salt and pepper. Serve as a bed for grilled salmon or other dishes needing something sweet and colorful.

3 **Garlic pasta:** Cook up some pasta al dente. Drain and set aside, reserving some of the cooking liquid. Heat olive oil in the same pan, add a few cloves of garlic, and cook till fragrant. Return the pasta to the pot, and thin with a touch of pasta water. Toss well. Season with salt and pepper. Serve alongside protein and vegetables.

4 **Roasted any vegetable:** Think Brussels sprouts, cauliflower, mushrooms, eggplant, and even starchy ones like potatoes or sweet potatoes. Chop the vegetables, and spread them in a single layer on a baking sheet. Drizzle with olive oil, and season with salt and pepper. Bake in a 425°F oven until crisp (about 15 to 30 minutes, depending on the vegetable. Potatoes and heartier veggies will take longer). Stir about halfway through the cooking process.

5 **Roasted asparagus with fresh herbs and garlic:** Clean asparagus and snap off the woody ends. Spread the spears on a baking sheet. Season with fresh garlic and fresh herbs of your choice, salt, and pepper. Drizzle with olive oil. Bake at 425°F until crisp (about 15 minutes).

6 **Melt-in-your-mouth red cabbage:** Slice an onion, and fry it with a bit of olive oil until caramelized, about 20 minutes on medium-low; add shredded red cabbage, and stir to combine. Simmer on low until wilted, 30 to 40 minutes. Splash with lemon juice or balsamic vinegar, and serve with any dish needing color and texture.

7 **Chunky fruit and veggie salsas:** Make a quick salsa with roughly chopped vegetables and/or fruits tossed with olive oil and an acid of your choice (any type of vinegar or citrus juice works). Try mango, snap pea, and jicama tossed with rice vinegar; strawberries, cucumber, and parsley with white balsamic; cherry tomato, cauliflower, and yellow bell pepper with lemon juice. Add fresh herbs. The possibilities are endlessly seasonal.

8 **Skewer and grill:** Skewer a bunch of same-size cut veggies—like mushrooms, bell peppers, onions, or summer squash—marinate them in vinaigrette, and grill away!

9 **The chickpea solution:** Chickpeas are one of the most versatile items in your pantry. Not only can you use them to whip up hummus, you can turn them into a base, straight out of the can, for almost-instant side dishes—from salad tossed with your favorite vinaigrette and chopped veggies, to a warm chickpea side dish, quickly sautéed in herbs or with curry paste and coconut milk.

10 **Quick-cook veggie noodles:** Spiralize your favorite veggies (think zucchini, squash, or carrots), or in a pinch use a vegetable peeler to create ribbons. Sauté your veggies in olive oil or butter. Add garlic, fresh herbs, or Parmesan for flavor, with a hint of lemon juice at the end. Or toss with pesto at the end (page 272).

GUILTLESS ZUCCHINI FRITTERS

STEPS: GRATE, MIX, FRY! / **Makes about 20 small fritters**

In our house, this zucchini version of the classic potato latke (aka pancake) is a year-round staple. I put a healthified spin on these fritters by shallow-frying them in olive oil and reheating them before serving. We served a big hungry crowd the other night, and nobody even noticed that they were healthy. Now that's the test of a good dish!

1 small yellow onion grated (about ½ cup)

2 garlic cloves, minced

2 to 3 small to medium zucchini, grated (about 2½ cups)

2 large eggs

1 tablespoon all-purpose gluten-free flour (optional)

½ teaspoon salt

Pinch of freshly ground black pepper

2 tablespoons chopped fresh basil

Olive oil, for frying

1 Line a large plate with paper towels.

2 Grate the onion. Set the onion and minced garlic aside in a large bowl.

3 Grate the zucchini using the small holes on a box grater. Squeeze out any excess liquid from the zucchini (use a cheesecloth if you have one, or a kitchen towel), and transfer to the bowl with the onions.

4 Stir in the eggs, flour, if desired, salt, pepper, and basil, mixing thoroughly.

5 In a large skillet, heat 3 tablespoons of olive oil (or more, if needed, but just enough to shallow-fry the fritters) over medium-low heat until hot but not smoking. Working in a few batches, drop tablespoon-size scoops of batter into the pan about 2 inches apart. Cook, turning once, until golden and crisp, about 5 minutes total per batch. Set aside to drain on the paper towel–lined plate.

6 If you plan to make these in advance or want to have them piping hot, when you're ready to serve reheat them in a 350°F oven for a few minutes.

› *nail this*

As you fry, occasionally stir the batter in the bowl to reincorporate the eggs evenly (they tend to settle to the bottom).

Fry over a low flame so the fritters don't burn.

Resist the urge to make bigger fritters; because of the low amount of flour they are fragile and hard to flip if too big.

» *flip it*

Swap the zucchini with grated potato, sweet potato, broccoli, or cauliflower!

Make a quiche: Bake the fritter batter in a shallow, round baking pan. See page 32 for a quiche method. Add a handful of shredded cheese to top it off.

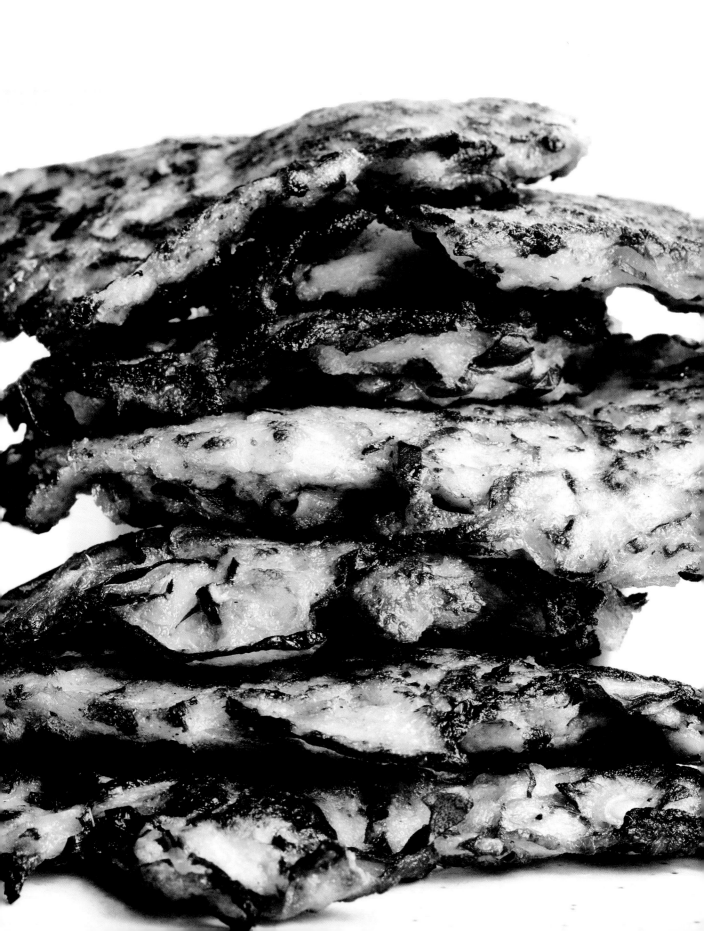

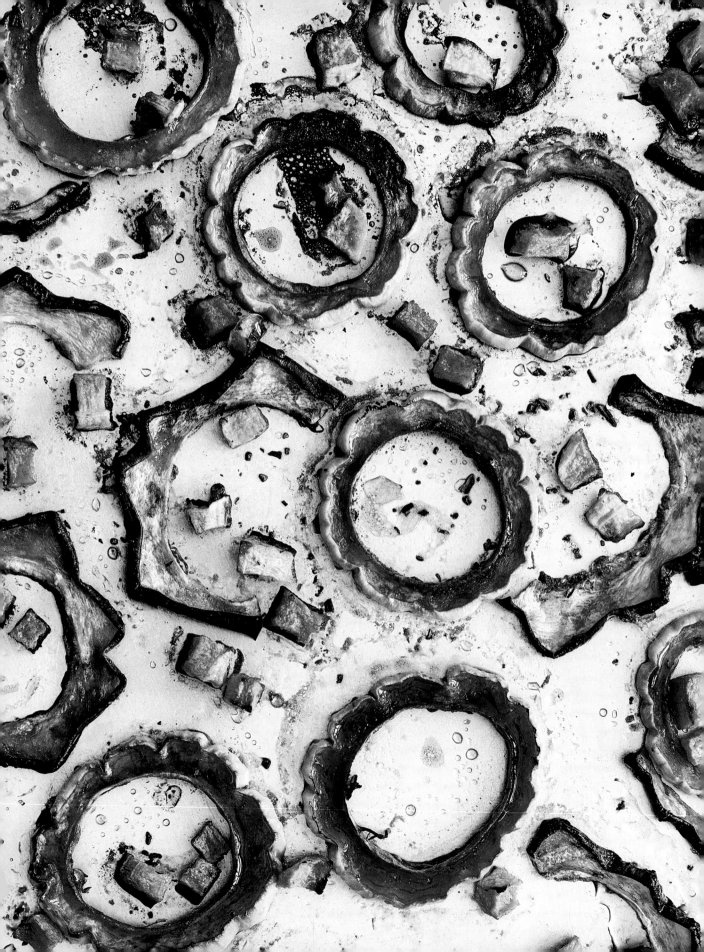

CANDIED WINTER SQUASH

STEPS: TOSS, ROAST! / **Makes 4 to 6 servings, depending on squash size**

Something magical happens when winter squash, maple, and vanilla marry. The edges of the squash caramelize and taste almost like candy! This side dish pairs well with chicken or other meat or as part of a dinner menu that's in need of a pop of color or a sweet balance to savory dishes.

1 small pumpkin, butternut squash, acorn squash, or kabocha, skin on, cut in half and seeds removed, then sliced into ¼-inch-thick slices

1 tablespoon olive oil (or enough to coat)

1 tablespoon maple syrup

½ teaspoon vanilla extract

¼ teaspoon sea salt or Rosemary-Infused Salt (page 268), or to taste

1 Preheat the oven to 400°F.

2 Toss the squash with the remaining ingredients on a large baking sheet.

3 Roast until the edges are caramelized and the mixture is bubbly, roughly 25 minutes. Carefully flip the slices and continue caramelizing the second side until browned, another 15 minutes (about 40 minutes total).

> *nail this*

For the sugars and the squash to caramelize, the key is to roast the squash on high heat.

Squash sizes vary, so use the measurements of the other ingredients as a loose guide. Add a bit more or less oil and maple syrup to coat, just enough for the squash to glisten and look well coated when raw.

>> *flip it*

Add ground cinnamon or pumpkin pie spice for the holidays.

Omit the maple syrup if you'd rather it be less sweet; squash is often sweet enough, depending on the season.

Serve as an accompaniment to savory chicken, turkey, or beef.

Mound the cooked squash in a small circular mold, then press the soft squash down into the mold to create a perfect circle. Top with a slice of grilled halibut and some fresh greens as a stunning appetizer.

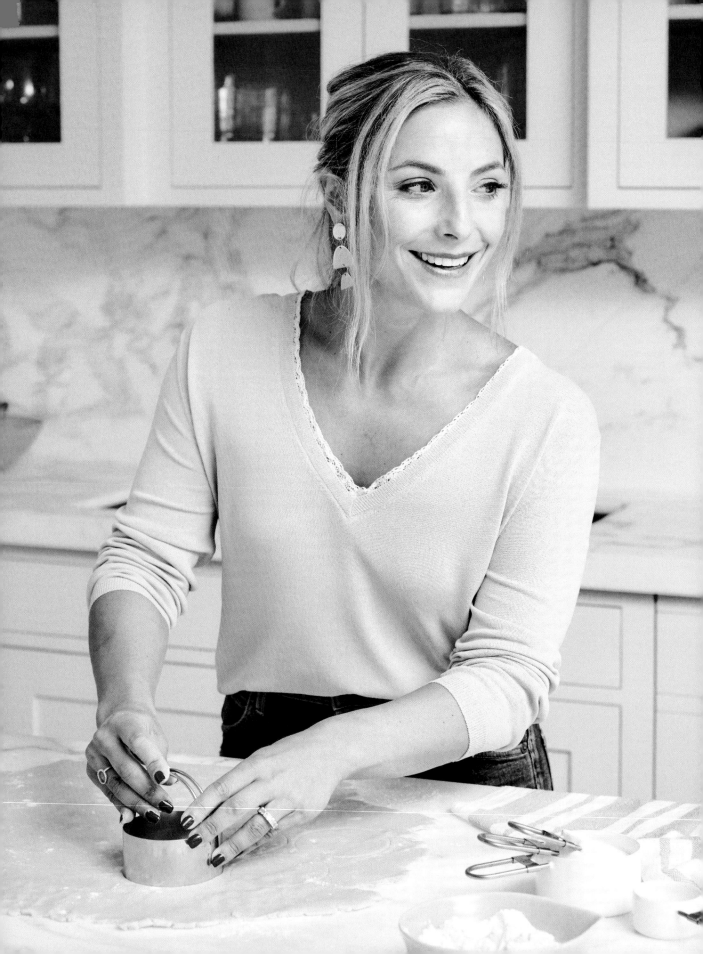

Chapter 8

INDULGENT DESSERTS

Do you ever say no to sweets for a while because you're being "good," and then polish off a whole box of chocolates? I've been there. Sensible indulging keeps us from overextending our willpower and eventually bingeing. A reasonable amount of sweets enriches our lives and keeps us sane and normal. And, frankly, girls who eat dessert really do have more fun. My sister Yael (mom of three and in superb shape), for example, says her life is happier if she allows herself a big slice of her favorite cake when the craving strikes. To compensate for her insatiable appetite for chocolate cake and brown buttercream frosting, she works out for an hour, six days a week. She eats clean most of the time but always saves room for dessert. In short, she embodies my definition of a fulfilled woman: She aspires for excellent health but is so attuned to her body and her desires that she has creatively found a way to have her cake and eat it too. Let's get baking!

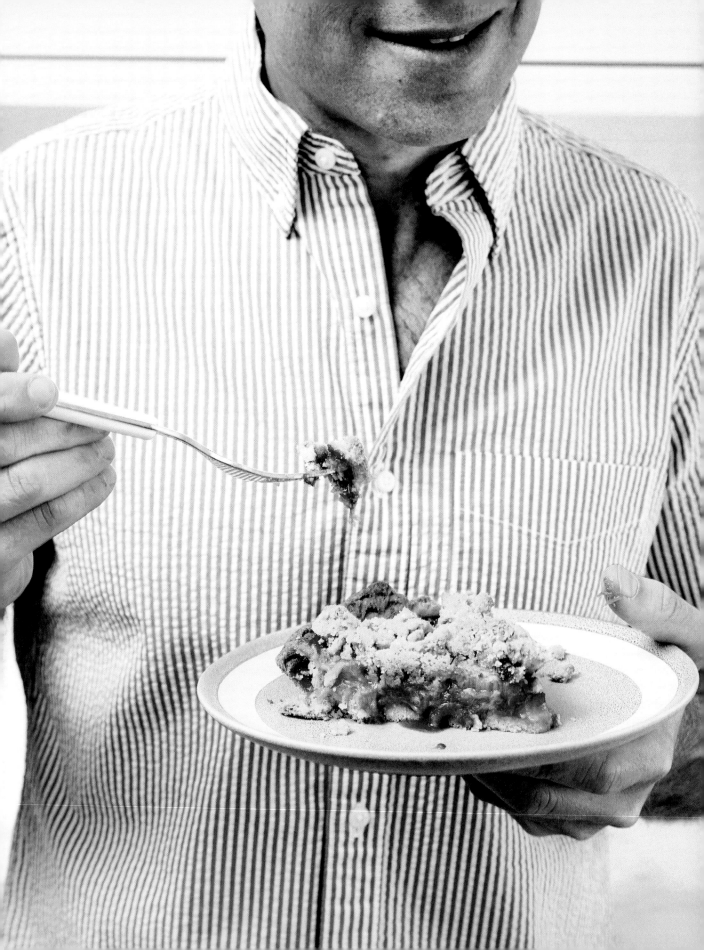

STRAWBERRY RHUBARB CRUMBLE PIE

STEPS: MIX, TOSS, FILL, BAKE! / **Makes 8 to 10 servings**

Sometimes, the most endearing part of baking is the feeling you give someone else when you bake them their favorite dessert. This strawberry rhubarb pie began as a tribute to Seth's love of rhubarb (he still gets giddy when I make it). The sweet, almondy crust is balanced with a fall-apart succulent berry filling and topped with a genius crumble that uses some of the crust dough as its base.

Tools: Food processor, 10-inch round glass pie dish)

Oil for greasing

CRUST

1 heaping cup sliced blanched almonds

1 cup all-purpose gluten-free flour

½ cup granulated sugar

⅓ cup butter or coconut oil

1 teaspoon baking powder

½ teaspoon xanthan gum (omit if already in flour)

1 large egg

1 teaspoon vanilla extract

⅛ teaspoon salt

TOPPING

⅓ cup reserved dough from crust

½ cup coconut oil

½ cup almond flour

½ cup gluten-free flour

½ cup granulated sugar

¼ cup sliced blanched almonds

1 teaspoon ground cinnamon

⅛ teaspoon salt

1 Preheat the oven to 350°F. Lightly spray or grease the pie dish with oil.

2 Make the crust: Process the almonds in a food processor until finely ground. Add the remaining crust ingredients, and pulse to combine.

3 Reserve ⅓ cup of the dough for use in the topping, and press the remaining dough into the pie dish, spreading it all the way up the sides. Set aside, or make in advance.

4 Make the topping: Place all the topping ingredients in the bowl of a food processor, and pulse to combine. Set aside.

5 Make the filling: In a medium bowl, mix together all the filling ingredients. Spread the filling over the crust.

6 Spread the crumb topping over the filling by grabbing fistfuls of topping to make big chunks that will hold together during baking— the best part.

7 Bake for 65 minutes, or until the fruit bubbles, the topping browns, and the crust is lightly golden but not overly brown. Tent the pie with foil if it is browning too quickly before it is cooked on top. Check the pie at the 55-minute mark—the exact baking time will depend on your oven.

CONTINUED

FILLING

2½ cups chopped (into ½-inch chunks) fresh rhubarb (about 10 9-inch stalks)

2½ cups sliced strawberries (about 1 pound)

¼ cup granulated sugar

1 tablespoon all-purpose gluten-free flour

Zest of one lemon

1 teaspoon vanilla extract

› nail this

Make sure the pie is baked enough that the rhubarb is soft. I once underbaked this pie for a dinner party, resulting in crunchy rhubarb—blah!

» flip it

Adding ground almonds to the crust imparts a unique texture. Use any shape—slivered, sliced, or whole—just make sure they're peeled (blanched). If you're pressed for time or only have almond flour on hand, that'll do.

Reduce the sugar in the crust to ¼ or ⅓ cup if you want it less sweet.

No food processor? Place the almonds in a Ziploc bag, and crush them with a rolling pin or wooden spoon. Mix the topping and the crust by hand.

Double the topping, and freeze the extra in a Ziploc bag to use as a crumble for any quick bread or muffin.

Turn Your Baking Flops into Successes

A few of my go-to dishes have come from experimenting with things that didn't go my way—successes from flops. Rather than throwing up your hands or getting frustrated, pause and figure out plan B.

Flopped brownies? Make a chunky-monkey ice cream! Simply chop the brownies and fold them into ice cream to compose one of the most requested desserts in my house. Or fold them into Decadent Frozen Almond Brownie Pie (page 213).

Overbaked cake? Make a trifle! Remove any burnt edges, cut the cake into bite-sized pieces, and layer them in a glass bowl with whipped cream and chopped fresh fruit. The cream will add moisture, and the presentation is stunning.

Underbaked cake? Cakes that drop in the center are common. Just ice the top and nobody will know.

Cracked cheesecake? Top with sour cream mixed with sugar, open a can of your favorite jam or pie filling to spread over the top, or cook up fruit and sugar into a compote and spoon it on!

Misshapen cookies? Maybe you baked your cookies too close together and they spread into each other. Or perhaps they baked up into odd and undesirable shapes. It happens. Grab a cookie cutter and make them round again. Save the trimmed bits to fold into ice creams and frozen pies, or add them to nuts for a cookie trail mix.

Ugly-looking pies or crumbles? If your pie doesn't come out the way you'd hoped, slice it in the kitchen and serve it plated, with whipped cream or whipped coconut cream or a scoop of ice cream on top, and a mint or berry garnish for color.

ANYTIME NEW YEAR'S APPLE CAKE

STEPS: SOFTEN, BEAT, WHISK, BAKE! / **Makes 10 servings**

For over a decade I've been baking Susie Fishbein's absolutely divine New Year's apple cake from her book *The Kosher Palette*. I've tweaked and played with my own gluten-free and flexible version. The dense batter bakes to buttery precision, and topped with honeyed apples it combines to make the ideal ending to a meal. (Truth: I never wait for New Year's to bake this—it's just too good to wait for.)

Tools: 10-inch springform pan

APPLES
3 Granny Smith apples, peeled, cored, and sliced into ¼-inch wedges

⅓ cup honey

3 tablespoons fresh lemon juice

WET INGREDIENTS
1 cup granulated sugar

½ cup dark brown sugar

¾ cup coconut oil, melted

2 teaspoons vanilla extract

4 large eggs

2 teaspoons minced lemon zest

DRY INGREDIENTS
2 cups all-purpose gluten-free flour

2 teaspoons baking powder

1 teaspoon xanthan gum (omit if already in flour)

½ teaspoon salt

TOPPING
2 tablespoons granulated sugar

1 teaspoon ground cinnamon

1 Preheat the oven to 350°F. Line the bottom of the pan with parchment. Spray the sides of the pan with oil spray.

2 Cook the apples, honey, and lemon juice in a saucepan over medium heat until softened, 5 to 7 minutes. Drain and discard the liquids from the cooked apples and set aside.

3 For the wet ingredients: With an electric mixer, beat the sugars, oil, and vanilla until blended. Add the eggs and zest, and beat until all is incorporated but not overmixed.

4 For the dry ingredients: In a separate bowl whisk together all the dry ingredients. Add the mixture to the wet ingredients, combining well with a spatula or large spoon.

5 Pour the batter into the prepared pan. Fan the apples in 2 concentric circles, overlapping the edges, to cover the batter. In a small bowl, combine the sugar and cinnamon for the topping, and sprinkle over the top of the apples and batter.

6 Bake the cake for about 1 hour, or until just set and lightly golden, checking it often toward the end of baking. Allow the cake to cool completely before removing it from the pan. Slice and serve!

> nail this

The batter will look scant. Don't freak out; it will rise.

You'll notice the edges starting to brown while the center is still soft. Watch carefully, and remove the cake from the oven when the center is just set so you don't burn the edges.

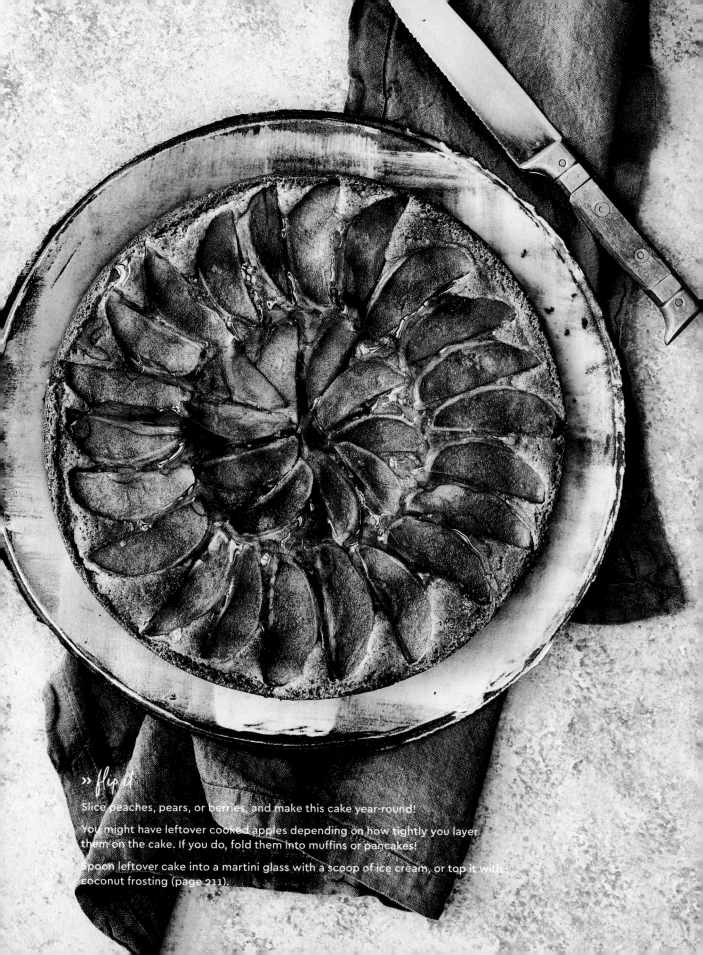

» flip it

Slice peaches, pears, or berries, and make this cake year-round!

You might have leftover cooked apples depending on how tightly you layer them on the cake. If you do, fold them into muffins or pancakes!

Spoon leftover cake into a martini glass with a scoop of ice cream, or top it with coconut frosting (page 211).

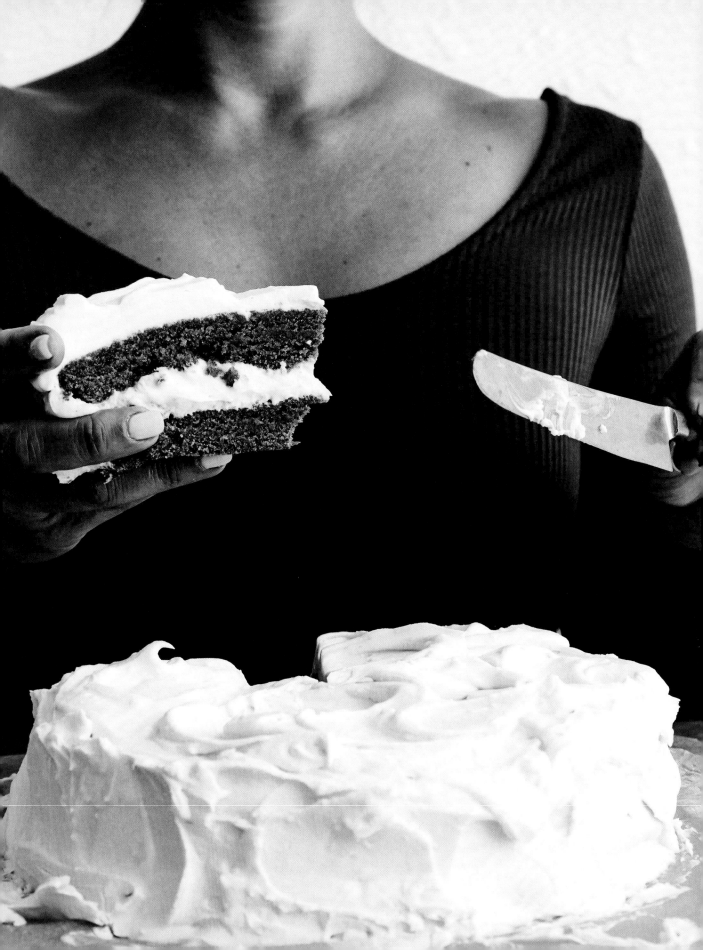

CARROT CAKE WITH MARSHMALLOWY FROSTING

STEPS: WHISK, MIX, BAKE, WHIP, FROST! / **Makes 1 layer cake or 12 cupcakes**

This carrot cake melts in your mouth and is as decadent as they come. It's super moist, just dense enough to be substantial, and iced with a light and velvety coconut frosting that complements all that richness. You can make this cake vegan, turn it into cupcakes, or use the versatile frosting on any other cake. If you are catering to coconut haters (it's a shame really, but I know some too), you can leave the cake naked or ice it with your favorite buttercream or cream cheese frosting.

Tools: Two 7- or 8-inch round cake pans or a 12-cup muffin pan, electric mixer

DRY INGREDIENTS
2 cups all-purpose gluten-free flour

2 teaspoons ground cinnamon

1 teaspoon baking powder

1 teaspoon baking soda

1 teaspoon xanthan gum (omit if already in flour)

½ teaspoon salt

¼ teaspoon nutmeg

WET INGREDIENTS
1¼ cups packed dark brown sugar

½ cup extra-virgin olive oil

½ cup full-fat coconut milk

2 teaspoons vanilla extract

1 teaspoon apple cider vinegar

1 large egg

1 cup finely grated carrots, packed

1 Preheat the oven to 350°F.

2 Grease the sides and bottom of pans, and line the bottoms with rounds of parchment paper. The cake is very moist, and the parchment eases its release later.

3 In a medium bowl, whisk together all the dry ingredients.

4 In a separate bowl, whisk by hand or use a mixer to beat together the brown sugar, oil, coconut milk, vanilla, and vinegar. Add the egg, stirring just to combine, then fold in the grated carrots.

5 Stir the dry ingredients, a third at a time, into the wet ingredients. Divide the batter between the two prepared cake pans.

6 Bake for 30 to 35 minutes if using 7-inch pans, 20 minutes if using 8-inch pans, and 25 minutes if making muffins, or until a toothpick inserted into the center comes out clean. Watch carefully, and do not overbake.

7 Allow the cakes to cool completely in their pans on a cooling rack. Once cooled, you could freeze the cakes for icing later.

CONTINUED

FROSTING

3 cups coconut cream, well chilled then drained (use solids only)

1 cup confectioners' sugar

1 tablespoon vanilla extract

8 While the cakes are cooling, prepare the frosting: Place all the frosting ingredients in an electric mixer bowl. Mix on high speed until soft peaks form. The mixture only beats well if it's really cold, so you may need to place it in the fridge to cool midway through, then beat it again. Chill to set, about one hour.

9 Remove the cakes from the pans, discarding the parchment. Set one of the layers on a serving platter, and spread a layer of frosting on top. Stack the other layer on top, and frost the top and sides of the cake.

› *nail this*

When making the frosting, chill the coconut cream until it's very cold— this is essential for it to beat well. And use only the solids from the can of coconut cream; discard any water, or the frosting won't thicken.

›› *flip it*

Vegan option: Replace the egg with 3 tablespoons flaxseed meal plus 6 tablespoons water, combined to make a paste. If the vegan cake drops in the center, see the next tip.

Cake flop help: In general, if your cake is underdone and flops in the center, you'll be okay; just use frosting to hide it. Or make a trifle with cream, cake, and berries.

Zucchini chocolate chip cake: Swap the carrot with zucchini, and add a few handfuls of chocolate chips.

Nutty cake: Add a handful of toasted chopped walnuts or pecans to the cake batter.

If you're making cupcakes and don't have time to prepare the frosting, pop a large marshmallow on top of each cupcake 5 minutes before they're done baking. Simple and yummy.

DECADENT FROZEN ALMOND BROWNIE PIE

STEPS: MIX, BAKE, STIR, FREEZE, DRIZZLE! / **Makes 10 to 12 servings**

This outrageous almond butter pie happened by accident one day while I stared down at a batch of flopped brownies. I decided to get my act together, chop them up, discard the burnt edges, and fold pieces of the underbaked center into ice cream. In this over-the-top recipe, I stretched that idea even further by using part of the brownie batter as the "pie crust" base and baking and folding the rest into a rich almond butter filling. On to more good news: Cheat your way to a tempting slice by using a boxed brownie mix!

Tools: 9- or 10-inch springform pan, 9 x 9-inch square baking pan, parchment paper, electric mixer (or bowl and whisk)

1 17-ounce box gluten-free brownie mix (your favorite brand!)

1½ cups dark chocolate chips, divided

2 13.5-ounce cans full-fat coconut milk

1 cup natural almond butter

⅔ cup confectioners' sugar

1 tablespoon vanilla extract

Pinch of salt

½ cup chopped unsalted almonds, toasted

1 Preheat the oven to 350°F. Line the bottom of the springform pan and the square baking pan with parchment paper.

2 Make the crust: Follow the directions on the box of brownie mix, jazzing up the batter by stirring in 1 cup of the chocolate chips. Spread half the brownie batter in the springform pan, about ½ inch deep. Bake the brownie crust just until set and slightly underbaked, about 8 minutes (usually a bit less time than the box says). Set the crust aside to cool for roughly 30 minutes. If you're pressed for time, cool the crust on the countertop for a few minutes, and then pop it in the refrigerator for 10 minutes.

3 Spoon the rest of the brownie batter into the square baking pan, and bake for about 10 to 15 minutes. The brownies should be underdone. (You can bake this pan of brownies at the same time as you do the crust; remove this pan from the oven earlier so the brownies for the filling are very mushy.) Let cool completely, then chop up the soft brownies to yield 1 cup (this will use about half the pan; freeze or eat any remaining bits).

4 Make the filling: Meanwhile, with an electric mixer (or by hand with a whisk), beat the coconut milk, almond butter, confectioners' sugar, vanilla, and salt until creamy. Pour the filling over the brownie crust in the springform pan.

5 Dot the filling with the chopped brownie chunks. Sprinkle in some chopped toasted almonds for crunch.

CONTINUED

6 Cover and freeze the pie for 3 hours, or overnight, to solidly set the filling.

7 Make the chocolate topping: Bring a small pot of water to a boil. Place a bowl on top of the pot to create a double boiler, and place the remaining ½ cup chocolate chips in the bowl to melt, whisking often to ensure even melting. Remove the bowl from the heat when the chocolate is fully melted and smooth, after just a few minutes.

8 Drizzle the melted chocolate over your pie to create a pretty pattern. Return the pie to the freezer to set the chocolate, about 15 minutes. To serve, gently release the springform mold, and cut the pie into thin slices.

9 If you're not serving it immediately, cover the pie with plastic wrap twice, to ensure that it's completely sealed. (See page 44 for more on preventing freezer burn.) It will keep for up to 2 months in the freezer.

› nail this

Don't overbake the crust. You want the texture of a fudgy, outrageously scrumptious brownie base.

This works best if you prepare it in a springform pan, so that when you release the sides the cake presents beautifully.

If your pie has been frozen for a while, let it thaw on your countertop for 10 minutes, or until it softens enough to slice. Transfer to a cutting board and slice with a sharp knife.

» flip it

Try any other butter: Peanut or cashew butter works well. Or ditch the nut-butter filling altogether, and just fill the pie with your favorite ice cream.

Consider additional fold-ins: chopped dark chocolate, cookie crumbles, or other nuts.

Crust substitute: 1 batch gluten-free Chocolate Chip Cookie dough (page 223; use only part of the dough). Or make your favorite homemade brownie recipe.

Ditch the brownie crust and use the filling to make chilled single-serve chocolate almond butter mousse in individual dessert glasses, or in ramekins topped with ganache.

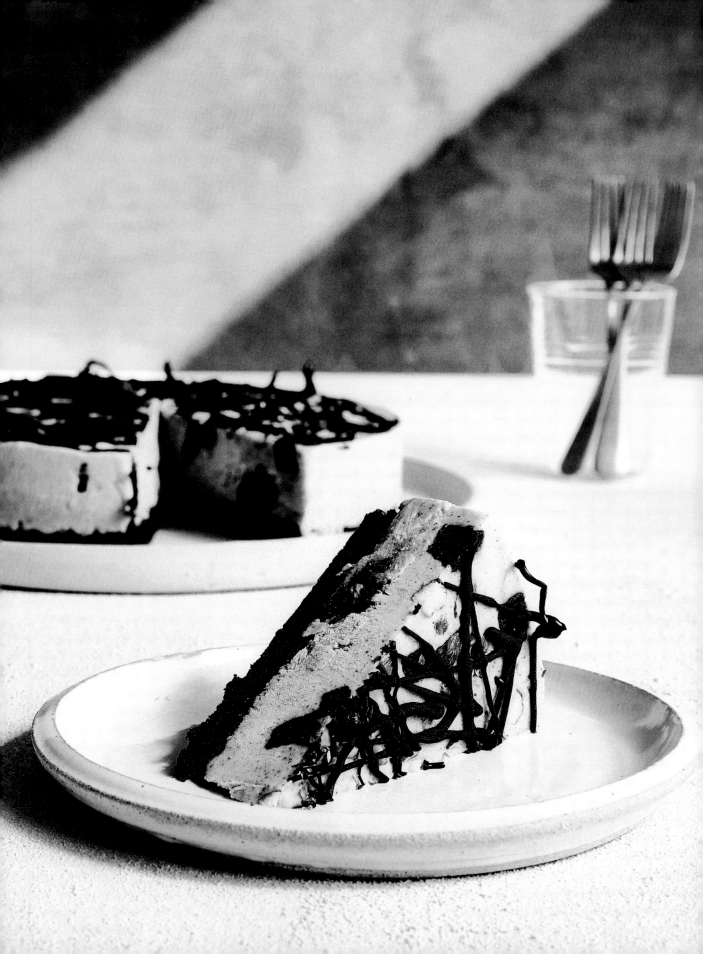

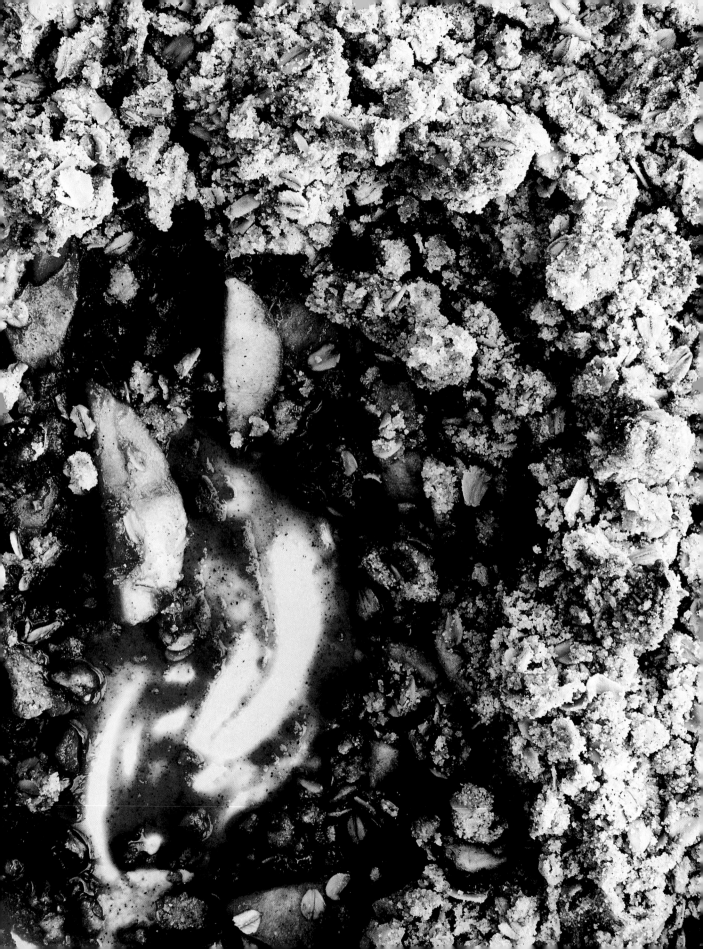

HOME-STYLE APPLE CRANBERRY CRISP

STEPS: MIX, CRUMBLE, BAKE! / **Makes 12 servings**

My Aunt Mindy used to make this comforting dessert for me when I was a teenager and visited her for a few weeks every summer. When I bake it, I'm taken back to those days when we'd lick our plates and sit around the table with smiles. One day she shared this simple recipe with me, and I've been making her apple crisp ever since. If you bake this dessert I promise you'll never have leftovers (although you might be compelled to go to the gym the next day).

Tools: 11 × 7-inch baking pan

FILLING

6 to 8 Granny Smith apples, peeled, cored, and cut into ½-inch slices

½ batch Apple Cranberry Sauce (page 158), or 1 14-ounce can whole-berry cranberry sauce

CRISP TOPPING

1½ cups old-fashioned rolled oats

1½ cups all-purpose gluten-free flour

1½ cups granulated sugar

1½ sticks unsalted butter or ¾ cup coconut oil, at room temperature

2 teaspoons ground cinnamon

Ice cream, for serving (optional)

1 Preheat the oven to 350°F.

2 Place the apples in the baking pan. Add the cranberry sauce, and stir it with the apples until incorporated.

3 Make the topping: In a large bowl, combine all the topping ingredients. Grab fistfuls of topping to form balls that hold together, then crumble the topping in big chunks over the fruit (the large chunks of baked topping are the best part).

4 Bake for about 45 to 50 minutes, uncovered, or until the filling is bubbling and the topping has browned to a crisp.

5 Let cool to room temperature. Serve with a scoop of ice cream, if desired.

> nail this

Not all apples are created equal in size! Start with 6 apples, and work up to 8 if the filling looks too skimpy in the baking dish—it should be substantially full, with room left for the topping.

If the topping is very soft once mixed, pop it in the fridge for 10 minutes to harden before crumbling it over the fruit.

» flip it

Use any apples you like, but Granny Smith apples work best because of their tartness, which balances the sweetness of the crumble.

Use crisp topping on muffins, breads, or any of your favorite fruit crisps or pies.

Make a peach, blueberry, or pear crumble. Prep the fruit, and add a hint of cinnamon, lemon juice, sugar, and flour to bring it together. Top with crumble.

For a non-oat-based topping, use the streusel on page 65.

UNBELIEVABLY DAIRY-FREE CHEESECAKE

STEPS: MIX, CREAM, BAKE! / **Makes 10 to 12 servings**

My diners are usually stunned that this cheesecake is dairy free—it's really that good. In truth, it's more decadent than I like to admit, and we serve it only occasionally (to my kids' dismay). I'm breaking my own flexible rules by sharing it with you because this cake contains one ingredient that's necessary without exception: nondairy "cream cheese." It is available in many supermarkets, but locating it can sometimes be a challenge. Still, some things are worth searching for.

Tools: 10-inch springform pan, electric mixer

CRUST

2 cups (8 ounces) graham cracker crumbs (I use gluten free—or use any cinnamon cookie, crushed into crumbs)

8 tablespoons coconut oil, melted

1 tablespoon granulated sugar

FILLING

3 8-ounce packages plain dairy-free "cream cheese," preferably Tofutti brand

1 cup granulated sugar

1 tablespoon fresh lemon juice

2 teaspoons vanilla extract

1 teaspoon minced lemon zest

3 large eggs

1 cup well-chilled coconut cream solids (drain before measuring)

3 tablespoons all-purpose gluten-free flour

Pinch of salt

Pineapple or cherry compote or seedless raspberry jam, for topping (optional)

1 Preheat the oven to 225°F. Line the bottom of the springform pan with parchment paper, and spray the sides with cooking spray (or the cake will stick).

2 Make the crust: In a medium bowl, mix together the crumbs, coconut oil, and sugar. Press the mixture into the bottom of the prepared pan; place it in the freezer while you prepare the filling.

3 Make the filling: In the bowl of an electric mixer, combine the cream cheese, sugar, lemon juice, vanilla, and lemon zest. Cream the ingredients together, scraping down the sides and bottom of the bowl and beaters. Continue mixing until well blended.

4 Add the eggs one at a time, beating well after each addition. Add the chilled coconut cream, and beat for one full minute.

5 Stir in the flour and salt, mixing until just incorporated.

6 Remove the pan from the freezer, and pour the filling over the crust. Bake for approximately 2 hours, or until the sides are set and the center still jiggles a little bit but springs back when touched.

7 Turn off the oven and open the door. The cake will continue baking as the oven cools down and should dry to a smooth finish on top, with no cracks. Refrigerate, covered, overnight.

8 Run a knife around the edge of the cake, then remove the springform. Top the cake with pineapple or cherry compote, if desired. If using jam, make a glaze by warming it in the microwave for 30 seconds, then cooling it to room temperature (so that it's runny and spreadable).

› nail this

Discard any clear water from the can of coconut cream, and use only the white, creamy solids.

You need to chill this overnight so it will set. Plan on making it a day ahead of serving. It can be made up to 2 days in advance.

Notice the low oven temperature? This helps the cake bake evenly, avoiding burnt edges or cracks on top.

» flip it

Make mini cheesecakes in individual springform pans; baking time will vary based on the pans' size.

If your cake does crack, just top it with berries and nobody will notice.

Save any leftover coconut cream for smoothies or curries. It can also be frozen for later use.

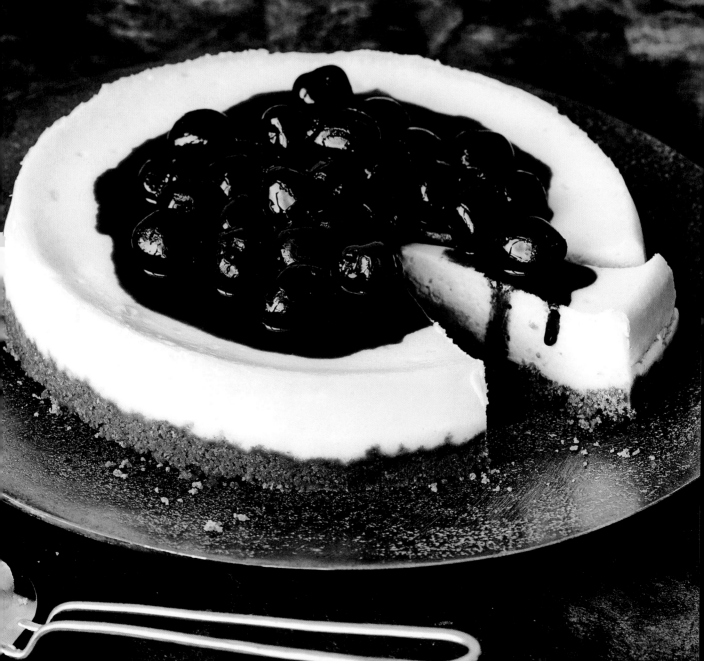

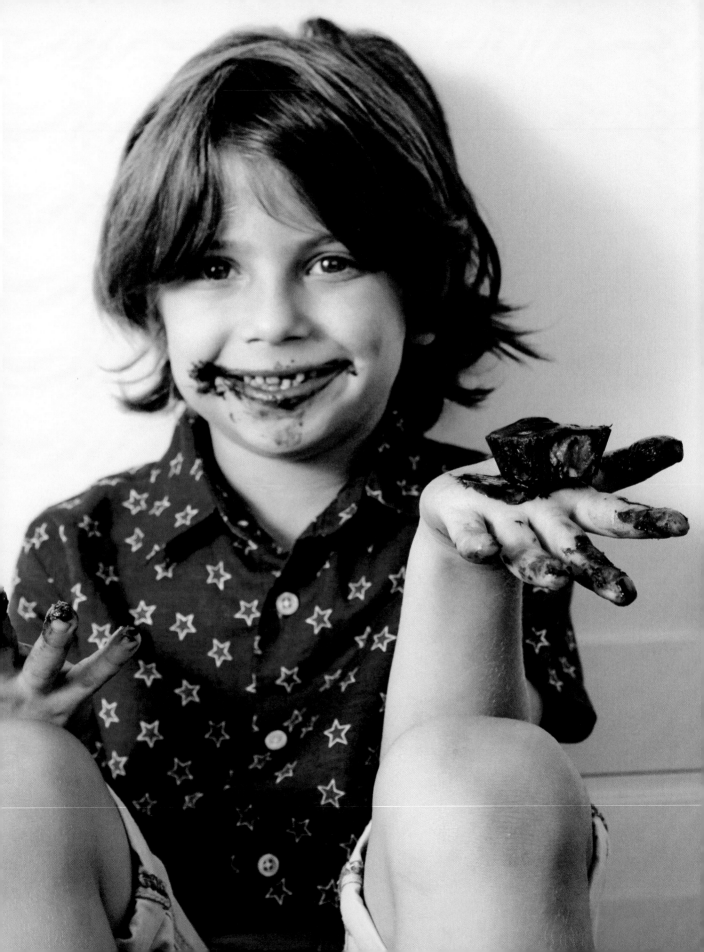

BETTER-THAN-BOUGHT CHOCOLATE PEANUT BUTTER CUPS

STEPS: MIX, MELT, BRUSH, FREEZE, FILL! / **Makes 32**

I grew up eating (arguably too many) chocolate peanut butter cups. These days, store-bought processed chocolates are generally off limits for me, but my craving for them continues to linger. Once I discovered this too-good-to-be-true way of making homemade peanut butter cups, my longing was fulfilled. These creamy, sweet, and salty chocolates are not only better than I remember the bought version to be, they are also a stunning (and convenient) way to wow a crowd. Make them in advance, and pop them onto a silver platter for dessert. That is, unless a kid sneaks few first.

Tools: Mini muffin pan and liners, small pastry brush

2 cups natural chunky peanut butter

½ cup raw honey

1 tablespoon coconut flour

1 teaspoon vanilla extract

2 teaspoons sea salt

2 10-ounce bags dark chocolate chips

1 In a medium bowl, mix the peanut butter, honey, coconut flour, vanilla, and salt. Refrigerate the mixture while preparing the chocolate.

2 Boil a few inches of water in a saucepan (or double boiler). Melt the chocolate chips in a metal bowl set above the water, stirring occasionally.

3 Place mini paper liners inside the muffin cups. This helps with transport and keeps the chocolates from moving.

4 Using a mini pastry brush, coat each liner with a thin layer of chocolate, enough to cover the sides and bottom of the liner. Place the muffin pan in the freezer to set the chocolate.

5 Remove from the freezer. Spoon about 1 teaspoon of the peanut butter mixture into each cup. Fill it almost to the top, but leave room for some chocolate. Press down on the peanut butter to flatten it.

6 Carefully, using a teaspoon, drizzle chocolate over the top of the peanut butter, to cover. I like to take the chocolate in my hand to do this last step, tilting my hand around to get the chocolate to spread.

7 Refrigerate the cups until they are set. They keep, sealed and refrigerated, for 1 month or frozen for 3 months.

CONTINUED

› nail this

Make these when you have ample time and patience. They are super easy but take time to assemble.

If you're using natural peanut butter, which separates, transfer the whole jar into a mixing bowl, and mix to incorporate the oil and remove clumps. Do this every time you open a jar of peanut or almond butter so that it's ready and stirred. Same goes for tahini (page 273).

Don't skip the step of setting each layer in the freezer.

Do not use the back of a spoon to spread the chocolate because you want the top flat and smooth, without spoon marks. Just drizzle!

»› flip it

Use almond or cashew butter instead of peanut butter.

You can omit the coconut flour, if desired.

Use half dark chocolate and half white chocolate: dark on the bottom layer and white on the top.

Add chopped pretzels to the peanut butter filling, and sprinkle the top of the candies with salt. Yummy!

Leftover chocolate? Make chocolate bark! Stir chopped nuts into the melted chocolate, spread it on a baking sheet, and chill it in the fridge to set.

Pressed for time? Make truffles: Place the peanut butter filling in the fridge to harden. Remove it, and roll it into balls. Coat the balls in melted chocolate or cocoa powder.

CHOCOLATE CHIP COOKIE ICE CREAM SANDWICHES

STEPS: MIX, BAKE, ASSEMBLE, FREEZE! / Makes about 26 to 30 cookies or 12 to 15 ice cream sandwiches

How many more cookie recipes does one need? Just one. A flexible one. I've been testing these bad (good) boys for close to ten years, and they are the most amazing gluten-free, chewy cookie ever. But why stop at a cookie? Make ice cream cookie sandwiches with this genius method for getting your ice cream to fit perfectly inside a cookie—no mess involved. And you can use this flexible cookie dough to make pie crust, cookie bars, and more.

Tools: 2½-inch round cookie or biscuit cutter, for sandwiches

WET INGREDIENTS

1½ sticks (¾ cup) unsalted butter, at room temperature

½ cup packed dark brown sugar

½ cup granulated sugar

2 teaspoons vanilla extract

2 large eggs

DRY INGREDIENTS

2¼ cup all-purpose gluten-free flour

1 teaspoon baking soda

½ teaspoon xanthan gum (omit if already in flour)

Pinch of salt

1 cup dark chocolate chips

½ cup chopped pecans, toasted (optional)

4 pints ice cream (select a variety of flavors, e.g., vanilla, chocolate, coffee)

1 Make the cookies: Preheat the oven to 350°F. Line baking sheets with parchment paper.

2 In a large bowl, cream together the butter, sugars, and vanilla. Add the eggs, and beat well.

3 In a separate bowl, combine the flour, baking soda, xanthan gum if needed, and salt. Stir the blend into the wet mixture, then fold in the chocolate chips and nuts, if desired. The dough will be wet.

4 Use a spoon or a mini ice cream scoop to mound a heaping tablespoon (or 1½ tablespoons) of dough into your hand. Roll into a round. Repeat with the remaining dough. If making sandwiches, the baked cookies must be big enough to fit your cookie cutter (note that they will spread while baking). Arrange the rounds on a baking sheet, leaving space between them. Press them gently, until they're about ½ inch thick.

5 Bake the cookies until set and slightly underdone, about 8 to 10 minutes. Cool on a wire rack, then serve or freeze, if desired.

6 Make the ice cream sandwiches: Cut the cookies into rounds using the biscuit cutter. Pour the toppings into separate shallow bowls.

7 With a very sharp chef's knife, slice the pints of ice cream (including their containers) horizontally into 4 rounds, each about ¾ inch thick. Remove the paper, and cut the ice cream into smaller rounds, using the biscuit cutter. (Work quickly!)

CONTINUED

TOPPING IDEAS

Sprinkles

Chopped nuts

M&M's

Chopped chocolate-covered coffee or espresso beans

Toasted coconut

Melted chocolate

Mini butterscotch or caramel chips

Shaved white, milk, or dark chocolate

8 Slide each of the ice cream rounds onto a cut cookie, and top it with a second cookie to create a sandwich.

9 Roll each sandwich on its side in your chosen toppings. Serve. Or freeze, wrapping each sandwich individually in plastic wrap to keep well frozen.

› nail this

For ultra-chewy cookies, remove them from the oven before you think they're ready. The top will be set, but don't wait for browned edges—or you'll enter crunchy-cookie land.

The key to making these visually stunning is to cut the cookies and the ice cream using the same-sized cookie cutter, so the ice cream fits exactly onto the cookie.

Work quickly during assembly so the ice cream doesn't melt.

»› flip it

Swap chocolate chips with peanut butter chips or white chocolate chips. Cut up fancy chocolate-covered nuts to replace the chips; this version comes out divine.

Press half the batch of dough into a 10-inch springform pan and bake it to make a cookie-crust base (instead of a brownie base) for the Decadent Frozen Almond Brownie Pie (page 213).

Use the cookie dough to make small, edible bowls for serving ice cream. Press the dough into greased muffin tins, and bake for about 10 minutes or until set.

To lighten up your cookies, try this flour combo: 1½ cups all-purpose gluten-free flour plus ¾ cup almond flour.

Dip half of each sandwich in melted chocolate—glorious.

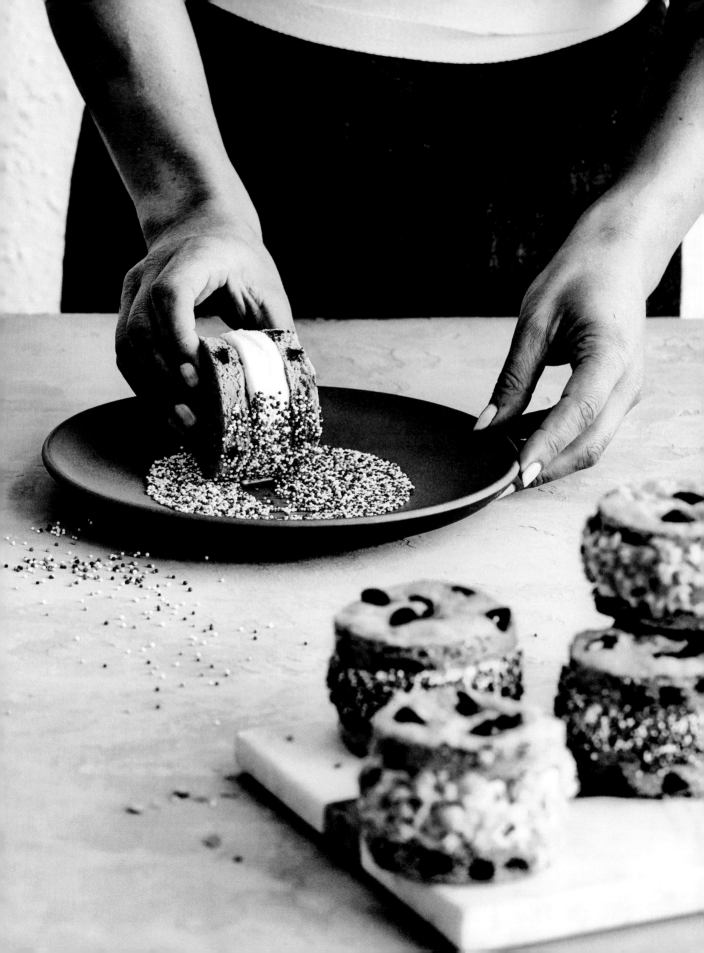

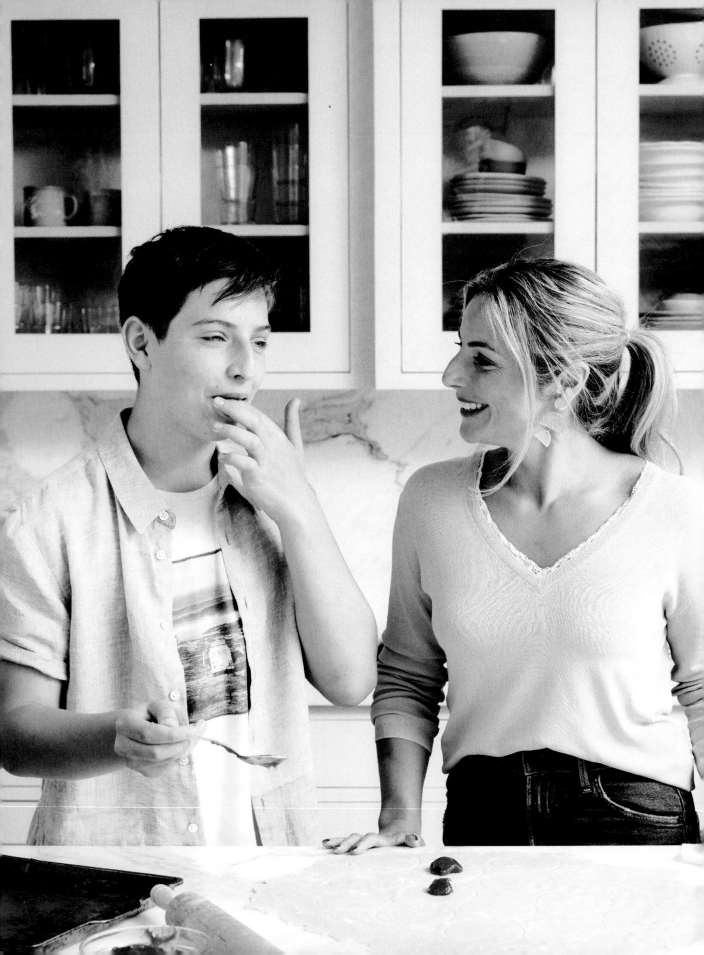

ROCKIN' RASPBERRY HAMENTASCHEN

STEPS: MIX, SHAPE, FILL, BAKE! / **Makes 45 hamentaschen**

My friend Michal taught me how to make hamentaschen nearly twenty years ago on the Jewish holiday of Purim, when the task of rolling and shaping the popular triangle-shaped filled cookie treat seemed far too daunting—especially as a new mom to a five-month-old. Michal's recipe is foolproof, her method precise—and, as it turns out, it's also supremely flexible. Over the years, I've adjusted it slightly and made it gluten free, but the deliciousness of the original remains. You can make infinite varieties of filling, and the dough is great for everything from pie crusts to endless cookie variations.

Tools: Electric mixer (optional), 3-inch round cookie cutter, wire cooling racks

RASPBERRY FILLING

1 cup seedless raspberry jam

1½ teaspoons cornstarch

1 teaspoon vanilla extract

Zest of 1 lemon

DRY INGREDIENTS FOR DOUGH

2½ cups all-purpose gluten-free flour, plus more for rolling

2 teaspoons baking powder

½ teaspoon xanthan gum (omit if already in flour)

½ teaspoon salt

WET INGREDIENTS FOR DOUGH

½ cup butter or coconut oil, at room temperature

1 cup granulated sugar

1 large egg

2 teaspoons vanilla extract

2 tablespoons orange juice

1 Make the raspberry filling: In a bowl, stir together all the filling ingredients. Stir well to incorporate, getting rid of all lumps. Refrigerate to set while you make the dough.

2 Preheat the oven to 350°F. Assemble a rolling pin, plastic wrap, a 3-inch round cookie cutter, and baking sheets lined with parchment paper.

3 Carefully measure all the dry ingredients, and whisk together in a medium bowl. Set aside.

4 Cream the butter and sugar together with an electric mixer in a separate large bowl. Add the egg and vanilla, and beat to combine.

5 Add the orange juice and the dry ingredients, alternately, to the wet batter. This step helps prevent the dry ingredients from flying everywhere during mixing. Stop the electric mixer when the dough is 90 percent combined, then finish mixing by hand, just until all is incorporated to avoid overmixing. Refrigerate the dough for 10 minutes.

6 Clean and dry your countertops well, and, if desired, cover them with plastic wrap or a silicone pastry mat. Keep a bit of flour nearby to lightly dust the rolling surface and to add to the dough if it is too sticky. Be careful not to add too much flour because you want the dough sticky enough to pinch together. If your dough is a tad gummy, you can cover it with plastic wrap before rolling—this method works really well.

CONTINUED

TOPPING
Confectioners' sugar
(optional)

7 Roll out the dough to about ¼ inch thick, or as thin as you can while still being able to work with it. Sometimes on your first batch you'll realize you rolled the dough too thin or too thick. Adjust the next batch accordingly.

8 Cut the dough into rounds with a 3-inch cookie cutter. Spoon about 1 teaspoon of the chilled raspberry filling into the center of each. Fold the edges of the dough toward the center to create three sides of a triangle, and pinch the edges together to seal tightly, leaving a very small amount of filling exposed in the middle. Transfer the cookies to the prepared baking sheets, spacing them 1½ inches apart.

9 Bake for 10 minutes, or until just set and barely golden on the bottom. Allow to cool for 1 minute, then use a spatula to transfer the cookies to wire cooling racks. Let cool completely.

10 Dust the cookies with confectioners' sugar, if desired, before serving.

> *nail this*

Make the dough the night before you bake the cookies. Roll it into a large disc, cover it with plastic wrap, and place it in the refrigerator. Remove the dough from the fridge two hours before rolling.

I like my hamentaschen soft, so I underbake them. If you prefer yours a tad crunchier, bake them for a few extra minutes.

You'll be tempted at first to roll the dough too thick—don't! These cookies are more delicate and light when the dough is thinner. But if the dough is too thin, it will fall apart when you try to pinch it into a triangle, so find the sweet spot.

This dough is forgiving; you can roll it and reroll it multiple times, and it still rolls beautifully.

>> *flip it*

Swap out the orange juice with almond milk.

Cut the cookies with the top of a wine glass or drinking glass if you don't have a cookie cutter.

For lemon curd hamentaschen: Use the curd from my lemon mousse recipe (page 233) as the filling. It produces a flatter cookie that opens up more in the center, but it is delicious.

For date hamentaschen: Make the date filling from my Date-Bar Bites (page 229).

This dough is my go-to pie crust. Not only can you roll it but you can also press it into a pan. Or make sugar cookies, using different-shaped cookie cutters.

DATE-BAR BITES

STEPS: BOIL, MIX, LAYER, BAKE! / **Makes 32 to 36 squares**

Dates and oats marry happily in this old-fashioned, childhood-favorite bar treat. Use the delectable date filling for hamentaschen, and the crust to top other breads and muffins. Slice the bars into mini bites, and serve them with a scoop of vanilla ice cream, or as a component of a well-presented fruit and cookie platter.

Tools: 13 × 9-inch baking pan

FILLING
1 pound Medjool dates (or other moist date), pitted and chopped

¼ cup maple syrup

Juice and zest of 1 orange

⅔ cup coarsely chopped raw walnuts or pecans

1 teaspoon ground cinnamon

1 teaspoon vanilla extract

CRUST AND TOPPING
1¾ cups all-purpose gluten-free flour

1½ cups old-fashioned rolled oats

1 cup packed dark brown sugar

¾ cup coconut oil, at room temperature

½ teaspoon baking soda

⅛ teaspoon salt

1 Make the filling: In a saucepan over medium-high heat, combine the dates with ½ cup water, maple syrup, and orange juice. Bring to a boil.

2 Remove the pan from the heat, and stir in the orange zest, nuts, cinnamon, and vanilla. Set aside.

3 Preheat the oven to 350°F. Grease the baking pan or line it with parchment paper.

4 Make the crust and topping: In a food processor, mix together all the crust ingredients until the combination is crumbly but still holds together.

5 Press ⅔ of the dough into the baking pan (reserve ⅓ for the topping).

6 Spread the filling evenly over the crust. Sprinkle the remaining ⅓ of the topping over the filling. Bake for 30 minutes, or until lightly golden.

7 Cool completely, then refrigerate it until cold (to make the cutting easier). Cut into 1½-inch squares.

> nail this

Before serving, invert the pan to transfer the bars to a cutting board.

You'll notice that other recipes for baked items usually call for melted coconut oil. Since this is going in a food processor and it's for a crumble, don't melt the oil—just soften it.

>> flip it

If you don't have a food processor, use quick-cooking oats, melt the coconut oil, and mix by hand.

PUMPKIN AND WHITE-CHOCOLATE COOKIES

STEPS: WHISK, BAKE, MELT, DIP! / **Makes 36 cookies**

One of my favorite childhood memories is returning home from school to the smell of freshly baked cookies. To this day, my mom bakes her classic soft and chewy, cake-textured pumpkin spice cookies. Here's my spin, a you-wouldn't-know-it's-good-for-you version that mimics Mom's original recipe. I purposely avoid oversweetening these cookies because after they are baked they get dipped in white chocolate. If you prefer a sweeter cookie (yes please, says my daughter), add some extra maple syrup or a few tablespoons of sugar.

Tools: Parchment, wire cooling racks

DRY INGREDIENTS

1 cup all-purpose gluten-free flour

½ cup sorghum flour

½ cup tapioca starch or potato flour

¼ cup granulated sugar

1½ teaspoons baking powder

1½ teaspoons pumpkin pie spice

1 teaspoon ground cinnamon

1 teaspoon baking soda

½ teaspoon xanthan gum (omit if already in flour)

¼ teaspoon salt

WET INGREDIENTS

1 cup puréed fresh pumpkin or canned pumpkin

¾ cup butter or coconut oil, at room temperature

½ cup maple syrup

2 large eggs

1 tablespoon vanilla extract

TOPPING

1 10-ounce bag white chocolate chips

1 cup chopped pecans, toasted

1 Preheat the oven to 350°F. Grease a baking sheet with oil spray, or cover it with parchment.

2 Whisk together all the dry ingredients in a large bowl.

3 Separately, with an electric mixer or a whisk, beat together the wet ingredients. Fold the wet mixture into the dry ingredients.

4 Using a tablespoon, scoop the dough into balls. Use your hands to coax them into rounds. The dough will be a little sticky.

5 Arrange the dough balls on the prepared baking sheet, and bake for 10 minutes or until the cookies are set. Cool them on a wire rack.

6 For the topping: Boil a few inches of water in a saucepan (or double boiler). Melt the white chocolate in a bowl set over the pan, stirring occasionally. Dip each cookie halfway into the melted white chocolate, turning to complete the coverage. Use as much as you like, and coat as much of the cookie as you desire. You can also just drizzle the white chocolate on top.

7 While the chocolate is still gooey, sprinkle the pecans on top. Allow them to cool completely on parchment-lined baking sheets or a cooling rack.

> *nail this*

The absolute key to success is to avoid overbaking these—you don't want them to be dry.

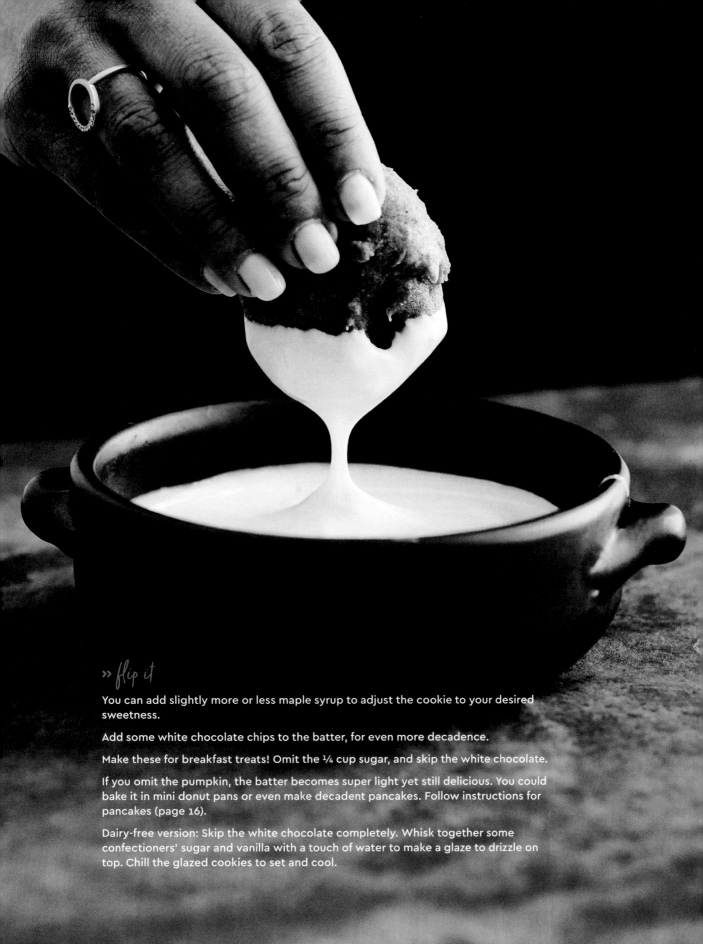

» flip it

You can add slightly more or less maple syrup to adjust the cookie to your desired sweetness.

Add some white chocolate chips to the batter, for even more decadence.

Make these for breakfast treats! Omit the ¼ cup sugar, and skip the white chocolate.

If you omit the pumpkin, the batter becomes super light yet still delicious. You could bake it in mini donut pans or even make decadent pancakes. Follow instructions for pancakes (page 16).

Dairy-free version: Skip the white chocolate completely. Whisk together some confectioners' sugar and vanilla with a touch of water to make a glaze to drizzle on top. Chill the glazed cookies to set and cool.

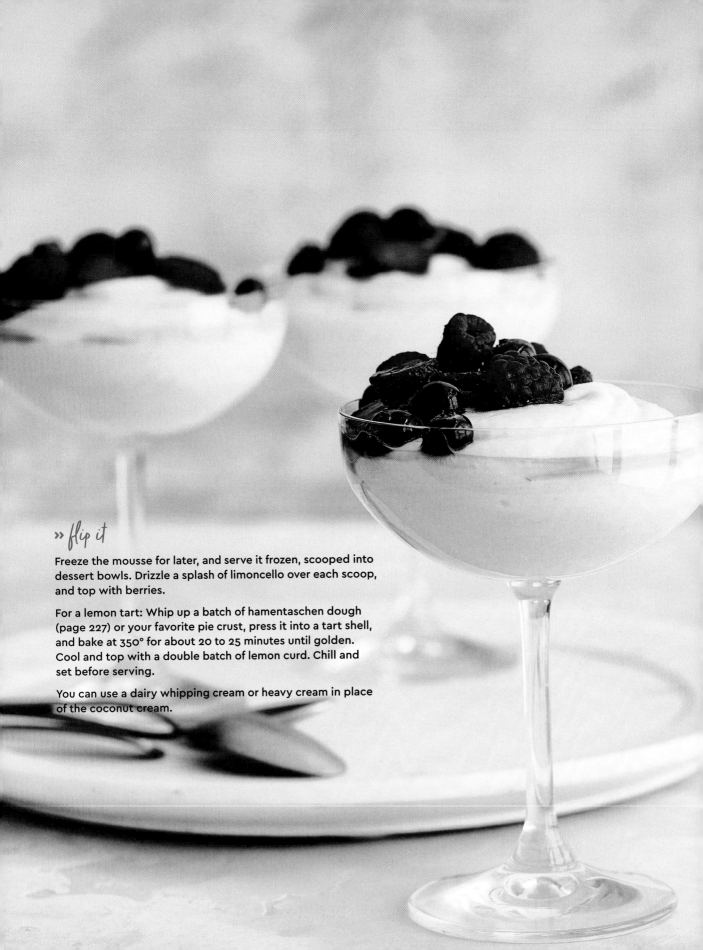

» flip it

Freeze the mousse for later, and serve it frozen, scooped into dessert bowls. Drizzle a splash of limoncello over each scoop, and top with berries.

For a lemon tart: Whip up a batch of hamentaschen dough (page 227) or your favorite pie crust, press it into a tart shell, and bake at 350° for about 20 to 25 minutes until golden. Cool and top with a double batch of lemon curd. Chill and set before serving.

You can use a dairy whipping cream or heavy cream in place of the coconut cream.

LIGHTENED-UP LEMON MOUSSE WITH DRUNKEN BERRIES

STEPS: WHISK, CHILL, BEAT, FOLD, MARINATE! / **Makes 8 to 10 servings**

Ah, the simplicity and lightness of lemon mousse and berries! Sometimes (and especially) after a big meal, the last thing you want is a heavy dessert, and this delicate mousse fits the bill. It's creamy, super citrusy, and no fancier than jazzed-up lemon curd—whipped with egg whites and coconut cream—topped with limoncello-infused berries. For all you lemon lovers, this mousse will be love at first lick.

Tools: Electric mixer

LEMON CURD

½ cup (1 stick) unsalted butter or ½ cup coconut oil

¾ cup granulated sugar

2 large eggs, plus
2 large egg yolks (whites reserved for mousse)

6 tablespoons fresh lemon juice

1 packed tablespoon grated lemon zest

Pinch of salt

LEMON MOUSSE

1 batch lemon curd

2 large egg whites (reserved from above)

¾ cup drained coconut cream, well chilled (solids only)

DRUNKEN BERRIES

1 cup raspberries

1 cup blueberries

1 cup sliced strawberries

⅓ cup limoncello

1 Make the lemon curd: In a medium saucepan over medium-low heat, combine all the curd ingredients, and cook, whisking, until thickened, about 5 minutes. Be sure to whisk constantly so the curd doesn't curdle. Once the mixture starts to boil, continue whisking and boiling for 1 minute, to thicken it further. Allow it to cool completely, then refrigerate it to set, at least 3 hours.

2 Make the mousse: In a bowl, using a hand or stand mixer, beat the egg whites until soft peaks form, 3 to 5 minutes. If they don't form massive peaks, don't worry—they will firm up as they chill. In a separate bowl, beat the coconut cream until soft peaks form, 3 to 5 minutes.

3 Assemble the mousse: Add the whipped coconut cream to the cooled curd, and beat until incorporated, about 1 minute. Using a spatula, fold the beaten egg whites into the curd mixture until they're fully incorporated.

4 Make the berries: Mix together the raspberries, blueberries, and strawberries in a medium bowl, and stir in the limoncello. Marinate in the refrigerator for a few minutes or up to 1 hour (they will absorb more alcohol the longer they sit—your call).

5 To serve: Divide the mousse into 8 to 10 martini or champagne glasses, spooning a few tablespoons into each. Transfer them back to the fridge until ready to top with berries and serve, or immediately top with berries and serve.

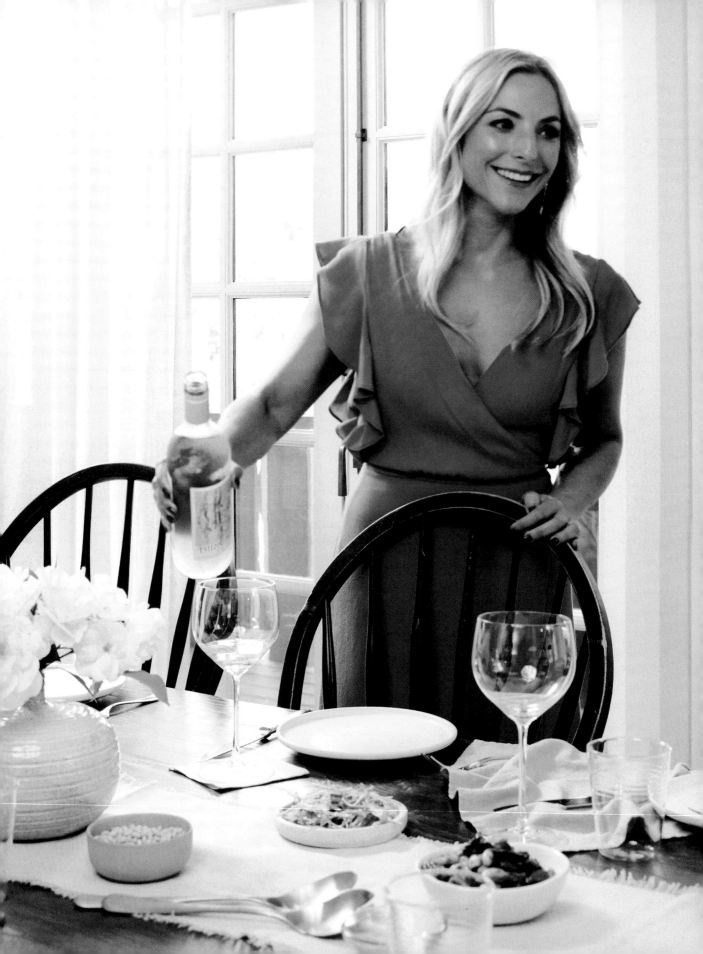

Chapter 9

DRINKS AND NIBBLES FOR FRIENDS

Some of our most cherished, magical moments happen at home with good friends, a drink in one hand and a nibble in the other. Entertaining is a great way to build and deepen friendships. Barriers fall, conversation flows, and real connections are made. I used to fuss when friends came over, stressing out to make perfect home-cooked bites. But I've since learned that people are just thrilled to be welcomed, home-cooking or not. I know that dinner parties can sometimes feel intimidating to host. It's okay; you'll get there. Why not take the pressure off and plan for a casual get-together instead? Invite friends over for a drink, a predinner bite, or a weekend hello. In this chapter, I've shared my most coveted and delectable foods—dishes that pass the finger-food test and drinks that make the evening a fun celebration. If you're looking for more inspiration, head over to the small plates chapter—every one of those recipes is interchangeable as party food and doesn't require a fork (my personal prerequisite for effortless stand-up hosting).

Flexible Hosting with Flair

Hosting a dinner party can be daunting and time-consuming. Between the planning, shopping, and chopping, the person who usually gets squeezed is you. But with a few simple preparation tricks, you'll be able to put on your party hat and host an uncomplicated party your guests will never forget.

Plan a smart menu.

Plan your menu around your life, not your life around your menu. Think of how much time you have and what ingredients are available in your pantry. Grocery shop and make sure you balance more time-consuming main dishes with easier things, like salads and sides. Don't take on more than you can handle.

Cook and freeze things ahead of time.

Consider making your dessert in advance and freezing it. You can also make salad dressings a few days before the big event, and chop your veggies in advance. Do as much as you can as early as you can.

Set your table the night before.

Set the table when you have downtime. Lay out serving dishes and serving utensils for each dish, and if you're planning a big feast label each bowl with what's going in it (in case you're like me and forget those sorts of details). If you're serving buffet style, arrange your table early with any decorations or food labels you might want to use.

Make your home a sanctuary.

Create a playlist of mood-appropriate songs in advance, light candles, set out flowers, and get your house ready to greet your guests. If you don't entertain a lot, it can be hard to have friends in your personal space. Get over it, though, because people are just happy to come over for home-cooked food. It doesn't have to be perfect.

Plan your seating.

I always find it stressful when I have a slew of dinner guests and haven't thought about where everyone is going to sit—it can sometimes get awkward. Take the guesswork out of it for everybody, and get creative with place cards for each guest. Personalizing the seating makes guests feel welcome and at ease.

Enjoy a glass of wine during meal prep.

Cooking is way more fun with music and wine. Pour yourself (and whoever you've enlisted to help you in the kitchen) a glass. Or, if you plan well, take your glass to the bathtub, and soak in some bubbles before your feast. You'll arrive as a mellowed-out, happy hostess!

If all else fails, fake it.

Just because you host the party doesn't mean you need to make everything from scratch. Check out my cheats and hacks on page 151. Doctor up some store-bought goodies like guacamole, hummus, or other spreads and dips. Boil some frozen edamame. Buy the bread. Mix and match pre-prepared dishes with a few homemade ones—and if you pour your guests a glass or two of champagne before they eat, they may never even notice!

LYCHEE MOJITO YOUR WAY

STEPS: FREEZE, BLEND OR STIR, CUSTOMIZE! / **Makes 2 to 4 drinks**

This crowd-pleasing drink will wow your guests and calm their worries. Warning: Sipping on this cocktail may transport you to your favorite island. The recipe below is the way I like my mojito, but I urge you to play with the balance of alcohol, sugar, acid, and mint to arrive at your perfect sip. Make these mojitos in advance (and drink one first) so that when your guests arrive you're greeting them with a smile instead of slaving over the blender.

Tools: Blender, martini or cocktail glasses

8 to 10 lychees (about half of a 20-ounce can), or use fresh ones!

½ cup lychee liqueur

½ cup light rum

⅓ cup fresh lime juice

A few sprigs of fresh mint, chopped, plus more for garnish

1 cup crushed ice

1 12-ounce can soda water, chilled

Lime wedges, for garnish

1 Drain the lychees, reserving the syrup. Freeze the lychees until hardened. (In a pinch skip this step if you must.)

2 When the lychees are frozen, place 8 to 10 of them in the blender along with the liqueur, rum, lime juice, and chopped mint leaves. Blend, but don't overdo it! Keep a few chunks in there. This is your base mixture.

3 For a frozen version: Add the desired amount of ice to the blender, and blend with the base mixture. Start with ½ cup of ice if you prefer the drink stronger; more ice will dilute it.

4 For a nonfrozen version: Pour soda water into a glass, and add the desired amount of base mixture. Stir in some ice.

5 Adjust the flavors: If you prefer your drink sweeter, add a touch of the canned lychee syrup. If you prefer it both stronger and sweeter, add more lychee liqueur. Adding more lime will make it more sour, and adding ice will dilute the strength.

6 Garnish each glass with 2 lychees, a sprig of mint, and a wheel of lime on the edge.

» flip it

Make it virgin: omit the alcohol.

Swap lychee for mango, pineapple, passion fruit, strawberry. For an awesome hack, make puréed-fruit ice cubes (page 266).

If you don't have the time to freeze the lychees and need this drink now, just blend it with a bit of extra ice.

You can prepare the mix ahead of time and freeze it for an hour or two to have a slushy base when guests arrive.

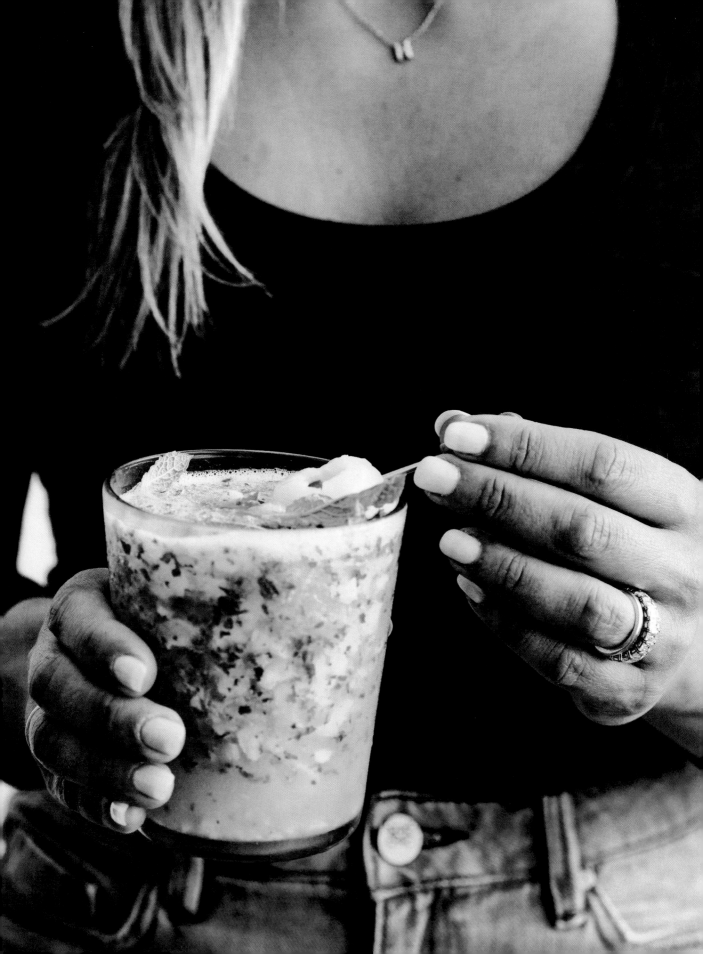

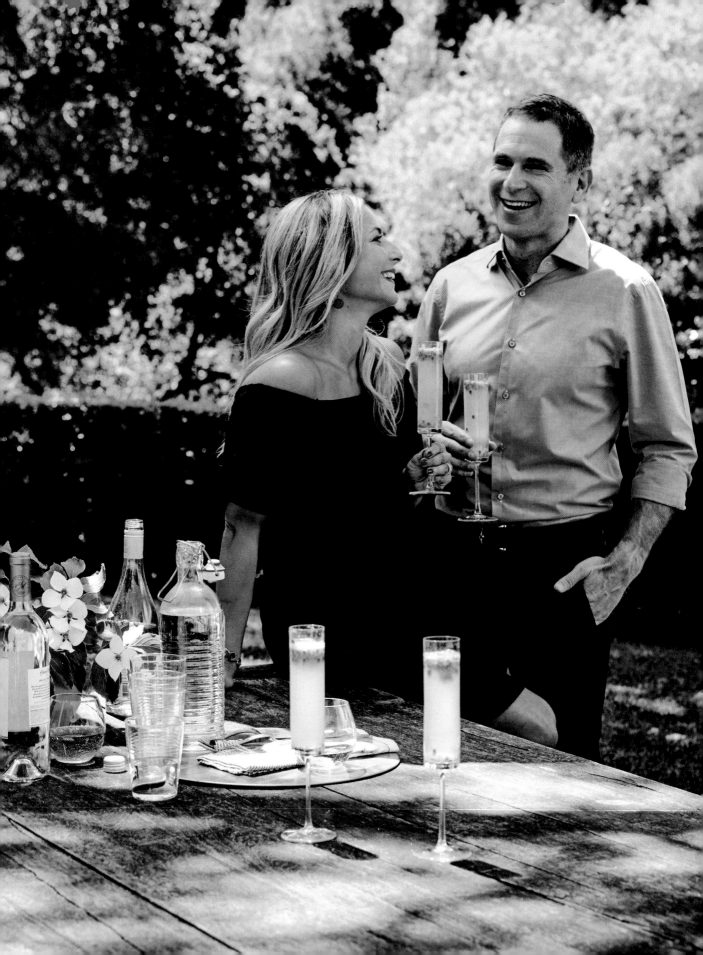

PASSION FRUIT BUBBLY

STEPS: SCOOP, STIR, BUBBLE! / **Makes 6 drinks**

Seth and I love to serve and sip on this elegant drink to add passion to any party. Tart and textured passion fruit is balanced by peach liqueur, then finished with prosecco or champagne. Serve this at your next party, and it won't even matter how good the rest of your food tastes.

6 to 8 fresh passion fruits

½ to ¾ cup peach liqueur

1 750 ml bottle prosecco, chilled

1 Set out 6 champagne glasses. Slice the passion fruits open, and scoop the meat from one passion fruit into each glass, about 3 teaspoons per serving—or less, depending on how much passion you like in your drinks!

2 Add 1 to 2 tablespoons of peach liqueur to each glass, or more depending on how sweet you like it.

3 Top with the desired amount of prosecco, and serve.

> *nail this*

These are always better if you taste as you go.

>> *flip it*

Swap lychee liqueur for the peach liqueur—love the tropical flavor!

Use as much or as little liqueur or prosecco as you like to balance sweet/strong.

No passion? No problem! Try this with ripe mango pieces or pineapple instead.

Virgin: Mix sparkling grape or apple juice with the passion fruit. Or try sparkling water for a less sweet option.

Make puréed mango, passion fruit, and pineapple ice cubes (page 266).

SPARKLING FRUIT SPRITZER

STEPS: SQUEEZE, STIR, SPLASH! / **Makes 2 drinks**

Ah, the perfection of a fruity soda! I prefer mine unsweetened, but if you like yours sweet, add a touch of juice or an indulgent splash of fruity liqueur. This drink tastes like an over-the-top fresh lime soda and makes for an impressive beverage to serve friends. Can't find guava or fresh mango? Who cares? Add whatever fruit makes you happy. This fruity refresher keeps on giving; just add soda water—the longer it sits the more aromatic it gets.

4 slices orange

2 small limes, cut in half

6 thin slices guava or mango

4 strawberries

4 slices pineapple

2 small handfuls fresh mint, stems on

1 12-ounce can soda water, chilled

2 splashes fruit juice, limoncello, or fruit liqueur (optional)

1 Squeeze the juice from the orange and limes into two tall (highball) glasses; divide the rinds between the glasses.

2 To each glass, add 3 slices guava or mango, 2 strawberries, 2 slices pineapple, and a small handful of mint, and stir together.

3 Top each glass with soda water, and add an optional splash of fruit juice—or spike each glass with limoncello or liqueur.

» flip it

Create a flavored-sparkling-water bar with a variety of fruits to squeeze or stir in, soda presented in a decorative pitcher, and an array of juices or alcohols to choose from for the final splash!

Vodka, rum, or a sugary liqueur like peach brandy make for great spiked-soda options.

Serve with iced-tea spoons to make it easy to retrieve the fruit from the glass once the liquid is gone.

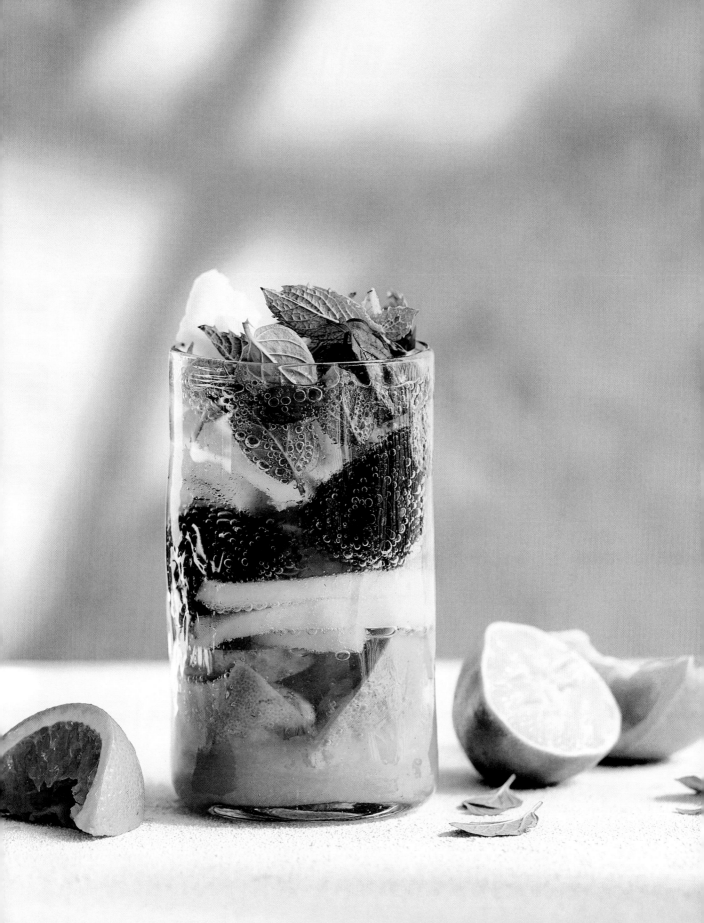

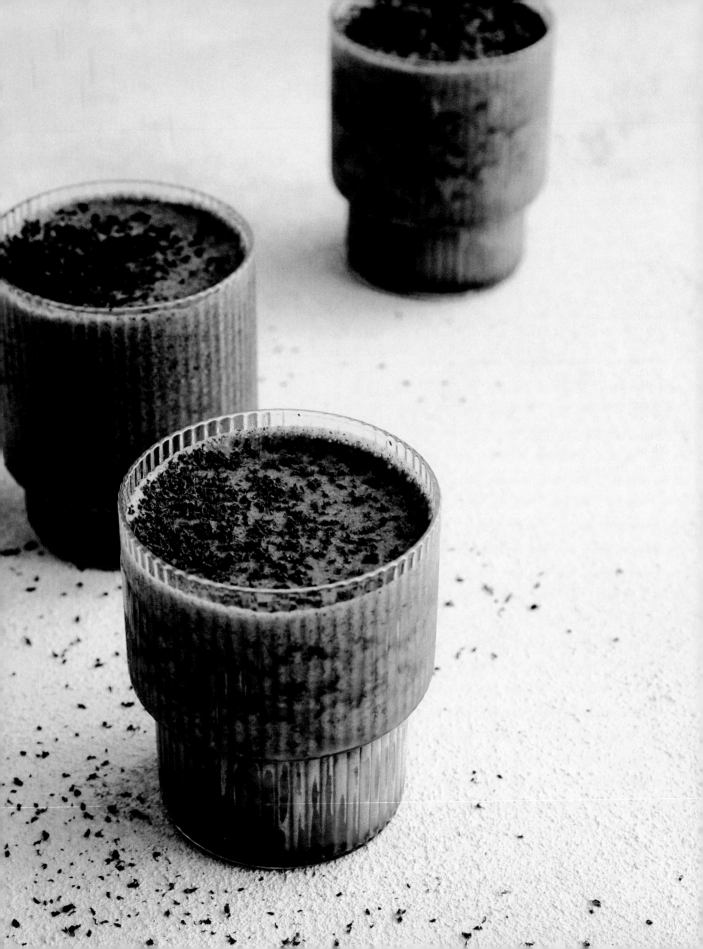

CREAMY COFFEE BOMB

STEPS: FREEZE, BLEND, SIP! / **Makes 4 servings**

This boozy frozen milkshake is truly the bomb. With only five sinfully indulgent ingredients and a slew of flexible options you really can't go wrong. Serve it as a party drink, or freeze and dish it into small glasses as a coffee granita with chocolate shavings for dessert.

Tools: Blender

4 coconut milk ice cubes (page 266), or use ⅓ can (½ cup) full-fat coconut milk

4 espresso ice cubes (about ½ cup of brewed coffee before freezing)

½ cup espresso vodka or coffee tequila

2 tablespoons chocolate chips

Chocolate shavings, to garnish

1 Place the coconut milk ice cubes, espresso ice cubes, espresso vodka or coffee tequila, and chocolate chips in a blender, and blend until smooth.

2 Divide between 4 glasses (each with a straw), and serve immediately. Or transfer to a container and freeze. When ready to serve, use a spoon to transfer the mixture to a party glass, and top with shaved chocolate.

» *flip it*

Transform this into a coffee granita and serve it for dessert, frozen with extra chocolate for a boozy, caffeinated treat.

CHEESY CAULIFLOWER POPPERS

STEPS: STEAM, MIX, COAT, BAKE! / **Makes 30 to 40 poppers**

Holy wowzers! The idea for these yummy, creamy, and crunchy mouthfuls came to me as I was menu planning for my five-year-old's birthday party. I was looking for healthy finger food that both kids and adults would devour, and this recipe went beyond satisfying that criterion—it blew everyone's socks off! Make these for your next party or to take to a potluck, or serve a few as a side dish for a meal.

Tools: Food processor, small scoop (optional)

Olive oil, for greasing pan

1 medium head cauliflower (about 2 pounds 6 ounces), cored and cut into florets

½ medium yellow onion, cut into chunks

2 garlic cloves, crushed

1 teaspoon sriracha sauce (optional)

¾ teaspoon salt

¼ teaspoon freshly ground black pepper

1 cup shredded Cheddar cheese

¾ cup almond flour

2 large eggs, beaten

COATING

½ cup Gluten-Free Cracker Crumbs (page 276)

½ cup grated Parmesan cheese

Salt and freshly ground black pepper, to taste

1 Preheat the oven to 400°F. Generously oil a large baking pan.

2 Bring about 2 cups of water to a boil in a medium to large pot fitted with a steamer. Steam the cauliflower until slightly softened, about 7 minutes.

3 Place the onion and garlic into the bowl of a food processor, and pulse briefly to combine. Add the cauliflower, in batches if needed, and pulse until crumb-like in consistency.

4 Add the sriracha, if desired, and the salt and pepper. Pulse briefly to combine.

5 Transfer the mixture to a bowl. Add the Cheddar and the almond flour, and combine well. Taste the dough for seasoning, then mix in the eggs.

6 To make the coating, stir together the cracker crumbs, Parmesan, and salt and pepper in a shallow bowl and set aside.

7 Place the oiled pan in the oven to heat it. If the steps below take you more than 10 minutes, check on the pan so the oil doesn't burn.

8 To make the poppers, I like to create an assembly line with the bowl of dough, the bowl of coating, and a sheet of parchment paper. Roll a heaping tablespoon (about a generous-sized mouthful) of dough in the coating, then place on the parchment. Repeat until all the dough is used up.

CONTINUED

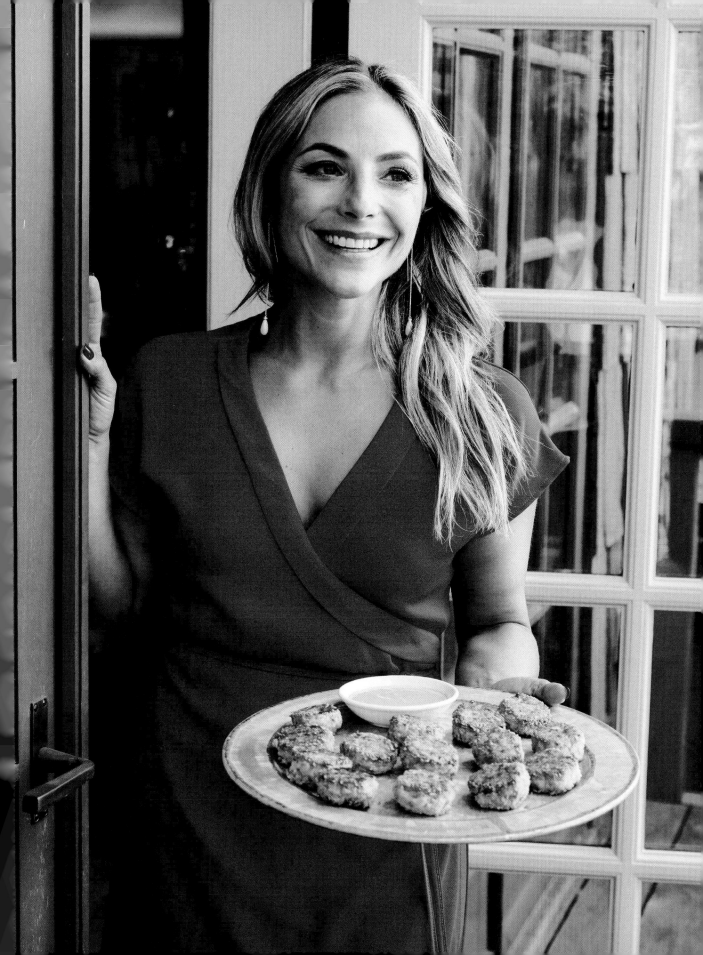

9 Remove the hot pan from the oven (be careful!). Arrange the coated poppers on the hot pan, and return them to the oven. Bake until golden, about 15 minutes, then flip them and continue cooking until all sides are golden-brown, about 15 minutes more. Gauge the timing based on your oven, and check frequently. These are best eaten immediately, but you can make them ahead and warm them in a hot oven to recrisp them.

> *nail this*

Every cauliflower is different. You need roughly 5 cups of florets. If yours is a smaller or larger cauliflower, adjust the seasonings accordingly.

>> *flip it*

For outrageous cauliflower fritters, add 4 eggs to the batter. Omit the coating. Lightly oil a skillet, and follow the instructions for frying Guiltless Zucchini Fritters (page 198).

Save some cauliflower florets and roast them simply with olive oil, salt, and Parmesan cheese.

Flip the coating—use crushed cornflakes, bread crumbs, almond flour, or ground nuts.

CARROT CROQUETTES

STEPS: STIR-FRY, CHILL, DIP, ROLL, FRY! / **Makes about 40 (8 appetizer servings)**

These curried carrot nibbles of heaven are crispy on the outside and perfectly soft and creamy on the inside. They are small enough to enjoy as a single bite but satisfying enough to coat your stomach for that extra glass of wine. They are what you'd call in Yiddish a *patchka*—which to me translates as a labor of love, but for special friends they're worth the effort. I can't make enough of these, and in twenty years I've never had one left for kitchen snacking after the party. Bummer for me.

Tools: Wok or deep frying pan, small scoop (optional)

6 tablespoons unsalted butter or olive oil, divided

2 cups shredded carrots

1 small yellow onion, finely chopped

1 garlic clove, minced

1½ teaspoons curry powder

1½ teaspoons salt

¼ teaspoon ground coriander

Dash of cayenne

¼ cup all-purpose gluten-free flour

1 cup whole milk

2 large eggs, yolks and whites separated

1½ cups cornflake crumbs (page 152)

¼ cup olive oil, for frying

1 Heat 4 tablespoons of butter in a wok or deep frying pan over medium-high heat. Add the carrot, onion, garlic, curry powder, salt, coriander, and cayenne. Cook, stirring, until the vegetables are tender, about 3 minutes.

2 Add the remaining 2 tablespoons of butter; stir in the flour until well blended. Remove the pan from the heat, and gradually stir in the milk.

3 Return the pan to medium-low heat, and cook the mixture, stirring constantly, until thickened, about 3 minutes. Add the 2 egg yolks and cook, stirring, just until bubbly, about 3 minutes. Reserve the whites for later.

4 Spread the mixture evenly onto an ungreased 8- or 9-inch square baking pan. Chill thoroughly, at least 3 hours or overnight. This helps set the carrot mixture so that the balls are easy to roll.

5 Put the 2 reserved egg whites in a shallow bowl and the cornflake crumbs in another shallow bowl.

6 Shape the chilled carrot mixture into 1-inch balls. Any bigger and they fall apart when cooking. Dip each ball into the egg whites, then roll it in the crumbs to coat completely.

CONTINUED

7 In a large frying pan coated with oil, fry the croquettes over medium heat in batches, turning them occasionally, until they are browned, 3 or 4 minutes. Remove them with a slotted spoon, and drain them on paper towels.

8 Serve immediately, or you can keep them warm in a 200°F oven until serving time. These can be made up to 2 days in advance and kept refrigerated. To reheat, arrange them in a single layer on a large baking sheet, and bake in a 375°F oven, uncovered, for 20 to 25 minutes, or until crisp.

> nail this

I always double this recipe. If I'm going to the trouble of making it, it pays to invest the time and have some extras handy in the freezer.

Don't attempt to form croquettes any larger than about 1 inch in diameter. And don't skip the chilling step because the carrot mixture needs to be firm to form the croquettes.

If you're prepping them in advance to fry the next day, cover the uncooked balls and refrigerate them overnight.

» flip it

Make these dairy free: swap the milk with a dairy-free milk and the butter with coconut oil.

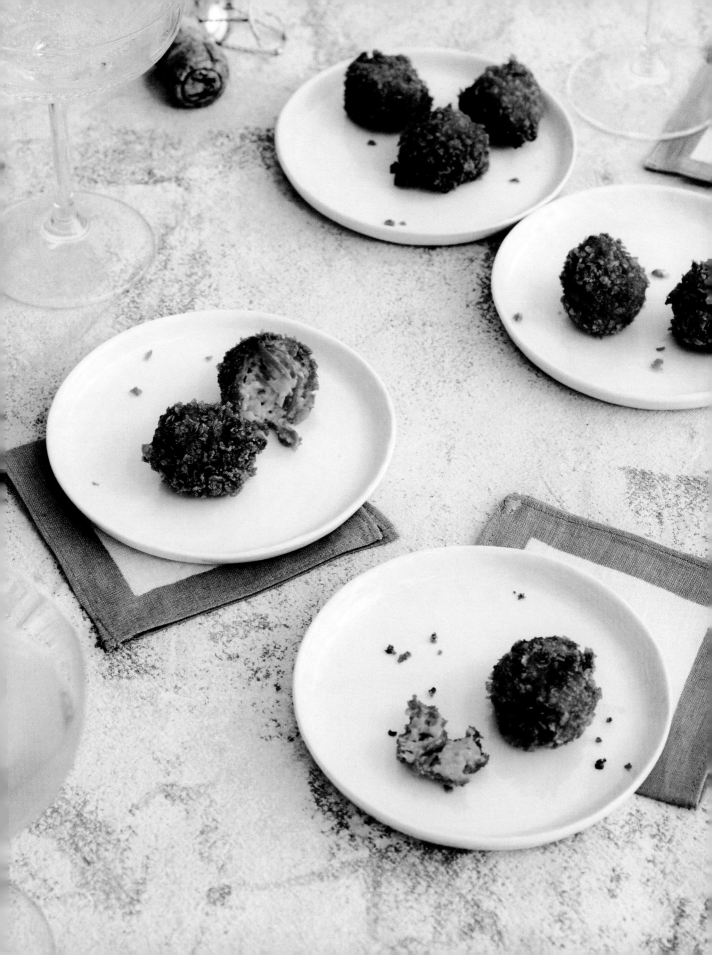

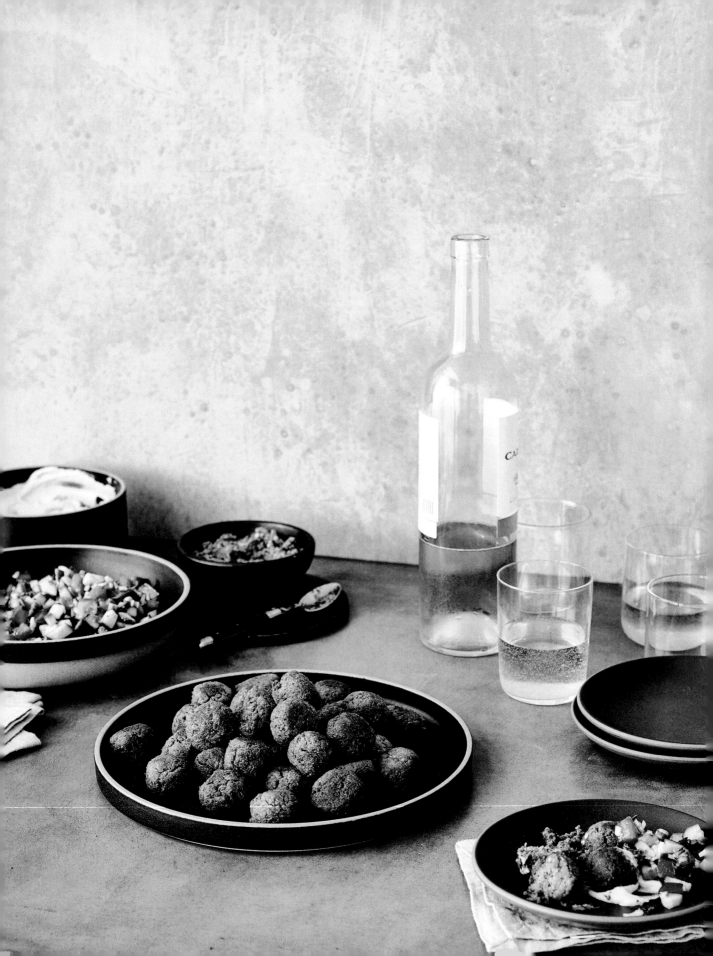

LEAN AND GREEN FALAFEL BITES

STEPS: BLEND, ROLL, BAKE! / **Makes 30 to 40 falafel balls**

It's hard to beat the real-deal, deep-fried falafel sold on every street corner in Israel. But I was determined to eliminate the fried mess at home while still maintaining the authentic crispy bite. I finally put my deep-fried versus oven-baked falafel balls to the test because I was not going to settle for second best. Lo and behold, after testing both, the oven-baked ones tasted better, stayed crispy longer, and rivaled my favorite street vendor's...uhhh...balls. Whoop! My secret is to preheat a fair bit of oil on a baking sheet until it sizzles, and then drop the falafel into the hot oil. Bonus: You won't smell like fried oil, risk an oil-splatter burn, or have to flip these falafel babies more than once. Score.

Tools: Food processor, rimmed baking sheet, small scoop (optional)

FALAFEL

1½ cups dried chickpeas

1 small onion, roughly chopped (about 1½ cups)

½ cup chopped fresh parsley

½ cup fresh baby spinach

5 garlic cloves

2 teaspoons cumin

1½ teaspoons salt

1 teaspoon ground coriander

Pinch of cayenne pepper, if desired

Freshly ground black pepper, to taste

Olive oil (about 1 cup), for oven-frying

1 In a large bowl, soak the chickpeas overnight in cold water.

2 Preheat the oven to 425°F.

3 Drain the chickpeas. Pulse in a food processor with the remaining falafel ingredients (except the oil), in batches if necessary, until well blended and finely chopped.

4 Roll the falafel dough into 1-inch balls; set aside.

5 Pour oil to a depth of ¼ inch on your baking sheet. This will seem like a lot, but it's necessary. Place the pan in the oven for 10 minutes or until the oil is sizzling (drop a tad of falafel dough on the pan to test).

6 Working quickly, line up the balls on the hot, oiled sheet pan (be careful of the hot oil). The falafel balls should sizzle.

7 Position the pan in the oven near the source of heat (top or bottom—not the middle of the oven).

8 Bake until the falafel balls are deep golden-brown (and look fried!), about 10 minutes, then turn them to finish browning, another 10 minutes. When done, transfer the balls to paper towels to absorb the oil.

CONTINUED

ISRAELI SALAD

3 large tomatoes, chopped

4 small Persian cucumbers, chopped

½ cup diced red onion

3 green onions, whites and greens chopped

Juice of one lemon

⅓ cup extra-virgin olive oil, or to taste

Handful of parsley, chopped (optional)

Handful of fresh mint, chopped (optional)

Salt and freshly ground black pepper, to taste

TO SERVE

1 16-ounce can or jar Israeli or kosher pickles

The Ultimate Flexible Tahini (page 273)

Green Schug (page 278; optional)

Leaves from 1 head butter lettuce

9 While the falafel is baking, make the salad: In a large bowl, combine the tomato, cucumber, red onion, green onion, lemon juice, and olive oil. Toss the mixture with the parsley and mint, then season with salt and pepper.

10 Serve the falafel with the bowl of Israeli salad, pickles, tahini, Green Schug if desired, and lettuce cups. Show your guests how to stuff a lettuce cup like they would a falafel in a pita.

› *nail this*

You might be tempted to use canned chickpeas instead of dried. Don't! It won't work. But you're not cooking the dried chickpeas anyway, so using canned isn't a time-saver.

You'll be tempted to skimp on the oil for the baking pan—again, don't. It's how the falafel sizzles and takes on that real-deal falafel flavor.

Watch the falafel carefully while it's cooking, and check the doneness by flipping one or two.

Placing them near the source of your oven's heat delivers the best result. If your oven has a setting to adjust the heat to the lower part, use that; the bottom of the falafel balls will sizzle first, just like they would if pan-frying.

» *flip it*

Serve Israeli salad on a stick! Skewer chunks of cucumber and halved cherry tomatoes to serve with the falafel.

You can completely play with the seasoning in the falafel dough, making it spicier or more robust, adding more or less parsley or spinach. Or omit the parsley altogether (my kids won't eat falafel that contains herbs, shame but true).

Pan-fry these, if you prefer.

UPGRADED BABA GHANOUSH

STEPS: ROAST, CHOP, MIX! / **Makes 6 to 8 servings, as a nibble**

Most baba ghanoush calls for charring the eggplant over a flame or broiling the eggplants and watching them diligently, so they can produce a smoky flavor. This version eliminates this step, and is mild and deliciously chunky but smooth on the palate. I go unorthodox here and use small Japanese eggplants, with their tender skins left on. Chop the eggplant by hand instead of using a food processor to maintain some chunks (and to save on washing dishes). The addition of parsley, pomegranates, and nuts make this a colorful celebration, perfect in a bowl, on a mezze platter, or spooned on top of cucumber rounds.

3 Japanese eggplants

Olive oil, for roasting

Salt and freshly ground black pepper, to taste

3 tablespoons tahini

2 tablespoons fresh lemon juice

2 garlic cloves, minced

¼ cup chopped parsley

¼ cup pomegranate seeds

Extra-virgin olive oil, for serving

Pine nuts, to garnish

Sliced cucumbers, for serving

1 Preheat the oven to 400°F. Lightly grease a baking sheet.

2 Slice the eggplants in half lengthwise, and arrange them on the baking sheet, skin-side up. Drizzle them with olive oil, season with salt and pepper, and roast for 30 minutes (longer if you use regular eggplants) or until the sides are charred and the eggplant is very soft and cooked all the way through. Remove the pan and allow the eggplants to cool.

3 In a large bowl, combine the tahini, lemon juice, 1 tablespoon of water, and garlic. Season with salt and pepper and whisk well.

4 Using a large chef's knife, finely chop the eggplants (leaving the skin on). Use the spine of the blade to mash the pieces together slightly. Transfer the eggplant to the bowl with the tahini mixture and stir well, using a spoon to achieve the desired consistency: slightly chunky rather than completely smooth. Taste and add more lemon, garlic, or salt if desired.

5 Stir in the parsley and pomegranate seeds. Or you could add only the parsley, reserving the pomegranate seeds to use as a garnish.

6 If serving in a bowl, drizzle with oil and garnish with pine nuts. For pretty party bites, spoon some baba ghanoush on top of a cucumber round. Garnish with more pomegranate seeds, parsley, and pine nuts to make it look pretty and colorful.

CONTINUED

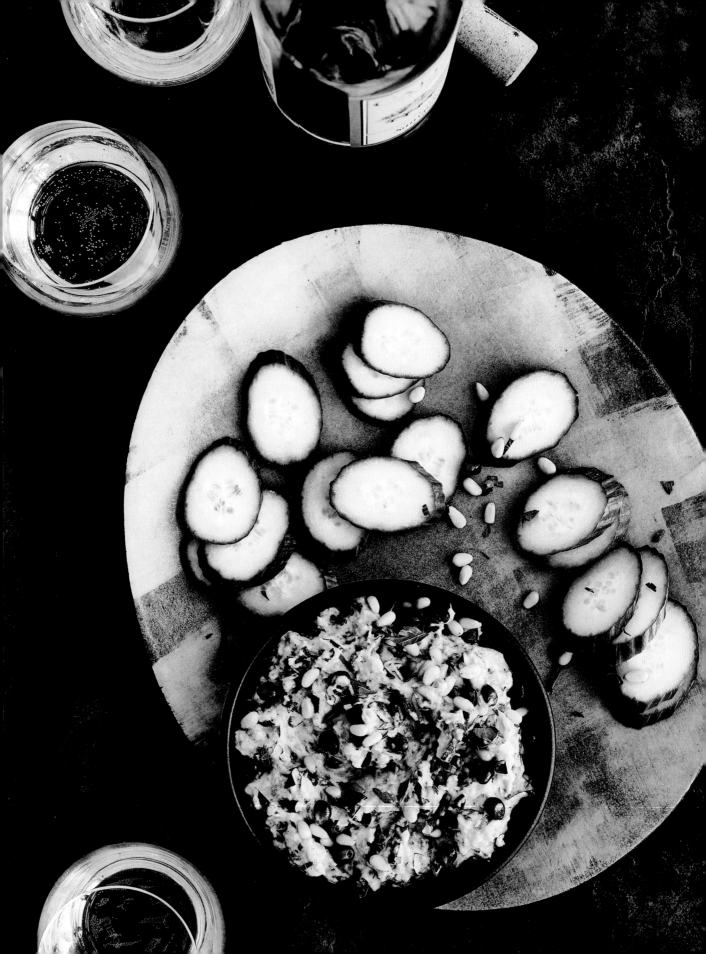

› nail this

This recipe produces a slightly lemony and garlicky dip. Taste and season as you go—you might want to start with less garlic and then add more if it's needed.

The dip is best eaten immediately. If it sits for a little while, mix thoroughly and taste to adjust the seasoning.

Make sure the eggplant has no hard spots when you remove it from the oven. It should be soft and easily choppable.

»» flip it

Japanese eggplants are long and skinny and lighter purple in color. They have mini seeds, and the skin is soft enough to eat. You can use a larger, darker eggplant; if you do, cook it for a few extra minutes to ensure softness, and peel it once it's cooled and before chopping, as the skin tends to be tough.

If you prefer, cook the eggplant more traditionally, with tongs over an open stovetop flame until the skin is charred and easily removable and the flesh soft. Cool, remove the skin, and proceed as described in the recipe.

SPICED BEEF LOLLIPOPS

STEPS: SAUTÉ, MIX, MOLD, BAKE! / **Makes 30 pieces**

Ground beef gets fancy here! *Oohs* and *aahs* are guaranteed when you present these spiced meatballs on cinnamon sticks. They are a ton of fun to eat (no fork needed) and look absolutely stunning on a party platter, served with bright green tahini. Swap the beef with ground lamb or turkey, and consider serving them as a plated appetizer for a dinner party.

30 cinnamon sticks

FOR VEGETABLES
3 tablespoons olive oil, for frying

2 medium yellow onions, finely chopped

1 cup grated carrots

1 cup grated zucchini

2 garlic cloves, minced

½ teaspoon salt

¼ teaspoon freshly ground black pepper

FOR BEEF
2 pounds lean or grass-fed ground beef

1½ teaspoons cumin

½ teaspoon salt

¼ teaspoon freshly ground black pepper

¼ cup minced fresh parsley

2 large eggs, beaten

⅓ cup chopped pine nuts, toasted (optional)

¼ teaspoon cayenne pepper (optional)

Green Tahini, for serving (see Tahini Flip, page 273)

1 Soak the cinnamon sticks in water for at least 15 minutes so they won't burn while baking.

2 Make the vegetables: Heat the oil in a skillet over medium heat, and cook the onions, stirring, until translucent, about 5 minutes. Add the carrots, zucchini, garlic, ½ teaspoon salt, and ¼ teaspoon pepper, and cook until the vegetables are softened and cooked through, about 10 minutes. Set the veggies aside to cool.

3 Prepare the beef: Place the beef in a medium bowl, and season it with the cumin, salt, and pepper. Mix in the parsley, eggs, and cooked veggies until well combined. Add the pine nuts and cayenne pepper, if desired.

4 Chill the mixture for one hour (or less if you're in a pinch) to firm it up before shaping.

5 Preheat the oven to 400°F. Lightly grease a large baking sheet with oil.

6 Roll about 2 tablespoons of the chilled beef into a football shape and mold it onto the cinnamon stick, leaving one end of the stick free as a handle.

7 Arrange the beef sticks on the baking sheet. Bake for 12 minutes, or until the meat is browned and cooked through. Serve at once.

› *nail this*

It will seem like a lot of vegetables, but they will cook down and add a lot of flavor to the beef.

» *flip it*

No cinnamon sticks? Add a pinch of cinnamon to the mixture, and make meatballs served with toothpicks.

Prepare beef on sticks in advance. Chill until ready to bake.

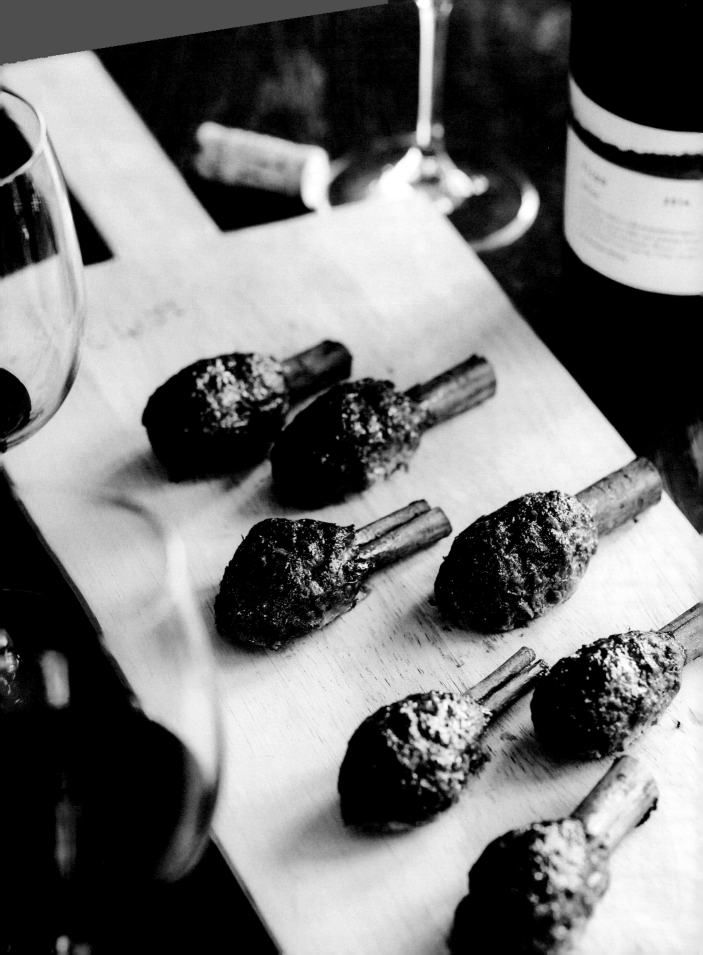

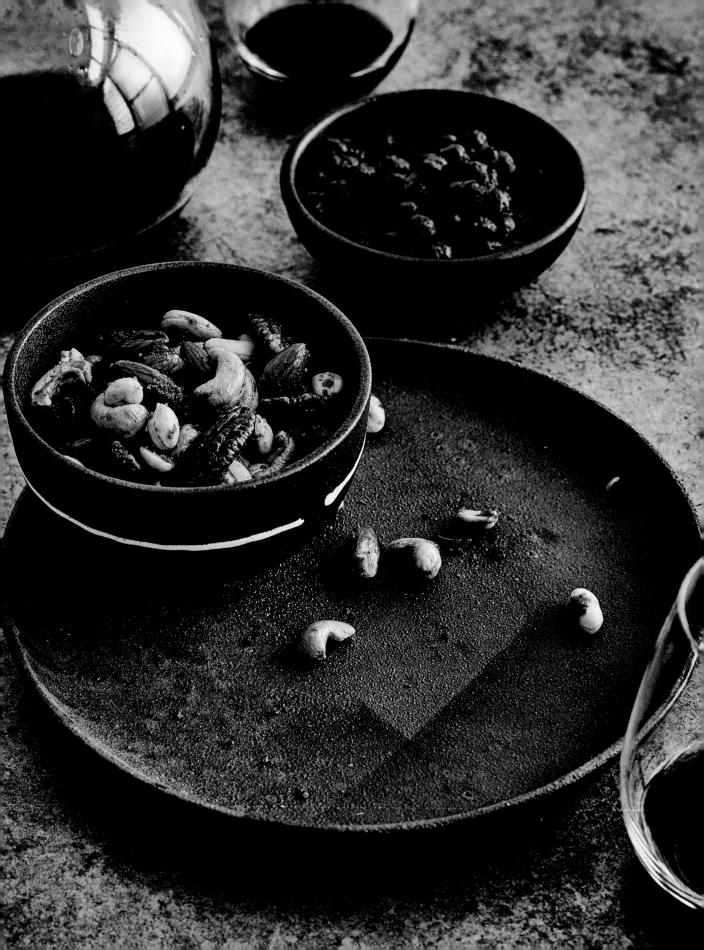

ROSEMARY PARTY NUT TRAIL MIX

STEPS: MELT, STIR, ROAST! / **Makes 3 cups**

I love making this nut mix in a dehydrator, to be certain not to burn it, but the oven method turns out a product that is equally delicious—and it means you can roast nuts and have them ready in 20 minutes or less, instead of 20 hours! Keep a batch in the fridge or pantry for unexpected visitors or snack attacks.

Tools: Baking sheet

2 tablespoons unsalted butter or olive oil

2 tablespoons maple syrup

2 tablespoons dark brown sugar

1 tablespoon plus 1½ teaspoons fresh or dried rosemary, chopped

2 teaspoons cumin

2 teaspoons salt

¼ teaspoon cayenne pepper

3 cups raw nuts (peanuts, cashews, pecans, almonds)

TRAIL MIX ADD-INS (OPTIONAL)

2 cups popped popcorn

1 cup dried cherries

1 Preheat the oven to 350F°. Line a baking sheet with parchment paper.

2 Melt the butter or olive oil in a large saucepan over low heat. Stir in the maple syrup, brown sugar, rosemary, cumin, salt, and cayenne. Add the nuts and toss for 30 seconds, until fragrant. Do this quickly so you don't burn the sugar and spices.

3 Transfer the nuts to the prepared baking sheet and spread into an even layer. Bake for 15 to 20 minutes, or until fragrant and starting to lightly brown. Check and toss frequently, every 5 to 7 minutes, to avoid burning. Don't leave the room while the nuts are in the oven!

4 Once the nuts are cool, stir in optional ingredients to make a trail mix, if desired.

> *nail this*

It's always a good idea to premeasure your ingredients before you begin to cook or bake. In this case, the spices need to be added quickly, so it's helpful for them to be ready.

>> *flip it*

If making in a dehydrator, omit the butter or oil, and simply toss the spices and the nuts with maple syrup and brown sugar. Dehydrate for 1 to 2 days.

Serve these in a bowl for party snacks, or add them to salads.

Chop the nuts and fold them into ice cream, or use them for Decadent Frozen Almond Brownie Pie (page 213).

Add 1½ cups total of pretzels, chocolate chips, and dried mango.

For a result that's almost like a brittle, use slivered almonds, but they burn faster, so adjust the oven time to 10 minutes total, checking every few minutes.

SWEET AND SALTY CHICKPEAS

STEPS: DRAIN, TOSS, ROAST! / **Makes about 2 cups**

Ditch the peanuts in favor of a protein-rich, good-for-you party snack to pair with that glass of red wine—without compromising your craving for a delectable sweet and salty bite. I can never make enough of these crunchy chickpeas, so I often prepare more than one batch. Or just serve the peanuts and don't beat yourself up, because salty peanuts are pretty awesome too.

2 15.5-ounce cans chickpeas, drained

¼ cup maple syrup

2 tablespoons olive oil

2 teaspoons tamari

1 teaspoon paprika

1 teaspoon garlic powder

1 to 2 teaspoons sriracha sauce

1 teaspoon salt

¼ teaspoon freshly ground black pepper

1 Preheat the oven to 400°F.

2 Spread the chickpeas on a baking sheet, and toss them with the rest of the ingredients. (No need to mess up a separate bowl to measure out the sauce.) The mixture will be runny—this is good! The chickpeas will absorb all the flavors and dry out.

3 Bake for 10 minutes, then lower the oven temperature to 225°F and continue baking until the chickpeas are dry and crispy (taste them occasionally to test), about 2½ hours. Toss the chickpeas every once in a while. The edges tend to brown faster. If you're impatient, raise the heat to 350°F toward the 1-hour mark, and diligently watch them (so they do not burn) as they finish crisping. Once they're done, turn the oven off, open the door slightly, and allow the chickpeas to cool slowly in the oven to achieve maximum crispness.

4 These keep in the fridge for up to a week when stored in an airtight container. You might want to pop them in the oven (or in your dehydrator if you have one) to recrisp before serving.

> *nail this*

Patience is a virtue. Let these slowly dry and absorb the marinade on low heat in the oven. If you rush, they will still be good, but more chewy than crispy.

Not crispy enough? Increase the baking time by 10 minutes, and remember to leave them in the oven after you turn it off to dry them out further.

» *flip it*

If you have leftover chickpeas, add them to a salad (this might be my favorite way of eating them).

Make a chickpea and veggie side dish: Chop some mushrooms, cauliflower, and fresh ginger, and toss with all the ingredients listed above. Roast at 400°F for approximately 30 minutes or until crisp.

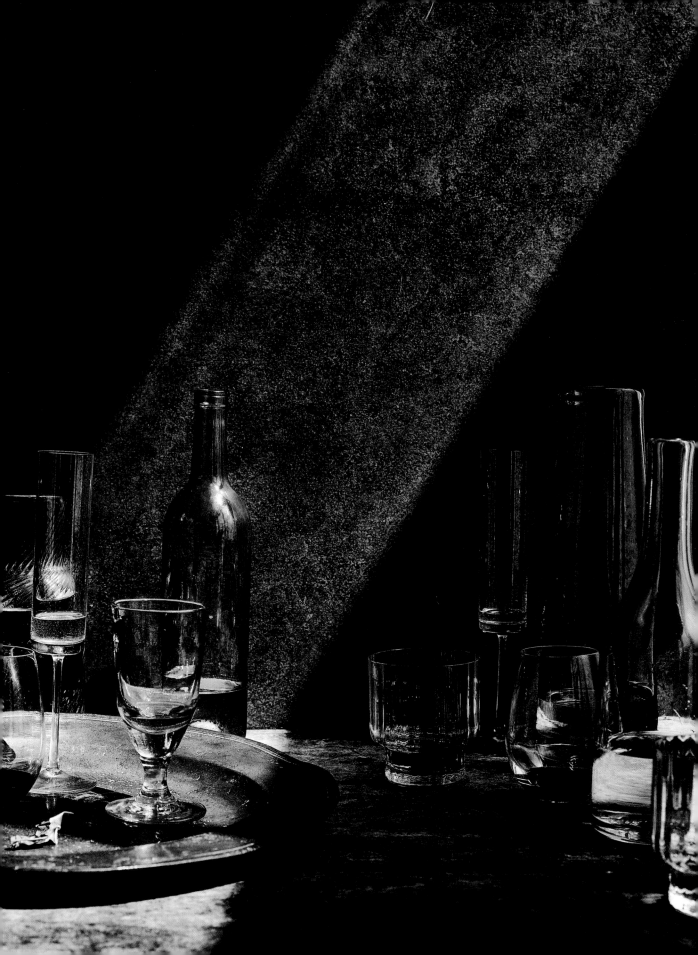

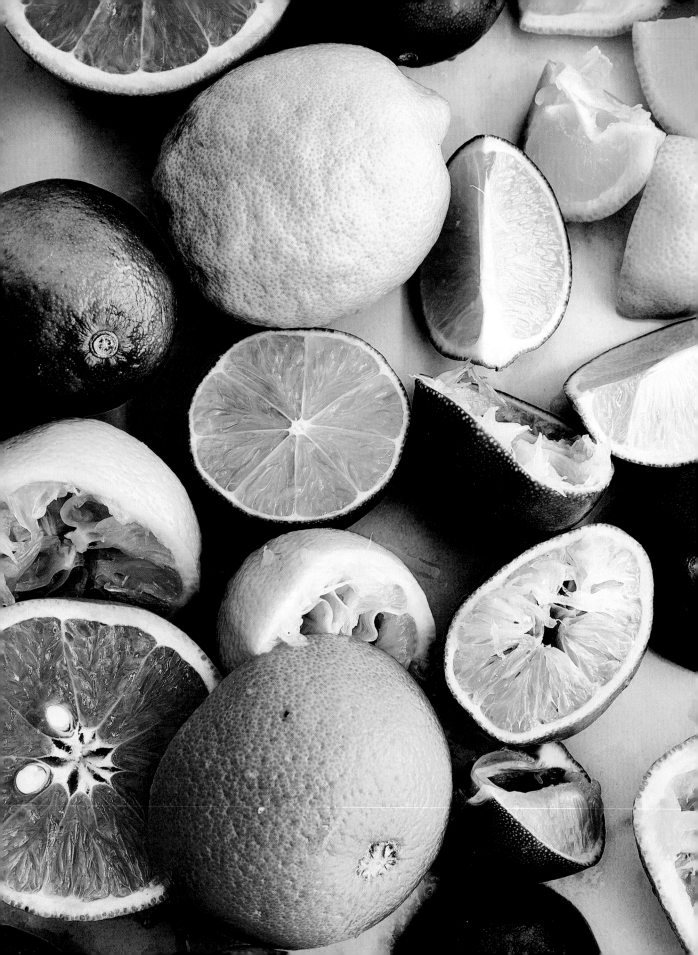

Chapter 10

CONDIMENTS AND PANTRY ESSENTIALS

Your pantry is your backbone. Keeping a well-stocked kitchen and home is essential to being less frazzled and guarantees that you are always a step away from whipping up a meal in minutes. It takes some initial planning, but I promise it will pay off in the end. Many of the items in this chapter are things I make in big batches and keep for months on end (like crispy onions, seasoned salt, schug, and ice-cubed everything). Or condiments that complement many dishes (like tahini, hummus, sautéed veggies, or sriracha mayo). They can't be kept as long but are so popular they quickly disappear from the fridge. Then there are the items that you can make with the intention of freezing them (pesto, marinara, or juice cubes). But don't stop at *my* pantry essentials. What are the go-to's that you make all the time? Consider allocating one day a month or a weekly time slot to preparing food in batches so you always have your favorite things on hand.

ICE CUBE INFUSIONS

STEPS: FREEZE! / 4 cubes = ½ cup liquid / 8 cubes = 1 cup liquid / 1 tray = 14 cubes

Ice cube trays are my current gadget obsession. They are a genius way of freezing just about anything into bite-size servings. After you freeze your cubes, remove them from the ice cube tray and transfer them to a freezer container or Ziploc bag, labeled for easy access.

WINE CUBES

Make white or rosé wine cubes to keep your white or rosé wine chilled, or add red wine cubes to sangria.

JUICE CUBES

Pour juice into trays and freeze—it's that simple! Add fresh orange and pineapple juice cubes to slushy cocktails, or to Sparkling Fruit Spritzer (page 242).

FRUIT CUBES

Purée mango or pineapple in the blender, and freeze into cubes. Serve with Passion Fruit Bubbly (page 241), use as a base for smoothies, or just add to still or sparkling water for a flavor boost.

COCONUT MILK ICE CUBES
1 15.5-ounce can full fat coconut milk (about 1½ cups)

Coconut milk separates in the can. Shake the can well before opening it, or pour the coconut milk into a small bowl and whisk it to incorporate the solids into the liquids. Add coconut cubes to fruit smoothies or to my Creamy Coffee Bomb (page 245).

SAVORY CUBES
Flexible Green Pesto (page 272)

Family Secret Red Spread (page 271)

Curry paste (page 143)

Gravy, saved from Island Chicken Adobo (page 149) or Maple-Brined Turkey (page 155)

Freeze sauces or gravy into cubes, and defrost one or two cubes to add as a flavor enhancement to a soup, stew, stir-fry, or Cauliflower Fried Rice (page 176)—possibilities abound!

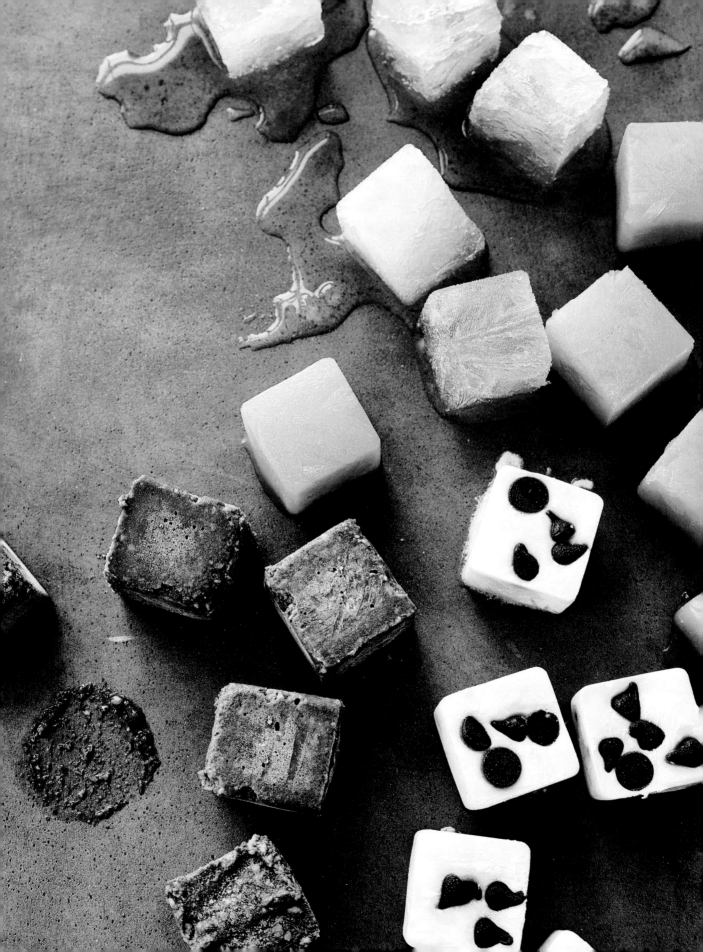

ROSEMARY-INFUSED SALT

STEPS: GRIND! / **Makes ½ cup**

Infused salt adds a hint of flavor and a layer of depth to anything you make. The process of grinding rosemary with a mortar and pestle takes just minutes and helps to blend the flavors. Store this spiked salt in a small jar right by your stovetop, and use it to enhance all your cooking. It will keep for as long as it lasts on your shelf.

Tools: Mortar and pestle or spice grinder

½ cup of your favorite salt

1½ teaspoons dried rosemary

1 Grind the rosemary using a mortar and pestle or spice grinder until aromatic, 30 seconds or so.

2 Add a few tablespoons of salt, a little at a time, grinding and incorporating it into the rosemary. Stir in the rest of salt. That's it!

3 Store in a sealed container on your countertop, and use on everything!

» flip it

Use your favorite dried herb if rosemary is not your thing—basil, sage, thyme… you get the picture.

No mortar? No problem. Place the ingredients in a Ziploc bag and use a rolling pin to crush them.

CRISPY ONIONS

STEPS: SAUTÉ, DEHYDRATE! / **Makes 2 cups**

I find happiness in the simplest of things. You'd never know that onions, sautéed and then dehydrated to a crisp, could be such a delicacy. I keep these better-than-fried onions in an airtight container, always, and sprinkle them on top of salads, dips, fried rice, meat dishes, and more. Quite frankly, these surprisingly sweet, candy-like onions might be the best thing in this book! They are ideally made in a dehydrator, but if you don't have one I've created an almost equivalent oven version that's decadent.

Tools: Dehydrator (optional)

2 large or 3 medium yellow onions

3 tablespoons olive oil

Salt and freshly ground black pepper, to taste

1 Cut the onions in half lengthwise, then thinly slice into half-moon slices.

2 Heat the oil in a large nonstick skillet over medium heat. Add the onions to the pan and cook, stirring frequently to ensure even cooking, until the onions are translucent, about 5 to 7 minutes.

3 Spread the onions in a single layer on a dehydrator sheet, and set the dehydrator to the maximum setting (150°F).

4 Dehydrate overnight or for around 10 hours, until the onions lose all their moisture and crisp up. Season with salt and pepper. Store for up to one month sealed and refrigerated, or up to 3 months in the freezer.

OVEN METHOD

1 *Note:* These become a deeper brown than the dehydrated version.

2 Preheat the oven to 160°F, or your oven's lowest setting.

3 Sauté the onions according to the instructions above, then spread them out on a baking sheet. Bake for 10 hours (yes that long), or until the onions crisp up. Season with salt and pepper. Add seasoned salt for additional oomph. If oily, blot with paper towels. Store for up to 1 week in an airtight container in the refrigerator.

» *flip it*

Try this with shallots, Vidalia onions, or red onions. Shallots cook quicker, so watch closely to avoid burning.

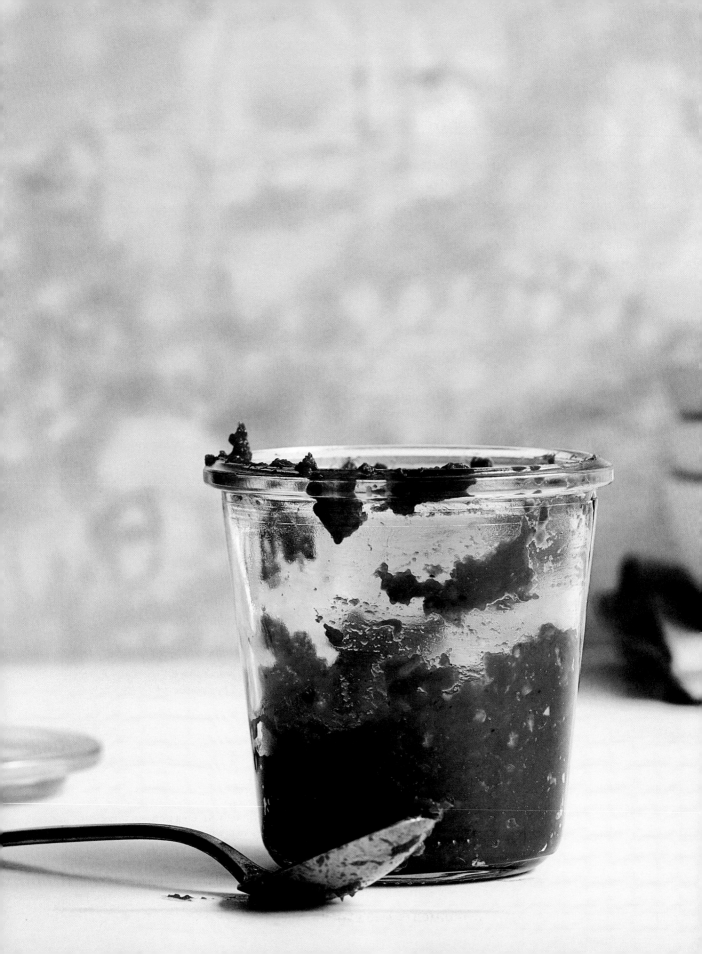

FAMILY SECRET RED SPREAD (SALAT ADOM)

STEPS: BOIL, PEEL, SIMMER! / **Makes 2 cups**

When I was growing up, our neighbor Zahava would deliver a weekly jar of this coveted spicy, rich tomato spread to our table (and eager mouths). I always thought that her Moroccan home and heart, both full of love, poured something secret into this delicacy. But after years of trying, I think I've captured her essence. Add a touch to soups, curries, and omelets for a flavor boost; serve as a spread with fish or chicken or as a mezze platter accompaniment. Anything that calls for tomato paste will be happily enhanced with a dash of this magic. It cooks all day, so start it in the morning and it will be done by dinnertime.

10 ripe tomatoes
(about 6 pounds)

1 whole head of garlic, each clove peeled and minced

½ cup olive oil, divided

1 tablespoon red pepper flakes

1 teaspoon salt

¼ teaspoon freshly ground black pepper

1 Boil a large pot of water. Add the tomatoes, and boil for 2 to 3 minutes until the skins start to separate from the flesh.

2 Peel the tomatoes (a breeze after boiling), discarding the skins, and chop the flesh into small chunks.

3 Heat about 3 tablespoons of oil in a large saucepan over high heat (I usually start with a generous coating on the bottom of the pan and add more as needed throughout the cooking process). Add the tomatoes and garlic, and bring to a boil. Reduce the heat to the lowest setting possible, and slowly simmer until the liquid from the tomatoes is reduced by half, about 3 hours. The mixture should still look very wet and soupy.

4 Season with the red pepper flakes, salt, and black pepper, and add more olive oil if the pan looks dry. Keeping a watchful eye, allow the sauce to simmer until the water completely evaporates, an additional 5 to 7 hours. (The amount of time depends on the juiciness of the tomatoes and the climate where you're cooking.) Toward the end of cooking, watch carefully and stir as needed to prevent the bottom from burning. It is ready once the mixture has reduced by half and thickened to a paste.

> *nail this*

I know that 8 to 10 hours sounds like a long time to watch a pot, but if it is kept truly on a very low simmer, you can safely leave it alone for the first two-thirds of the cooking time. Later, as it thickens, you should be close by to watch in case of burning.

FLEXIBLE GREEN PESTO

STEPS: BLEND, SERVE! / **Makes about 2 cups**

Oh, for the love of pesto. Despite its overpopularity, I still think it makes simple food seem rather fancy. I spread this green infusion on literally everything. I almost never add Parmesan cheese immediately because the sauce will keep longer without it. I usually keep a pesto dressing in the fridge ready to dress up a plain old bowl of greens.

Tools: Blender

3 cups fresh basil leaves (or leaves of other herbs), packed

½ cup spinach leaves, packed

¼ cup walnuts or pecans

¼ cup pine nuts

2 garlic cloves

1 tablespoon fresh lemon juice

½ teaspoon salt

Freshly ground black pepper, to taste

¾ cup extra-virgin olive oil

½ cup grated Parmesan cheese (optional)

1 In a blender, purée the herbs, spinach, nuts, garlic, lemon juice, salt, and pepper until well combined.

2 Continue blending, adding the oil in a thin stream until incorporated.

3 Stir in Parmesan before serving, if desired.

VARIATION: PESTO DRESSING

Purée the pesto with 1 small shallot and 1 tablespoon lemon juice in a blender. Taste and add salt and pepper as needed.

> *nail this*

Too much oil? Add more herbs or lemon. Too much lemon? Add more herbs and oil. Too flat? Add salt. Too herby? Add nuts, or oil and lemon.

When you store pesto in the fridge it might be solidified when you take it out. To soften, bring it to room temperature, or add a touch of hot water and stir.

>> *flip it*

Swap any herbs you like for the basil, like cilantro or parsley.

Swap arugula for spinach for a punchier pesto, or kale if you have it on hand.

Omit spinach completely for an herb-only pesto.

Don't go nuts finding the right nut! Use cashews or macadamia nuts in place of pine nuts.

If time allows, toast your nuts slightly to add extra flavor.

Swap Parmesan with nutritional yeast for a vegan version.

THE ULTIMATE FLEXIBLE TAHINI

STEPS: BLEND! / **Makes about 1¼ cups**

Tahini is one of the staples in our fridge that never goes to waste. This recipe works as a dip and a dressing—and also as the base for my Hummus Any Way Any Day (page 274). I like mine with a generous amount of garlic, lemon, and salt, but adjust the seasonings to make *your* version of the ultimate tahini. Get your hands on Israeli or Lebanese tahini if you can—the quality makes a difference.

Tools: Blender

1 cup raw tahini
¼ cup fresh lemon juice
3 small garlic cloves
1 teaspoon salt
Freshly ground black pepper, to taste

1 In a blender, combine the raw tahini with ¾ cup water and the remaining ingredients. Blend until smooth. Keeps in the fridge for up to 5 days.

VARIATION: GREEN TAHINI

1 Add 1½ cups chopped fresh parsley and ½ cup chopped fresh chives to the blender. Keeps for up to 3 days in an airtight container in the refrigerator.

2 Serve with Spiced Beef Lollipops (page 258).

> *nail this*

When you open a jar of tahini, oil lingers at the top, and the bottom is thick and clumpy. Stir your raw tahini in a separate bowl to combine, then return it to the container. Raw tahini keeps, opened and refrigerated, for a few months.

This recipe makes tahini of a thicker consistency, so feel free to add more water if you prefer (but not too much—it's easier to dilute than to thicken!).

» *flip it*

I usually add a splash more lemon juice because I'm a lemony girl.

No blender? No problem. Crush the garlic as finely as possible to avoid garlic chunks, and then whisk by hand.

HUMMUS ANY WAY ANY DAY

STEPS: BLEND, SERVE! / **Makes about 1½ cups**

After years of eating lip-smacking-good hummus in Israel, and obsessively testing my version of this Middle Eastern essential (which gets spread on just about anything), I present: the ultimate customizable chickpea dip. The essence of a great hummus lies in the liberal addition of tahini, the right balance of garlic, a generous amount of lemon, and enough patience to achieve a creamy and smooth texture. Your favorite ratio of flavors may be different from mine, and that's okay. Eat hummus your way.

Tools: Blender

2 tablespoons fresh lemon juice

1 15-ounce can chickpeas, drained and rinsed

⅓ cup tahini

1 garlic clove

1 teaspoon cumin

¼ teaspoon salt

¼ teaspoon freshly ground black pepper

1   In a blender, combine ¼ cup water with all the ingredients. Blend until smooth, adding a few more tablespoons of water, if needed, to thin the mixture to your desired consistency.

2   Adjust the seasoning to taste. Keep in the refrigerator, covered, for 2 days.

> *nail this*

Blend your hummus really well. The creaminess is an integral part of this dish's success.

>> *flip it*

For green hummus: Add ½ cup parsley leaves.

For sundried tomato hummus: Add 5 to 6 oil-packed sundried tomatoes.

For pesto hummus: Add 1 tablespoon Flexible Green Pesto (page 272).

For chunky hummus: Top with canned chickpeas or Sweet and Salty Chickpeas (page 262).

If you already have a batch of The Ultimate Flexible Tahini (page 273) whipped up, blend about ⅓ to ½ cup of it with the drained chickpeas, and season with additional lemon juice, garlic, salt, and pepper.

If you prefer to use dried chickpeas, soak ½ cup chickpeas overnight, rinse, and drain. Boil in water with a pinch of salt and baking soda (to soften the peas), and cook for up to 2 hours, or until very tender.

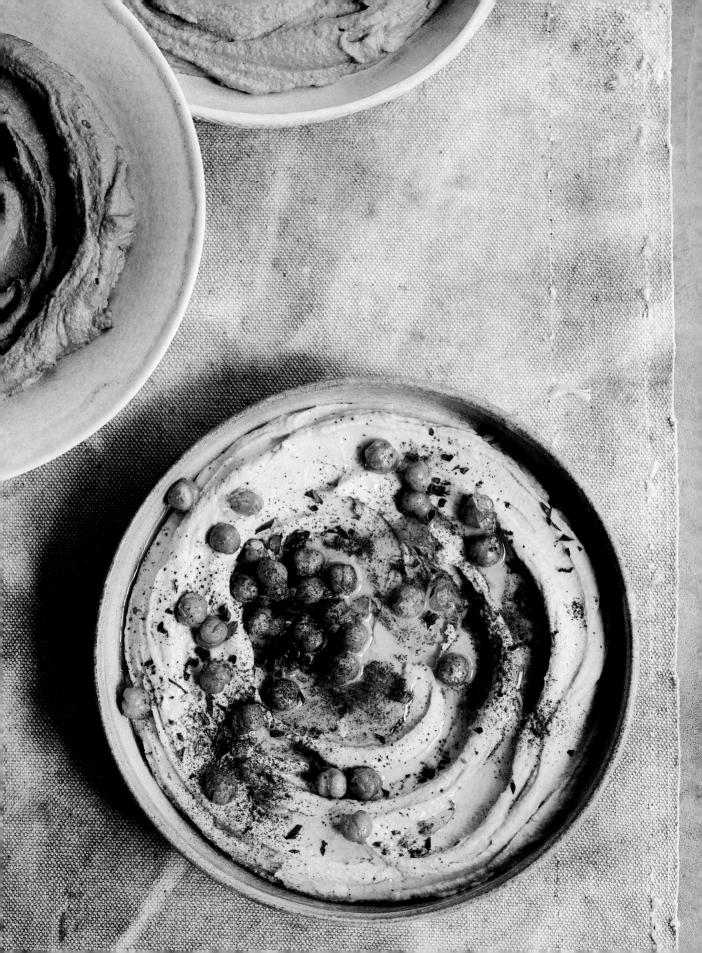

GLUTEN-FREE CRACKER CRUMBS

STEPS: CRUSH! / **Makes about 2 cups**

This is my new genius way of saying good-bye to breadcrumbs for (almost) ever. These cracker crumbs lend an unparalleled crunch to Cheesy Cauliflower Poppers (page 246), Showstopping Herb-Crusted Salmon (page 134), or any other dish that calls for crunchy breading. Keep crumbs labeled in space-saving Ziploc bags in the freezer so they are always available.

Tools: Food processor (optional)

1 4.25-ounce box of your favorite gluten-free crackers

2 teaspoons dried herbs, your choice

Salt and freshly ground black pepper (optional)

1 Put the crackers and herbs in a food processor, and pulse to crush them into fine crumbs. If you don't have a processor (or the patience to clean one), slip the crackers into a Ziploc bag, and use a rolling pin, knife sharpener, or any other tool you have to pound them into crumbs.

2 Season with salt and pepper, if necessary. (Crackers are often salted, which will probably eliminate the need to add more.)

> *nail this*

Use crackers that are super crunchy and taste good on their own. A dish is only as good as the raw materials behind it.

>> *flip it*

For quick, crispy, oven-fried fish: Dip a fish fillet in egg and then in cracker crumbs. Bake on a lightly oiled baking sheet in a 425°F oven for 15 to 20 minutes, turning once, or until both sides are golden-brown and crispy.

Breadcrumbs will have a place in a recipe on occasion when you want something spongier, for example in a filling rather than as a crispy coating. In that case, toast slices of bread in the oven or pop-up toaster till crisp, and then process to crumbs in a food processor.

SPICY SRIRACHA MAYO

STEPS: MIX! / **Makes about 1 cup**

This recipe is so simple it's hardly even a recipe! But spicy sriracha mayo is a staple in my kitchen, and it will elevate any dish you drizzle it on, too. The mustard lightens up the mayo and gives the sauce extra pizzazz. I usually prefer a two-to-one ratio of mayo to mustard, but if I'm feeling mustard-y I'll add more mustard. Experiment with more or less of each ingredient to suit your taste buds.

Tools: Plastic squeeze bottle

½ cup mayonnaise

¼ cup Dijon mustard

3 tablespoons sriracha sauce

1 In a bowl, mix the mayonnaise, mustard, and sriracha until well combined. I keep mine in a plastic squeeze bottle in the fridge and drizzle it everywhere to add kick.

> nail this

Use a good-quality Dijon mustard.

Authentic sriracha sauce is vital. No other spice or hot sauce will replace the complexity of sriracha's flavor.

Look for an olive oil mayo at your health food store.

» flip it

Replace the mayo with mashed avocado or half avocado and half mayo. It's not as decadent, but it's a good healthy twist.

Use more or less sriracha depending on the heat level you like. The quantities here are just suggestions.

Serve with Sesame Salmon Bites (page 87), Sneakily Good-for-You Beef Burgers (page 160), Hot and Crispy Sushi Rolls (page 93), or any seared salmon or chicken dish.

GREEN SCHUG

STEPS: BLEND! / **Makes 1½ cups**

Seth adds a dash of this piquant Israeli chile condiment to everything from soups to salads. He even eats it by the spoonful alongside chicken or mixed into omelets. I like to serve this pesto-like dip with my Lean and Green Falafel Bites (page 253). Add it to marinades for beef, chicken, and vegetables, but only use a touch! Beware: It's spicy, and that's the point. Lemon juice isn't traditionally added to schug, but I like how it balances the flavors.

Tools: Rubber gloves, food processor

10 jalapeño chiles (or another spicy green chile)

2 cups loosely packed fresh cilantro, leaves and small tender stems only (discard the long, thicker stems)

8 garlic cloves

1 teaspoon fresh lemon juice

½ teaspoon cumin

¼ teaspoon ground cardamom

¼ teaspoon salt

¼ teaspoon freshly ground black pepper

¼ cup extra-virgin olive oil

1 Wear gloves when handling the peppers because they are spicy! Remove the stems from the peppers. I like to keep the seeds in because they increase the spiciness—and I hate the hassle of removing them.

2 Place all ingredients except the olive oil in a food processor, and pulse to combine to a chunky paste. Continue processing, and slowly drizzle in the olive oil.

3 Taste and adjust the seasoning. The spice level will depend on the size of the peppers used. If it's far too spicy, add more cilantro; if it isn't hot enough, add more peppers. Add more salt and black pepper if desired.

4 Keeps for 1 week in the fridge or 3 months in the freezer. Freeze in ice cubes or small batches for easy access.

> *nail this*

Adjust and customize—resist the urge to measure exact quantities. The size of your peppers and garlic cloves, as well as the pungency of your cilantro, will always vary.

>> *flip it*

Add more oil and lemon, and serve this with Vietnamese Veggie Spring Rolls (page 88). Consider using it to spice up soups, omelets, Spaghetti Squash Pad Thai (page 171), quiches, or marinades.

Add a handful (or a cup) of fresh parsley leaves into your schug, in addition to the cilantro, to make it even more flavorful.

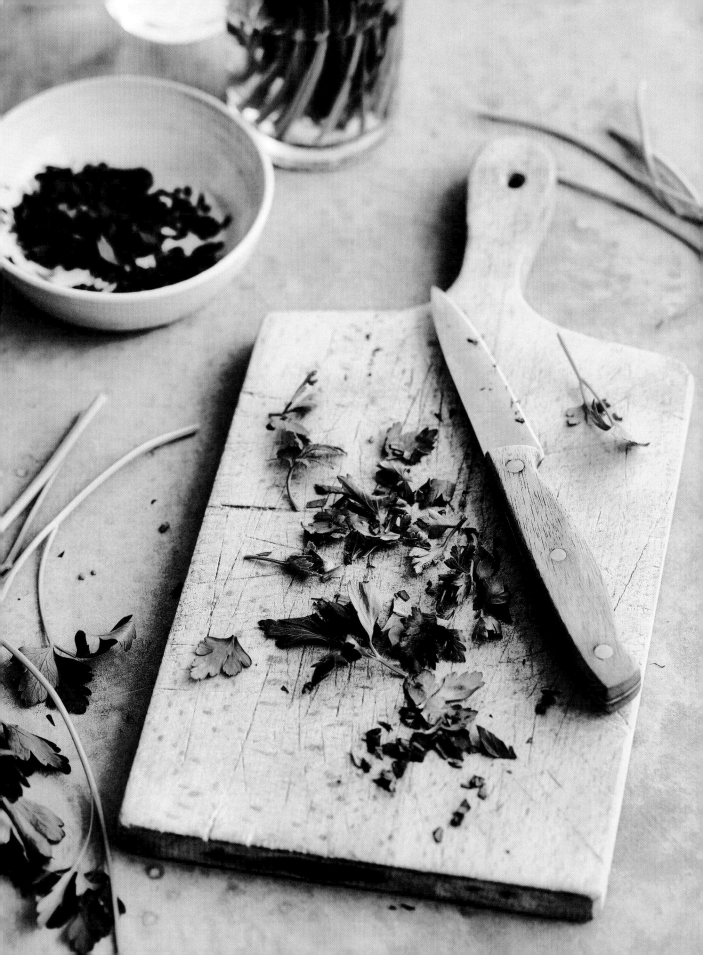

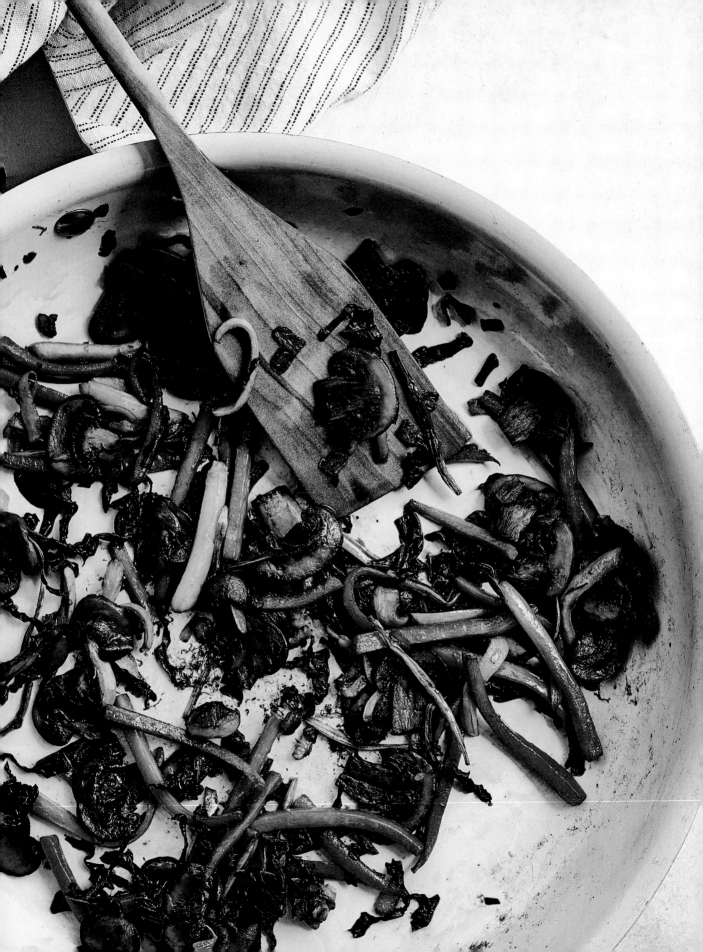

ANY VEGGIE SAUTÉ

STEPS: CHOP, SAUTÉ! / **Yield will vary based on vegetables used**

The key to eating more vegetables is to have them readily available. That's why we always keep a version of these all-purpose sautéed veggies on hand in the fridge. Incorporate them into your morning omelets, and swap them in for the veggies in Kid-Approved Breakfast Quesadillas (page 29), Sunny-Side Mushroom Bake (page 33), Sneakily Good-for-You Beef Burgers (page 160), Vietnamese Veggie Spring Rolls (page 88), Tuna and Veggie Cakes (page 139), or Hot and Crispy Sushi Rolls (page 93). See what I mean? Endlessly useful.

a large skillet, heat the olive oil over low to medium heat. Add the
ion and cook, stirring until translucent, about 10 minutes.

d the mushrooms and assorted veggies and cook, stirring, until
ey've begun to brown and the mushrooms have released their
ces, roughly 20 minutes. (If you want the veggies to wilt and get
happy and buttery, just make sure they sweat long enough; don't
imp on the time!) Set aside to cool. They will keep, in a sealed
container in the refrigerator, for up to 2 days.

spinach

» *flip it*

Use different veggies, or add some herbs or other seasonings to your liking.

VEGGIE-FULL MARINARA

STEPS: SAUTÉ, SIMMER, BLEND! / **Makes 6 to 8 cups (depending on how thick you want it)**

This outrageously good marinara is chock full of veggies that marry well with tomatoes. The thick sauce forms the foundation for my Noodleless Lasagna (page 180) and can be blended smooth for pizza or pasta occasions. Add sautéed ground beef to make a Bolognese, or use it to make a pizza version of the quesadillas (page 28). Sometimes for a super-quick and simple dish, I'll toss it with raw cauliflower in a saucepan and finish it with some cheese, so it tastes like pasta minus the noodles. Make a big batch, and you'll find endless uses for this tomato sauce.

Tools: Hand blender

2 tablespoons olive oil

1 medium yellow onion, finely chopped

3 to 4 garlic cloves, minced

1 large carrot, grated

1 medium zucchini, grated

½ cup chopped mushrooms, any kind

1 teaspoon dried oregano

1 teaspoon dried thyme

1 28-ounce can tomatoes, with juice

1 6-ounce can tomato paste

¼ cup chopped fresh basil

Salt and freshly ground black pepper, to taste

1 In a large saucepan over medium heat, heat the olive oil and cook the onions, stirring, until translucent, about 5 minutes.

2 Add the garlic, carrot, zucchini, and mushrooms, and cook, stirring, until the vegetables are soft and aromatic, about 5 more minutes. Stir in the oregano and thyme.

3 Add the canned tomatoes and cook, covered (but stirring occasionally), until very soft, about 20 minutes.

4 Whisk in the tomato paste and ¾ cup water. Cook, uncovered, until the sauce is thickened, 15 more minutes. If you're making it for lasagna, continue to cook until it's almost spreadable, with very little liquid left, to maximize flavor.

5 Remove the sauce from the heat and use a hand blender to finish.

6 Stir in the fresh basil, and season with salt and pepper to taste.

7 Transfer the marinara to jars. It keeps for 2 days in the fridge, or you can freeze it for up to 2 months.

> nail this

Don't skimp on the cooking time. The combo of tomatoes plus time is a must, to allow the flavors to intensify.

If using fresh herbs, always add them at the end of cooking. If using dried herbs, add them toward the beginning.

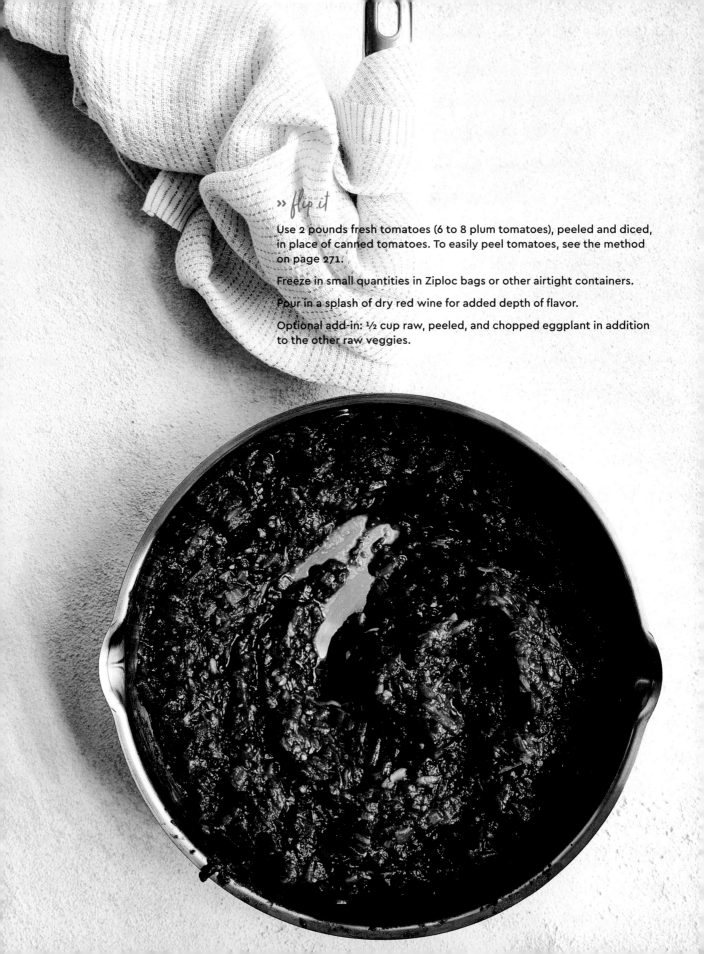

» flip it

Use 2 pounds fresh tomatoes (6 to 8 plum tomatoes), peeled and diced, in place of canned tomatoes. To easily peel tomatoes, see the method on page 271.

Freeze in small quantities in Ziploc bags or other airtight containers.

Pour in a splash of dry red wine for added depth of flavor.

Optional add-in: ½ cup raw, peeled, and chopped eggplant in addition to the other raw veggies.

How to Adapt Any Recipe to Make It Your Own

The freedom to open any cookbook and customize any recipe in it is within your reach! I used to flip through cookbooks and pass over so many cool ideas because I didn't know what to do with them. Now I can read a cinnamon bun recipe and make it gluten free, lower the sugar content in an apple pie without sacrificing flavor, swap out hard-to-find ingredients, or replace something obscure with something I already have in my pantry. Having the tools to understand and navigate any recipe takes time, but with practice it gives you ultimate freedom, and that makes cooking more fun and your options limitless. Go back to your other cookbooks now for inspiration, and follow some of these navigation guidelines.

Read the recipe from top to bottom to understand the method. Reading through the full recipe gives you the full picture. As you read, visualize the steps, and see yourself making it. This will allow you to really comprehend what's involved, how much time it will take, and any methods you might be unfamiliar with.

Identify what's essential and what's not. You'll soon learn what the essentials are for each recipe and what can be skipped over. I've tried to highlight this practice in these recipes by noting what's most important and what you can modify. Chances are you'll learn how to do this from trial and error ("Oops, I guess eggs are pretty essential in that lemon curd," or, "Actually, hoisin sauce can easily be replaced by BBQ sauce"). The more you cook, the more you'll learn.

Learn how to make substitutions. Google is your friend here. If you can't find an ingredient, look up what you can substitute. I once went on a wild-goose chase for mango chutney, then later discovered that apricot jam could stand in just fine. Get resourceful!

Modify any recipe to make it gluten free. My general rule is to replace 1 cup all-purpose wheat flour with 1 cup all-purpose gluten-free flour plus ½ teaspoon xanthan gum. That said, many flours on the market today (like Cup4Cup) already have xanthan gum included and can be replaced one-to-one. In many dishes, like quiche crusts or fritters, you can omit flour entirely by adding another egg or two to help the mixture bind.

Healthify any recipe. I almost exclusively pan-fry instead of deep-frying. In almost all baked goods you can reduce the sugar content by 10 percent or more without major ramifications or any sacrifice in the flavor. Consider enhancing baked goods with hemp, chia, or flax seeds, and replacing some of the grain flour with almond flour (proceed cautiously, as successfully replacing flour takes a few attempts, especially with baked goods). Sneak vegetables into recipes like savory pancakes, pasta, burgers, sauces, soups, and more.

Consider time-savers and hacks. Check out page 151 for ideas and methods that you can apply to any recipe to make it faster or easier. If a salad calls for glazed nuts, buy them in the supermarket ready-made. Instead of marinating and grilling the meat for chicken Caesar salad, use a rotisserie bird.

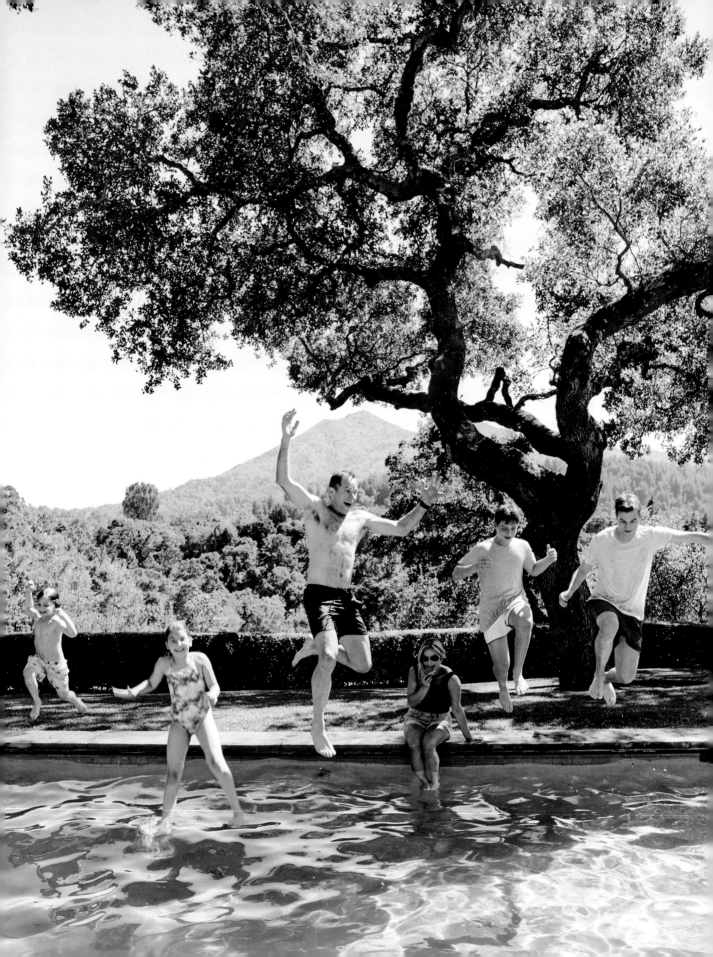

FLEXIBILITY BEYOND THE KITCHEN: YOUR TRANSFORMATION FROM COOK TO CHEF

It is my sincerest hope that this book has inspired you to become more chef-like in the kitchen and in your life. The fun of cooking and living begins after you've mastered the rules—and can then do things *your* way.

Flexibility as a concept might have begun here, with your relationship to food. But don't let it stop here. Becoming more chef-like in all areas of life means becoming more self-directed and self-motivated, possessing the ability to weave through the noise and conflicting information that come your way every day. These are the keys to finding your happy place. Navigating your way forward begins with getting organized, staying resourceful, and zigging and zagging in daily life to carve out your unique path. Next year, when you encounter the latest superfood, the trendiest diet, or the thing that someone else has that you want, stay focused on what you know to be true. Continue seeking, learning, experimenting, failing, and improving. Live a life that matters, on your own terms. There's no fast track to success, but if there were it would take the fun out of the game. Remain persistent, and aspire for *attainable* excellence.

If all else fails, and when you feel overwhelmed, pour yourself a glass of wine with a good friend, count your unique blessings, and exhale, because there's always tomorrow.

Tell me more about the food you want and share your cravings with me! Post your creative adaptations of the recipes in this book and share your journey by using the hashtag #foodyouwant and tag me @theflexiblechef on Instagram. For more recipes and inspo head over to my blog www.theflexiblechef.com I'm always just a message away. Stay hungry and stay flexible!

Nealy

CONVERSION CHEAT SHEET

Weights and Measures:

- A pinch = less than ⅛ teaspoon
- 3 teaspoons = 1 tablespoon = ½ ounce
- 4 tablespoons = 2 ounces = ¼ cup
- 16 tablespoons = 8 ounces = 1 cup = ½ pound
- 1 cup = 8 ounces (liquid) = ½ pint
- 4 cups = 32 ounces (liquid) = 2 pints = 1 quart

Temperatures, Fahrenheit to Celsius:

150°F = 65.5°F

325°F = 162.8°C

350°F = 177°C

375°F = 190.5°C

400°F = 204.4°C

425°F = 218.3°C

450°F = 232°C

475°F = 246.1°C

Approximate Equivalents:

- 8 tablespoons = 4 ounces = ½ cup = 1 stick butter
- 1 cup all-purpose pre-sifted flour = 5 ounces
- 1 cup granulated sugar = 8 ounces
- 1 large egg = 2 ounces = ¼ cup = 4 tablespoons

DIY Conversion Calculations

- Ounces to grams: multiply ounces by 28.3
- Grams to ounces: multiply grams by .0353
- Pounds to grams: multiply pounds by 453.59
- Pounds to kilograms: multiply pounds by 0.45
- Cups to liters: multiply cups by 0.24
- Fahrenheit to Celsius: subtract 32 from the Fahrenheit, multiply by 5, then divide by 9
- Celsius to Fahrenheit: multiply Celsius by 9, divide by 5, then add 32

ACKNOWLEDGMENTS

I always knew I was going to write a book, but if it weren't for the guidance and support of the following individuals, my idea would have remained a dream.

Mom, thanks for greeting me with a homemade lunch every day after school, and for teaching me everything I know about being a good cook and a good mother.

Abba, thank you for our Montana paradise, which has been the playground for testing and filming so many new recipes. You'll always be the bird on my shoulder.

Melissa, you're a trooper for handling everything else in the TFC world over the past year so I could type and test away in a cave. Thank you for being a killer video editor, writer, and gatekeeper, and also a loving confidant. And for inspiring me to wear more makeup.

Susan, thanks for being the best support and friend for the last fifteen years, and for your meticulous behind-the-scenes organization. Lisa, thank you for your exceptional proofreading skills, record turnaround time, and attention to detail beyond compare. Kim, you're awesome for flexibly jumping in at the last minute to edit with precision on deadline.

Marlita and Marilyn, your hard work has enabled this book. Thank you each for waking up with a smile, inspiring many of the recipes, and cooking them even better than I do.

Michael, your way with words has transformed my writing. Thank you for your guidance in shaping my "why" for this book.

Steve Troha and Dado Derviskadic, thanks for believing in me before I gave you enough of a reason to, and for putting up with my thousandth email and my still-perfectionist tendencies in my desire to make this book outstanding.

Renee Sedliar, I'll never forget our first call at six a.m. when I was in my pajamas in Hong Kong. I loved you at hello! We just jived, and you have since been nothing less than a dream editor. Thank you for the freedom you provided me and for your unwavering support. I'm forever your fan.

To the entire Da Capo team who worked tirelessly on the book.

Aubrie Pick, thank you for this beautiful work of art; I am so grateful to have had your eye to the lens. Fanny Pan, thanks for letting me into your kitchen and for styling the most exquisite dishes. Kristene Loayza, your idea to add pretzels to the peanut butter cups was genius, and your cooking skills are fierce. Josefine Wissenberg, thanks for your stunning makeup, which I'm still having trouble re-creating without your magic wand. Jennifer Bonnet, I loved our time together, your gorgeous blue jumpsuit, and your impeccable styling skills. Bessma Khalaf, thank you for your set assistance and happy spirit, and thanks to Natasha Kolenko for weaving the tapestry so seamlessly behind the scenes. Doug, thanks for welcoming us into your lovely home with such gracious hospitality.

Ashley Lima, you went so above your creative role. Thanks for letting me get involved in things you normally don't get bugged about, and for not smacking me when I changed the font for the fifteenth time. You are supremely talented, and it has been an honor to work with you.

To all my testers, thanks for burning a few edges and helping highlight the flaws until we got things right. Amber, Andi, Carla, Keren, Malka, Marci, Mira, Orah, Rebecca, Sandrella, Steve, Yael.

Ann Volkwein, your wisdom and precision guided this project from start to finish. Thank you for it all and more. Your expertise was obvious, and our friendship was a bonus. I already miss you, so let's get busy on the next book!

Ben, Eitan, Ayla, Liam, thanks for agreeing to eat the same foods all year as I tested these recipes. Thanks for (usually) eating salmon and broccoli and for (mostly) not complaining when I worked too much. You're my daily inspiration.

Seth, thank you for all the surprise dinner guests you brought home, which helped put my flexible approach to the test. Most importantly, I love you for the great adventure you've taken me on over the last twenty years. This book—and all of my dreams—is only complete with you by my side.

And finally, to all of you amazing friends who read my blog, watch my videos, attend my events, or have joined me for a homemade meal, your unwavering support has been the impetus for sharing these recipes.

INDEX